Elsevier's Medical Assisting Exam Review

Elsevier's Medical Assisting Exam Review

SEVENTH EDITION

Deborah Barbier Holmes, BSN, RN, RMA (AMT), CMA-C (AAMA)

Former Assistant to the Dean of Health and Sport Sciences (ret),
Former Medical Assistant Program Director (ret)
Iowa Western Community College
Council Bluffs, Iowa

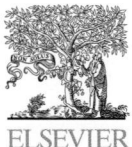

ELSEVIER

Elsevier
3251 Riverport Lane
St. Louis, Missouri 63043

ELSEVIER'S MEDICAL ASSISTING EXAM REVIEW,
SEVENTH EDITION

ISBN: 978-0-443-12666-6

Notice

Practitioners and researchers must always rely on their own experience and knowledge in evaluating and using any information, methods, compounds or experiments described herein. Because of rapid advances in the medical sciences, in particular, independent verification of diagnoses and drug dosages should be made. To the fullest extent of the law, no responsibility is assumed by Elsevier, authors, editors or contributors for any injury and/or damage to persons or property as a matter of products liability, negligence or otherwise, or from any use or operation of any methods, products, instructions, or ideas contained in the material herein.

Previous editions copyrighted 2022, 2018, 2014, 2011, 2007, and 2002.

Content Strategist: Yvonne Alexopoulos
Content Development Specialist: Laura Schmidt
Publishing Services Manager: Deepthi Unni
Project Manager: Manchu Mohan
Design Direction: Amy Buxton

Printed in India.

Last digit is the print number: 9 8 7 6 5 4 3 2 1

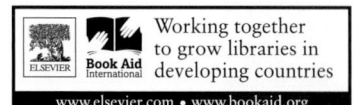

Working together
to grow libraries in
developing countries

www.elsevier.com • www.bookaid.org

To Granny and Jon,
my biggest fans and guardian angels.

Reviewers

Belinda Glover, M.Ed, CMA (AAMA)
Assistant Professor
Herzing University
Milwaukee, Wisconsin

P. Ann Weaver, MSEd, MT(ASCP)
Instructor, Medical Assistant Program (ret.)
Chippewa Valley Technical College
Eau Claire, Wisconsin

Previous edition reviewers

Tracie Fuqua, BS, CMA (AAMA)
Program Director and Instructor
Medical Assisting Program
Wallace State Community College
Hanceville, Alabama

Candace S. Dailey, MSN, RN, CMA (AAMA)
Dean Health Occupations,
Medical Assistant Program Director
Health Occupations
Nicolet College
Rhinelander, Wisconsin

Brigitte Niedzwiecki, MSN, RN, RMA
Medical Assistant Program Director and Instructor
Chippewa Valley Technical College
Eau Claire, Wisconsin

Julie Pepper, CMA (AAMA), BS
Professor Emeritus
Medical Assistant Program
Chippewa Valley Technical College
Eau Claire, Wisconsin

Preface

Skilled. Compassionate. Healer. Competent.

These are words that come to mind when describing the medical assistant. As the profession of medical assisting continues to evolve, the medical assistant must rise up to meet the new challenges. Earning a medical assistant credential is the first step toward a successful career.

There are many reasons to achieve medical assistant credentials. It shows that the student is recognized by a credentialing organization as having met predetermined qualifications. It shows proof of competency, and it shows others a commitment to the profession. A credential will be even more important in the coming years as medical assistants become more and more recognized for the versatile allied health professionals that they are.

Elsevier's Medical Assisting Exam Review was written to aid the student in studying for a medical assisting credentialing exam and was developed with today's busy student in mind. This textbook presents simplified study materials that focus on all the General, Administrative, and Clinical topics from the medical assisting curriculum in preparation for a range of popular medical assisting exams, including the CMA, RMA, CCMA, CMAS, CMAC, NCMA, and CMAA exams.

The book features the following:

- A single, comprehensive guide. This allows for information to be found easily in one text and eliminates the need for many big, bulky textbooks and stacks of notes.
- Up-to-date information about various important changes in the United States that have directly affected medical assisting, such as ICD-10 coding, the Patient Protection and Affordable Care Act, and the popularity of electronic health records.
- An easy-to-follow outline format. Information is organized and presented in this format to allow the student to identify key concepts and facts. All subject areas typically included in a Medical Assistant Program are covered.
- Three practice pretests and a posttest, complete with answers and rationales. These may help assess weak and strong areas.
- Access to the Evolve site (http://www.evolve.elsevier.com/Holmes/MAexam), which offers students 2500 practice examination questions for the CMA, RMA, CCMA, NCMA, CMAC, CMAS, and CMAA exams (to adequately prepare for whichever credentialing exam is on your to-do list), as well as flashcards and anatomy and physiology animations for some lighter, interactive practice.
- Simple pictures and diagrams to illustrate the text. These help to clarify concepts.
- Study and test-taking tips to help the student be successful. Included are suggestions on how to prepare to study, how to study, and how to take a multiple-choice exam.

As the practicing medical assistant moves on in his or her career, this text may be used as a source of reference. It is also useful as a reference for educators in creating lecture material, curriculum, or review courses.

I wish the best of luck to all who use this text to achieve their credential of choice. I hope it helps make the process a little easier.

Deborah Barbier Holmes

Acknowledgments

I am deeply grateful to the following people who have given me ideas, encouragement, praise, and support.

The Medical Assistant students that I have had the privilege of teaching over the years—they are THE reason for this project. They have been an endless source of ideas, criticism, support, and inspiration. I am so proud of being a part of their accomplishments and successes.

The Elsevier team—for supporting, understanding, listening to ideas, and helping tremendously. This project started as a discussion at a national convention, wound up as this book, and each edition has gotten better and better.

David (RN), Robert, Jennifer, and Scott—the loves of my life.

Maddie, Tyler, Aiden, Nolan, and Max—the other loves of my life—they call me "Housie."

Deborah Barbier Holmes

Contents

Study Tips: Taking Medical Assisting Examinations 1
Pretest 1 5
Pretest 2 11
Pretest 3 18

1 Medical Terminology 25
2 Anatomy and Physiology 36
3 Diseases and Disorders 73
4 Growth and Development 85
5 Communication 89
6 Law, Ethics, and Health Insurance Portability and Accountability Act 93
7 Professionalism and Career Development 102
8 Computer Concepts, Written Communications, and Mail Processing 104
9 Records Management 112
10 Patient Reception and Appointment Scheduling 120
11 Office Management 126
12 Finances 131
13 Coding 138

14 Health Insurance 141
15 Infection Control and Asepsis 146
16 Vital Signs and Anthropometric Measurements 150
17 Assisting With the Physical Examination 156
18 Assisting With Medical Specialties 162
19 Nutrition and Health Promotion 181
20 Therapeutic Modalities and Physical Agents to Promote Tissue Healing 189
21 Radiography and Diagnostic Imaging 193
22 Pharmacology, Medication Administration, and Intravenous Therapy 197
23 Minor Surgery 214
24 Clinical Laboratory 225
25 First Aid and Office Emergencies 241

Posttest 245
Pretest 1 Answer Key 251
Pretest 2 Answer Key 256
Pretest 3 Answer Key 262
Posttest Answer Key 268

Study Tips: Taking Medical Assisting Examinations

General Examination Descriptions

CMA Examination

The Certified Medical Assistant (CMA) examination is a computer-based examination. It is administered by appointment at testing sites throughout the United States. Individuals who meet the requirements set by the American Association of Medical Assistants (AAMA) are eligible to sit for this examination. The examination consists of 200 questions in multiple-choice format. Three subject areas are covered on the examination; the content of each area is broken down as follows:

General Medical Assisting Knowledge (28%)
- Psychology
- Communication
- Professionalism
- Medical law/regulatory guidelines
- Medical ethics
- Risk management, quality assurance, and safety
- Medical terminology

Administrative Knowledge (25%)
- Medical reception
- Patient navigator/advocate
- Medical business practices
- Establishing patient medical record
- Scheduling appointments
- Practice finances

Clinical Knowledge (47%)
- Anatomy and physiology
- Infection control
- Patient intake and documentation of care
- Nutrition
- Collecting and processing specimen
- Diagnostic testing
- Pharmacology
- Emergency management/basic first aid

The examination consists of 200 multiple-choice questions administered in four 40-minute segments. There is an optional 20-minute total for breaks between segments. The maximum time allowed for the examination is 3 hours and 15 minutes. All questions are assigned equal weight. Guessing at answers is not counted against you; the examination is scored according to the number of correct answers versus the total number of questions given. Before the examination begins, there is an optional tutorial that shows how to navigate through the exam. The maximum time for the tutorial is 15 minutes. The minimum passing score is 430. On successfully passing the exam, the medical assistant may wear the CMA (AAMA) credential. For more information on taking the CMA exam, visit the AAMA website at www.aama-ntl.org.

RMA Examination

The Registered Medical Assistant (RMA) examination is administered throughout the year either by paper and pencil or by computerized test. The paper test is administered at the school with a proctor; the school sets the time and dates. The computerized test is administered at Pearson Vue locations throughout the United States any day of the year except Sundays and holidays. Individuals who meet the criteria set forth by the American Medical Technologists (AMT) are eligible to sit for this exam. The examination consists of 210 questions in multiple-choice format, covering the same three general areas as the CMA examination. You are given 2 hours to complete the examination. The approximate percentage of material covered from each section and the content is broken down as follows:

General Medical Assisting Knowledge (41%)
- Anatomy and physiology
- Medical terminology

- Medical law
- Medical ethics
- Human relations
- Patient education

Administrative Medical Assisting (24%)
- Insurance
- Financial bookkeeping
- Medical receptionist/secretarial/clerical

Clinical Medical Assisting (35%)
- Asepsis
- Sterilization
- Instruments
- Vital signs
- Physical examinations
- Clinical pharmacology
- Minor surgery
- Therapeutic modalities
- Laboratory procedures
- Electrocardiography
- First aid

A minimum scaled score of 70 must be attained to pass the examination. On successfully passing the examination, the medical assistant may wear the RMA credential. For more information on taking the RMA exam, visit the AMT website at americanmedtech.org.

CMAS Examination (AMT)

The Certified Medical Administrative Specialist (CMAS) examination consists of 200 four-option, multiple-choice questions. The CMAS examination is administered throughout the year either by paper and pencil or by computerized test. The paper test is administered at the school with a proctor; the school sets the time and dates. The computerized test is administered at Pearson Vue locations throughout the United States any day of the year except Sundays and holidays. Individuals who meet the criteria set forth by the AMT are eligible to sit for this examination. The approximate percentage of material covered from each section and the content is broken down as follows:

Medical Assisting Foundations (13%)
- Medical terminology
- Basic anatomy and physiology
- Legal and ethical considerations
- Professionalism

Basic Clinical Medical Office Assisting (8%)
- Basic health history interview
- Basic charting
- Vital signs and measurements
- Asepsis in the medical office
- Examination preparation
- Medical office emergencies
- Pharmacology

Medical Office Clerical Assisting (10%)
- Appointment management and scheduling
- Reception
- Communication
- Patient information and community resources

Medical Records Management (14%)
- Systems
- Procedures
- Confidentiality

Health Care Insurance Processing, Coding, and Billing (17%)
- Insurance processing
- Coding
- Insurance billing finances

Medical Office Financial Management (17%)
- Fundamental financial management
- Patient accounts
- Banking
- Payroll

Medical Office Information Processing (7%)
- Fundamentals of computing
- Medical office computer applications

Medical Office Management (14%)
- Office communications
- Business organization management
- Human resources
- Safety
- Supplies and equipment
- Physical office plant
- Risk management and quality assurance

A minimum scaled score of 70 must be attained to pass the examination. On successfully passing the exam, the medical assistant may wear the CMAS credential. For more information on taking the CMAS exam, visit the AMT website at americanmedtech.org.

CCMA Examination (National Healthcareer Association)

The Certified Clinical Medical Assistant (CCMA) examination is administered in three formats: (1) paper and pencil; (2) school-administered, computer-based; and (3) commercial test center computer-based (PSI/Lasergrade). Paper and pencil and computer-based examinations are offered at most schools that are National Healthcareer Association (NHA) test sites. Candidates who wish to take the examination and may not currently be enrolled in a school program should first register for the examination at www.nhanow.com and then contact PSI online at www.psiexams.com to schedule an appointment to sit for the examination. The examination consists of 170 (20 pretest) multiple-choice questions. You have 2 hours and 50 minutes to take the examination. The approximate percentages from each section are as follows:

- Foundational knowledge and basic science (10%)
- Anatomy and physiology (8%)
- Clinical patient care (54%)
- Patient care coordination and education (5%)
- Administrative assisting (13%)
- Communication and customer service (5%)
- Medical law and ethics (5%)

For more information on taking the CCMA exam, visit the NHA website at nhanow.com.

CMAA Examination (NHA)

The Certified Medical Administrative Assistant (CMAA) examination is administered in three formats: (1) paper and pencil; (2) school-administered, computer-based; and (3) commercial test center computer-based (PSI/Lasergrade). Paper and pencil and computer-based examinations are offered at most schools that are NHA test sites. Candidates who wish to take the examination and may not currently be enrolled in a school program should first register for the examination at www.nhanow.com and then contact PSI online at www.psiexams.com to schedule an appointment to sit for the examination. The examination consists of 110 (20 pretest) multiple-choice questions. You have 2 hours and 10 minutes to take the examination. The approximate percentages from each section are as follows:

- Scheduling (17%)
- Patient intake (16%)
- Office logistics (11%)
- Compliance (15%)
- Patient education (10%)
- General office policies and procedures (14%)
- Basic medical terminology (17%)

For more information on taking the CMAA examination, visit the NHA website at nhanow.com.

CMAC Examination (AMCA)

The Clinical Medical Assistant Certification (CMAC) examination is offered as either pencil/paper or online through a proctored test site. The test consists of 200 questions and the examination time is 3 hours and 30 minutes. The approximate percentages from each section are as follows:

- Anatomy and physiology (12%)
- Phlebotomy (25%)
- EKG (11%)
- OSHA/infection control (19.5%)
- Medical law and ethics (11%)
- Medical office/patient care skills (14.5%)
- Health care systems (7%)

For more information on taking the CMAC examination, visit the AMCA website at www.amcaexams.com.

Study Tips for the Examination

Taking a certification examination is an important event in your career. This section will guide you in preparing for the examination by offering study techniques and tips and by describing the examination itself and what to expect when examination day arrives. A great deal of commitment is required on your part to study for the examination. Your performance on the examination will reflect your study habits. If you give an effort of 100%, you should do well; if you halfheartedly study for the examination, you will not do well. The earlier you begin studying for the examination, the better. It is up to you to determine what study methods work best for you. Once you have done this, discipline yourself and stick to your plan!

1. Assess your learning capabilities. This will help you to determine the amount of time you will need to study.
2. Request a content outline from your certifying agency. Review the outline and determine the amount of time you will need for your own learning capabilities.
3. Plot a study schedule. Divide the outline into subjects. Place the subjects into a study schedule. Allow extra time for subjects that are more difficult for you.
4. Set up a time schedule. Retention levels are higher when you study in short sessions.
5. Prepare to study.

- Create the environment.
- Select a place with a desk or table, straight-backed chair, and good lighting. Being too comfortable may encourage sleep.
- Keep the room temperature comfortable—not too warm or too cool.
- Avoid interruptions from family, friends, and telephone.
- Avoid unnecessary noise.
- Gather study tools.
- Gather all books, notebooks, and flashcards. Have extra pens, pencils, and flashcards handy.

6. Commit to study. You are preparing to take a national examination for your medical assistant credential!
7. Study!

- Study material you do not know. Do not waste time on the material you do know.
- Take a break halfway through each session.
- Study the subject you dislike or are weakest in first and the subject you like or are strongest in last.
- Do not study after a heavy meal.
- Take your review book, notes, or flashcards with you and answer questions at lunch time, coffee breaks, and in your spare time.
- Attend an examination review class or join a study group.

The Day Before the Examination

1. Be familiar with the directions and the route to the test site.
2. Review your notes briefly. Do not cram!
3. Go to bed early and get a good night's sleep.
4. Plan to arrive early at the test site. Doors will be locked to latecomers after a certain amount of time.
5. Have pencils and supplies ready to take with you to the examination.

The Day of the Examination

1. Eat a light breakfast.
2. Avoid caffeinated drinks. Caffeine can decrease the attention span and can overstimulate the metabolism. This reduces concentration.
3. Dress comfortably in layers.
4. Listen to traffic and weather reports beforehand.
5. Bring your flashcards for a last review while waiting to take the examination.
6. Bring test material, photo identification, admission card, and several No. 2 pencils with erasers. If you are taking the computerized examination at a testing center, you will not be allowed to bring anything into the testing area with you. The center will provide a locker for your belongings. The center will provide you with all the materials you will need for notes and computations.

Taking the Examination

As you sit down to take your exam, remember these important points.

1. Take a deep breath before starting.
2. Read all directions before starting.
3. If permissible, make notes on the examination booklet.
4. Read each question carefully and analyze what is being asked.
5. Pay attention to words that are emphasized by underline, capitalization, bold, or italics.
6. Concentrate on each question. Do not wander off to other questions.
7. Do not leave any blank answers. Guessing gives you a chance to get it right.
8. Be careful when marking answers on the answer sheet so that you do not skip a line or mark an incorrect circle.
9. Check your time periodically. Allow 1 hour per section.
10. Multiple-choice questions have one correct answer. Do not overanalyze. Give the best answer to the question as it is written.
11. If you do not know the answer immediately, start eliminating choices to at least two possibilities. Highlight or mark the question on the test booklet so you can return to it after finishing the rest of the test.
12. If taking the paper/pencil exam, check the answer sheet to make sure it is complete before turning it in.

Check your examination booklet for highlighted questions and return to them.

13. If taking the paper/pencil exam, make sure your identification information is on the answer sheet and that it is correct before handing in the test booklet and answer sheet.

Multiple-Choice Questions

1. Statements that contain words such as "always," "every," "never," and "all" are usually too broad and often incorrect.
2. If two choices have the same or almost the same meaning, they are both incorrect; eliminate both choices when you select your answer.
3. Be aware of directional words, such as "but," "except," and "however." They signal opposite meanings.
4. Try to answer the test question before looking at the options.
5. If you do not know the answer, eliminate the choices you know are wrong.
6. Read the question with the answer you selected to hear how they sound together.
7. To answer a multiple-choice question, you need to:
    a. Find the main idea
    b. Find and remember details that support the main idea
    c. Draw conclusions

General

Directions: Each of the following questions is followed by five possible responses. Select the *best* response.

1. The combining form for "joint":
   A. arthr/o
   B. ather/o
   C. cardi/o
   D. crani/o
   E. my/o
2. The abbreviation for "left eye" is:
   A. AD
   B. AS
   C. OD
   D. OS
   E. OU
3. Which of the following is a function of the liver?
   A. Bile production
   B. Detoxification
   C. Production of heparin
   D. Storage of glycogen
   E. All of the above
4. "Respondeat Superior" means:
   A. The Provider is superior
   B. The Thing speaks for itself
   C. Let the Master answer
   D. The Provider is responsible
   E. Speak only when spoken to
5. Excessive sugar concentration in the blood is:
   A. Hypoglycemia
   B. Hyperglycemia
   C. Hypernatremia
   D. Hyperglycosuria
   E. Hyperkalemia
6. The Provider-Patient relationship is legally considered a/an:
   A. Contract
   B. Professional Association
   C. Res ipsa loquitor
   D. Partnership
   E. None of the above
7. Which of the following respiratory disorders is characterized by a loss of lung capacity?
   A. Asthma
   B. Bronchitis
   C. Emphysema
   D. Turberculosis
   E. All of the above
8. Nonverbal communication may be conveyed by:
   A. Eye contact
   B. Body position
   C. Touch
   D. Silence
   E. All of the above
9. Bulimia is:
   A. A food mass
   B. Loss of appetite
   C. A blood condition
   D. A food allergy
   E. An eating disorder
10. Which of the following separates the heart into Right and Left Sides?
    A. Atrium
    B. Purkinje fibers
    C. Septum
    D. Aorta
    E. Foramen ovale

11. A nevus in the antecubital area is a:
    A. Mass on the shoulder
    B. Polyp on the lower back
    C. Wart on the ankle
    D. Scar on the knee
    E. Mole on the inside of the elbow
12. An inflammation of a joint is called:
    A. Arthrodesis
    B. Arthrodynia
    C. Arthroclasis
    D. Arthritis
    E. Arthrocentesis
13. The main function of the olfactory nerve is:
    A. Touching
    B. Tasting
    C. Smelling
    D. Seeing
    E. Hearing
14. Health is:
    A. Not attainable because of current lifestyles
    B. A disturbance in homeostasis
    C. An anomaly
    D. Physical, mental, and social well-being
    E. Organic in nature
15. The correct medical term for hives is:
    A. Urticaria
    B. Verruca
    C. A nevus
    D. Shingles
    E. Alopecia
16. The skin performs all of the following *except*:
    A. Temperature control
    B. Excretion of nitrogen-containing waste
    C. Perception
    D. Protection
    E. Synthesis of vitamin D
17. The membrane that surrounds the heart is the:
    A. Endocardium
    B. Endometrium
    C. Pericardium
    D. Perineum
    E. Myocardium
18. A mucous membrane:
    A. Lines closed cavities of the body
    B. Covers the lungs
    C. Lines the abdominal cavity
    D. Lines body cavities that open to the outside
    E. Surrounds the heart
19. The body cavity that contains the intestines is the:
    A. Thoracic
    B. Spinal
    C. Abdominal
    D. Pleural
    E. Peritoneal
20. Movement of a body part toward the midline of the body is:
    A. Supination
    B. Pronation
    C. Adduction
    D. Abduction
    E. Rotation

21. Reye syndrome:
    A. Can follow a viral illness in children
    B. Is caused by high fever
    C. Is a symptom of acquired immunodeficiency syndrome (AIDS)
    D. Causes muscular dystrophy
    E. Is the common cold
22. The vertebrae located in the lower back are the:
    A. Cervical
    B. Thoracic
    C. Lumbar
    D. Sacral
    E. Coccyx
23. The bone located in the posterior of the skull is the:
    A. Frontal
    B. Ethmoid
    C. Temporal
    D. Occipital
    E. Mandible
24. The peripheral nervous system is composed of how many pairs of spinal nerves?
    A. 2
    B. 5
    C. 12
    D. 20
    E. 31
25. The pons and medulla make up the:
    A. Brainstem
    B. Cerebellum
    C. Cerebrum
    D. Thalamus
    E. Right hemisphere
26. The failure of bone marrow to produce red blood cells results in which type of anemia?
    A. Aplastic
    B. Hemolytic
    C. Pernicious
    D. Microcytic
    E. Leukemia
27. Protrusion of a part of the stomach through the esophageal opening in the diaphragm is a(n):
    A. Esophageal aneurysm
    B. Esophageal varices
    C. Hiatal hernia
    D. Pyloric stenosis
    E. Gastroesophageal reflux disease (GERD)
28. Another name for the tympanic membrane is the:
    A. Ossicle
    B. Cochlea
    C. Auricle
    D. Eardrum
    E. Organ of Corti
29. The largest artery in the body is the:
    A. Brachial artery
    B. Temporal artery
    C. Radial artery
    D. Aorta
    E. Femoral artery

30. The sinoatrial node:
    A. Stimulates the diaphragm
    B. Is the same as the atrioventricular node
    C. Is the pacemaker of the heart
    D. Divides the heart into right and left sides
    E. Regulates blood flow to the brain
31. An x-ray taken to confirm a fracture of the distal forearm would include the:
    A. Tibia and fibula
    B. Radius and ulna
    C. Femur and trochanter
    D. Calcaneus and malleolus
    E. Humerus and scapula
32. Which of the following demonstrates an involuntary muscle action?
    A. Heartbeat
    B. Breathing
    C. Peristalsis
    D. Pupil dilation
    E. All of the above
33. Which of the following organs is located in the right upper quadrant?
    A. Liver
    B. Right ovary
    C. Appendix
    D. Uterus
    E. Stomach
34. Which of the following nerves stimulates the diaphragm?
    A. Trochlear
    B. Accessory
    C. Sciatic
    D. Phrenic
    E. Vagus
35. An abnormal lateral curvature of the spine is known as:
    A. Spondylosis
    B. Kyphosis
    C. Scoliosis
    D. Ankylosis
    E. Lordosis
36. The alpha cells in the pancreas are responsible for the production of:
    A. Insulin
    B. Glucagon
    C. Hydrochloric acid (HCl)
    D. Pepsin
    E. Gastrin
37. Which of the following is an example of "social" personal space?
    A. 12 to 15 feet
    B. Touching to 1½ feet
    C. 4 to 12 feet
    D. 1½ to 4 feet
    E. Private
38. How many permanent teeth does an adult have?
    A. 20
    B. 24
    C. 28
    D. 32
    E. 36
39. Legally, a physician:
    A. May not refuse treatment in an emergency situation
    B. May refuse to provide follow-up care after initial treatment
    C. Must provide a diagnosis to a patient's employer if requested
    D. Must provide a medical history to the patient's insurance company if the insurance company requests it
    E. May refuse to accept a patient if he or she chooses
40. Professionalism may best be displayed by:
    A. Keeping emotions to one's self
    B. Staying calm when dealing with angry patients
    C. Showing no consideration for other members of the team
    D. Referring all problems to the physician
    E. Arriving late or leaving early
41. The patient's medical record belongs to:
    A. The patient's spouse
    B. The physician
    C. The patient
    D. The patient's attorney
    E. The state medical board
42. A breast mass is found in a woman whose mother and sister have died of breast cancer. She cancels her next three follow-up appointments. Which defense mechanism is she using?
    A. Denial
    B. Anxiety
    C. Acceptance
    D. Isolation
    E. Suppression
43. Personality differences are due to:
    A. Age
    B. Experience
    C. Heredity
    D. Environment
    E. All of the above
44. Which of the following are characteristics desirable in a medical assistant?
    A. Adaptable
    B. Flexible
    C. Friendly
    D. Compassionate
    E. All of the above
45. Which of the following is *not* an example of stereotyping?
    A. Similar people have similar needs
    B. Elderly patients have hearing deficits
    C. Medicaid patients are lazy
    D. Educated patients have no fear of illness
    E. Young children react differently to stressful situations
46. To release medical information:
    A. The physician must sign a waiver
    B. The insurance company must make the request in writing
    C. The patient must sign a release form
    D. A certified record technician must be employed by the office
    E. The patient must deliver the records in person to the requester

47. Which of the following should be reported to the health department?
    A. Otitis media
    B. Strep throat
    C. Influenza
    D. Vaginal yeast infection
    E. Human immunodeficiency virus (HIV)

48. A patient complains of a sore throat. The provider takes a swab for a throat culture to diagnose and treat the complaint. The act is considered:
    A. Expressed consent
    B. Implied consent
    C. Invasion of privacy
    D. Informed consent
    E. Implied contract

49. Which of the following telephone calls should be given immediately to the physician?
    A. Another physician
    B. An angry patient
    C. A patient's family member
    D. A salesperson
    E. An insurance company

50. In Maslow's hierarchy of needs, the need to be loved and free from loneliness is a:
    A. Physiologic need
    B. Safety need
    C. Social need
    D. Self-esteem need
    E. Self-actualization need

51. If a patient refuses to consent to treatment, the medical assistant should:
    A. Schedule the patient for another appointment
    B. Force treatment on the patient
    C. Force the patient to consent
    D. Delay treatment and inform or consult with the physician
    E. Terminate the patient

52. An enforceable contract contains:
    A. An offer
    B. An acceptance
    C. A consideration
    D. A capacity
    E. All of the above

53. Blood is:
    A. The primary transport medium of the body
    B. Classified as a connective tissue
    C. Pumped by the heart
    D. Regulator of fluid and electrolyte balances
    E. All of the above

54. The opposite of anterior is:
    A. Distal
    B. Medial
    C. Proximal
    D. Posterior
    E. Lateral

55. Informed consent includes which of the following elements?
    A. Benefits and risks of the treatment
    B. Purpose of treatment
    C. Nature of the patient's condition
    D. Assessment of the patient's understanding of the treatment
    E. All of the above

56. All of the following are reasons for revoking a physician's license *except:*
    A. Mental incapacity
    B. Physical incapacity
    C. Conviction of a crime
    D. Unprofessional conduct
    E. Providing atypical care

57. The control center of a cell is:
    A. DNA
    B. Organelles
    C. Nucleus
    D. Ribosomes
    E. Cell membrane

58. Subcutaneous tissue:
    A. Is found under the skin
    B. Contains fat
    C. Is an injection site
    D. Connects the dermis to the muscle surface
    E. All of the above

59. Which of the following is *not* a bone of the lower extremity?
    A. Femur
    B. Humerus
    C. Tibia
    D. Fibula
    E. Metatarsals

60. The muscle in the upper extremity that is used as an injection site is the:
    A. Deltoid
    B. Biceps brachii
    C. Triceps brachii
    D. Trapezius
    E. Gluteus medius

61. The Health Information Portability and Accountability Act of 1996 was enacted to regulate all of the following *except:*
    A. Setting requirements for electronic transmission of health records
    B. Protection of patient privacy
    C. Improvement of continuity and portability in individual and group insurance
    D. Combating fraud and abuse
    E. Setting standards for employees with disabilities

62. Gas exchange in the lungs takes place in the:
    A. Pharynx
    B. Bronchi
    C. Trachea
    D. Bronchiole
    E. Alveoli

63. The liver:
    A. Makes bile
    B. Detoxifies harmful substances
    C. Produces heparin
    D. Stores glycogen
    E. All of the above

64. The largest portion of the brain is the:
    A. Cerebrum
    B. Cerebellum
    C. Medulla oblongata
    D. Brainstem
    E. Hypothalamus

65. There are _____ pairs of spinal nerves.
    A. 100
    B. 10
    C. 12
    D. 25
    E. 31
66. Gustatory receptors are located in the:
    A. Mouth
    B. Nose
    C. Eye
    D. Ear
    E. Skin
67. Insulin:
    A. Is produced by the liver
    B. Controls metabolism
    C. Increases blood sugar levels
    D. Decreases blood sugar levels
    E. Controls blood calcium levels
68. A decrease in the total number of white blood cells is called:
    A. Leukocyte
    B. Leukoderma
    C. Leukocytosis
    D. Anemia
    E. Leukopenia
69. The abbreviation meaning *immediately* is:
    A. prn
    B. STAT
    C. qod
    D. ad lib
    E. dc
70. The physician is legally obligated to report:
    A. Deaths
    B. Births
    C. Communicable diseases
    D. Abuse
    E. All of the above
71. The prefix "brady-" denotes:
    A. Slow
    B. Fast
    C. Hard
    D. Soft
    E. Difficult
72. The opposite of superficial is:
    A. Ventral
    B. Proximal
    C. Deep
    D. Distal
    E. Dorsal
73. An authorization in advance to withdraw artificial life support is:
    A. Assault
    B. Battery
    C. An advance directive
    D. Uniform Anatomical Gift Act
    E. Good Samaritan Act
74. The cell from which a muscle develops is called a(n):
    A. Myeloblast
    B. Osteoblast
    C. Myoblast
    D. Myoclast
    E. Erythroblast
75. Unconsciously avoiding the reality of an unpleasant event is:
    A. Regression
    B. Denial
    C. Repression
    D. Suppression
    E. Rationalization
76. "Tell me more about it" is an example of:
    A. An open-ended statement
    B. A closed statement
    C. Clarification
    D. Feedback
    E. Reflection
77. Communication with an adolescent patient includes all of the following *except:*
    A. Allowing for privacy
    B. Treating him or her with respect and dignity
    C. Answering questions honestly
    D. Lecturing
    E. Explaining procedures in terms he or she understands
78. Nonverbal communication may be conveyed by:
    A. Touch
    B. Eye contact
    C. Body position
    D. Silence
    E. All of the above
79. Bulimia is:
    A. A mass of food
    B. An eating disorder
    C. Loss of appetite
    D. A blood condition
    E. An arrhythmia
80. A mammogram is a radiograph of the:
    A. Chest
    B. Bladder
    C. Breast
    D. Lymph nodes
    E. Axilla
81. A cerebrovascular accident can also be called a(n):
    A. Arrhythmia
    B. Heart attack
    C. Aneurysm
    D. Stroke
    E. Thrombus
82. When interacting with a patient of another ethnic group or culture:
    A. Assume they have the same attitudes toward modern medicine that you have
    B. Never involve a family member
    C. Never allow yourself to make value judgments
    D. Never try to speak their language
    E. Never make eye contact
83. A sexually transmitted disease caused by a protozoal infestation is:
    A. Herpes
    B. Gonorrhea
    C. Trichomoniasis
    D. Crabs
    E. Syphilis

84. Which of the following respiratory disorders is characterized by a loss of lung capacity?
    A. Asthma
    B. Emphysema
    C. Bronchitis
    D. Tuberculosis
    E. Psoriasis

85. The type of membrane that lines cavities of the body that do not open to the outside is:
    A. Cutaneous
    B. Serous
    C. Mucous
    D. Pleural
    E. Peritoneum

86. Another name for an open fracture is a:
    A. Comminuted fracture
    B. Closed fracture
    C. Simple fracture
    D. Greenstick fracture
    E. Compound fracture

87. The Patient Self-Determination Act, which includes health care directives, ensures that patients are able to:
    A. Have health care insurance
    B. Have guaranteed confidentiality
    C. Control their own health care decisions
    D. Choose their own health care provider
    E. Donate their organs on their death

88. Fat is the main component of:
    A. The epidermis
    B. Adipose tissue
    C. Muscle tissue
    D. Tendons
    E. Lymphatic tissue

89. The ventral region of the body is described as:
    A. Superior
    B. Lateral
    C. Medial
    D. Anterior
    E. Posterior

90. This acute infectious skin disease is caused by staphylococci.
    A. Impetigo
    B. Psoriasis
    C. Athlete's foot
    D. Melanoma
    E. Eczema

91. The surgical removal of the gallbladder is a:
    A. Cholectomy
    B. Colostomy
    C. Cholecystectomy
    D. Laparoscopy
    E. Gastrectomy

92. The ability to imagine taking the place of the patient and accepting the patient's behavior is:
    A. Objectivity
    B. Empathy
    C. Sympathy
    D. Industry
    E. Subjectivity

93. Confidentiality of the patient's medical record is best demonstrated by:
    A. Discussing the information only among the office staff
    B. Allowing patients to read their own record at any time
    C. Never leaving records on counters or areas where other patients may see them
    D. Only the provider having access to the patient record
    E. Using a numeric filing system

94. This type of treatment reduces symptoms of a disease but does not cure the disease.
    A. Holistic
    B. Palliative
    C. Empirical
    D. Curative
    E. Definitive

95. When a patient is seen in the medical office, which of the following occurs first?
    A. Referral
    B. Examination by the provider
    C. Laboratory testing
    D. Instructions for follow-up care
    E. Prescription for medication

96. Which of the following professionals can manage routine patient care?
    A. Physician assistant
    B. Nurse practitioner
    C. Medical doctor (MD)
    D. Doctor of osteopathy (DO)
    E. All of the above

97. Which of the following is **NOT** an example of a patient advocate?
    A. Protecting patient's rights
    B. Completing insurance forms
    C. Diagnosing the patient
    D. Suggesting a community referral
    E. None of the above

98. Restrictions of confidentiality would apply to which of the following?
    A. A minor requesting confidential services
    B. Anything the patient tells the provider
    C. Information in the medical record
    D. Demographic information
    E. All of the above

99. The legal nature of the doctor-patient relationship is:
    A. A contract
    B. A professional association
    C. A professional partnership
    D. All of the above
    E. None of the above

100. In order for the medical office to release medical information to another source
    A. The patient must deliver the records in person to the requestor
    B. The patient must sign a release form
    C. The provider must sign a release form
    D. The insurance company must sign a release form
    E. All of the above

Administrative

Directions: Each of the following questions is followed by five possible responses. Select the *best* response.

1. Which of the following demographic information is included in a medical record?
   A. Chief complaint
   B. Date of birth
   C. Laboratory report
   D. Physical examination report
   E. Present illness
2. The portion of the fee that a patient with insurance must pay at the time of treatment is called the:
   A. Cost of coverage
   B. Premium
   C. Copayment
   D. Coordination of benefits
   E. Claim
3. HIPAA compliance in the medical front office refers to:
   A. Office policies
   B. Patient confidentiality
   C. Federal laws for patients with disabilities
   D. Registration of patients
   E. Insurance claims
4. EHR is an acronym for:
   A. Emergency health record
   B. Electronic hospital record
   C. Electronic health record
   D. External hospital research
   E. Extended health record
5. An electronic medical record software program can:
   A. Store a medical record
   B. Retrieve a medical record
   C. Create a medical record
   D. Edit a medical record
   E. All of the above

6. Which of the following methods can be used to enter a health history into an electronic record?
   A. The patient completes it on a computer
   B. The patient completes a paper form, and it is scanned into the record
   C. The provider enters the information while interviewing the patient
   D. None of the above
   E. All of the above
7. Both paper and electronic medical records:
   A. Include information from more than one source
   B. Provide for continuity of care
   C. Are legal documents
   D. Provide an ongoing record of the patient's health and treatment
   E. All of the above
8. During a routine physical examination, the provider decides to perform spirometry on the patient. How should this be coded?
   A. As a separate visit
   B. As a separate procedure
   C. Included as part of the office visit
   D. Only if the provider interprets the results
   E. Only if the medical assistant performs the procedure
9. How do insurance companies use procedure codes?
   A. To decide if there is enough information in the medical record
   B. To determine the level of care the patient received
   C. To determine if the patient is being cared for properly
   D. To decide whether the care being given corresponds to the patient's disease
   E. To bill the patient

10. When a patient has managed care insurance, who is the gatekeeper to authorize consultations with specialists?
    A. The primary care provider
    B. An employee of the insurance company
    C. The nurse practitioner
    D. The office referral coordinator
    E. The patient

11. Which of the following must *always* be completed on the insurance claim form?
    A. Referring physician name
    B. Employer's name
    C. Date of onset of illness
    D. If the physician accepts assignment of benefits
    E. All of the above

12. Which of the following types of scheduling allows for the most efficient use of staff, materials, and facilities?
    A. Open appointments
    B. Double-booking
    C. Wave
    D. Modified wave
    E. Grouping

13. An advantage of using the computer in the medical office is:
    A. Tasks can be performed repeatedly while maintaining accuracy
    B. Tasks can be performed with greater speed
    C. Tasks can be performed with greater accuracy
    D. A variety of tasks can be performed
    E. All of the above

14. Open punctuation is characterized by:
    A. Enclosure notation
    B. Absence of punctuation after the salutation and a comma after the complimentary close
    C. Modified block style
    D. Use of a colon after the salutation
    E. Block style

15. The federal insurance program that provides for the medically indigent is:
    A. CHAMPUS
    B. Medicare
    C. Blue Shield
    D. Medicaid
    E. HMO

16. A numeric filing system requires the use of:
    A. Lateral files
    B. An alphabetic cross-reference
    C. Color-coding
    D. A tickler file
    E. Subject headings

17. The file folder label for Jennie Holmes-Mathis should be:
    A. Jennie, Holmes-Mathis
    B. Mathis, Jennie Holmes
    C. Holmes, Jennie-Mathis
    D. Holmes-Mathis, Jennie
    E. Mathis, Jennie (nee Holmes)

18. Third-party participation in an office indicates the relationships among the:
    A. Physician, patient, and medical assistant
    B. Physician, medical assistant, and insurance company
    C. Physician, patient, and insurance company
    D. Physician, hospital, and insurance company
    E. Physician, patient, and hospital

19. A claim may be rejected by an insurance company because of the omission of:
    A. Complete diagnosis
    B. Policy number
    C. Patient birth date
    D. Itemization of charges
    E. All of the above

20. The first thing the medical assistant should do when answering the telephone is:
    A. Identify the practice and herself/himself
    B. Put the caller on hold
    C. Finish with the patient at the desk
    D. Ask the caller to identify themselves
    E. Ask for insurance information

21. The most formal of complimentary closings is:
    A. Very truly yours
    B. Warm wishes
    C. Sincerely
    D. Sincerely yours
    E. As always

22. When making an appointment, which of the following is *not* needed?
    A. Patient's name
    B. Telephone number
    C. Reason for visit
    D. Insurance information
    E. Availability

23. This type of call allows more than one person in more than one place to talk simultaneously.
    A. Person-to-person
    B. Conference call
    C. Three-party billing
    D. Appointment call
    E. Collect call

24. This procedure protects against the loss of data.
    A. Buffering
    B. Debugging
    C. Backing up
    D. Initializing
    E. Formatting

25. A tickler file is:
    A. A guide for processing insurance claims
    B. A list of procedures for equipment maintenance
    C. A type of color-coding
    D. A physician referral service
    E. Future events arranged in chronological order

26. All of the following would require a *Current Procedural Terminology* (CPT) code *except:*
    A. Diarrhea
    B. Mastectomy
    C. Otoplasty
    D. Hysterectomy
    E. Sigmoidoscopy

27. Which of the following characteristics of a receptionist might make an impression on a patient?
    A. Appearance
    B. Professionalism
    C. Manners
    D. Attitude
    E. All of the above

28. A direction to consider additional codes is:
    A. NEC
    B. NOS
    C. See also
    D. See condition
    E. See category
29. Which of the following is an addition to the ICD-10 compared with ICD-9?
    A. Greater number of codes
    B. More information on ambulatory care
    C. Expansion of injury codes
    D. Additional letters and digits
    E. All of the above
30. Which of the following pieces of correspondence is best sent by certified mail with return receipt requested?
    A. Patient records requested by another provider
    B. Fragile items with a high value
    C. Bill payments
    D. Letter informing a patient who has missed several appointments to find a new provider
    E. All of the above
31. Which of the following are Evaluation and Management (E&M) descriptors?
    A. Physical examination
    B. School physical
    C. Well-baby check-up
    D. Preoperative physical
    E. All of the above
32. Which is an example of a third-party payer?
    A. Health maintenance organization (HMO)
    B. Medicare
    C. Preferred provider organization (PPO)
    D. Patient's spouse
    E. Patient's parent
33. In the problem-oriented medical record (POMR) system, the initial database includes:
    A. A list of past medical problems
    B. A complete physical examination
    C. A numbered list of present problems
    D. The patient's progress
    E. A list of social problems
34. A trial balance is a comparison of:
    A. Cash on hand and cash received
    B. Daily charges and payments
    C. Balance sheet and income sheet
    D. Ledger card totals and account-receivable balance
    E. Owners' equity and liabilities
35. Which of the following calls require immediate transfer to the physician?
    A. A young child with a high fever
    B. A patient with a possible medical allergy
    C. Another physician
    D. An adult with a low-grade fever
    E. A patient with questions about a mammogram
36. Which is *not* part of basic information obtained at the patient's first visit?
    A. Insurance information
    B. Name, address, and telephone number
    C. Name of person who referred the patient
    D. Business address and business telephone number
    E. Diagnosis

37. Standard-size paper and envelope for business correspondence is:
    A. 8½ × 11; no. 10 envelope
    B. 7¼ × 10½; no. 7¾ envelope
    C. 5½ × 8½; 3½ × 6 envelope
    D. 6¼ × 9¼; no. 6¾ envelope
    E. 11 × 14; no. 10 envelope
38. The bank statement is reconciled with:
    A. The checkbook
    B. The day sheet
    C. Accounts receivable
    D. The payment record
    E. Both A and D
39. The record of the proceedings of a meeting is referred to as the:
    A. Agenda
    B. *Robert's Rules of Order*
    C. Itinerary
    D. Minutes
    E. Format
40. Most diseases or conditions are arranged in the tabular section of the ICD-10 manual:
    A. By age group
    B. By severity of symptoms
    C. Alphabetically
    D. By classification of disease or condition
    E. All of the above
41. The scheduling system based on scheduling similar appointments or procedures together is called:
    A. Wave
    B. Modified wave
    C. Grouping
    D. Double-booking
    E. Open scheduling
42. A new employee must complete which of the following?
    A. 501 form
    B. W-4 form
    C. W-3 form
    D. W-2 form
    E. FICA form
43. Patient information that is released without the patient's authorization might result in a legal charge of:
    A. Fraud
    B. Battery
    C. Invasion of privacy
    D. Abandonment
    E. Libel
44. A correctly addressed envelope includes:
    A. Omission of all punctuation
    B. Periods after abbreviation
    C. Periods after initials
    D. Comma between city and state
    E. Comma between street name and numbers
45. Which of the following circumstances would waive the need for a written release of medical records?
    A. Requested from other practices
    B. A subpoena
    C. Attorney request
    D. Hospital request
    E. Insurance company request

46. The term used to describe the bills the practice has to pay for rent, equipment rental, and salaries is:
    A. Outgoing accounts
    B. Accounts payable
    C. Cash due accounts
    D. Accounts receivable
    E. Double-entry accounts

47. The correct way to indicate an enclosure notation is:
    A. encl:
    B. Enclosure
    C. enclosure
    D. enc
    E. encl

48. An encounter form/superbill provides which of the following?
    A. Insurance claim
    B. Fee schedule
    C. Deposit slip
    D. Dictation
    E. Abnormal test results

49. Which of the following is the purpose of records management?
    A. Storage
    B. Arranging
    C. Accessibility
    D. Classifying
    E. All of the above

50. Which coding system is *not* associated with medical procedures?
    A. CPT
    B. *International Classification of Diseases*, 10th edition, Clinical Modification (ICD-10-CM)
    C. Health Care Financing Administration Common Procedure Coding System (HCPCS)
    D. Relative value scale (RVS)
    E. Resource-based RVS (RBRVS)

51. Which is *not* an indexing rule?
    A. Unit 1 is the surname
    B. A hyphen is disregarded
    C. Initials come after complete names
    D. Apostrophes are disregarded
    E. Names are divided into units

52. A provider who participates in Medicare performs a service for which she charges $250.00. How much should the provider charge Medicare?
    A. $0
    B. $100.00
    C. $250.00
    D. $350.00
    E. $500.00

53. The smallest piece of information that the computer can process is a(n):
    A. Output
    B. Bit
    C. Byte
    D. Font
    E. Icon

54. The index of files on a disk is the:
    A. Window
    B. Menu
    C. Byte
    D. Directory
    E. Icon

55. The appointment system of the office should take into account the needs of the:
    A. Staff
    B. Physician
    C. Patients
    D. A and B only
    E. B and C only

56. *Dear Mrs. May:* is an example of:
    A. Open punctuation
    B. Mixed punctuation
    C. Block punctuation
    D. Semiblock punctuation
    E. Modified block

57. A master list of equipment inventory includes all of the following *except:*
    A. Date of purchase
    B. Cost
    C. Operating manuals
    D. Estimated life of the piece
    E. Description

58. An illness that existed before an insurance policy is written is known as a(n):
    A. Special risk
    B. Exclusion
    C. Preexisting condition
    D. Waiting period
    E. Prior authorization required

59. A patient has not been seen in the office for 2 years. The patient's record would be found in the:
    A. Basement
    B. Active files
    C. Open files
    D. Inactive files
    E. Closed files

60. An important consideration when deciding how to position the computer monitor at the reception desk is:
    A. Patient confidentiality
    B. Staff access
    C. Lighting
    D. Position of the printer
    E. Availability of patient records

61. Which group of patients should be escorted to the examination room and given instructions on what they are to do?
    A. Children
    B. New patients
    C. Established patients
    D. Older adults
    E. All of the above

62. Which information is *not* essential for the surgery scheduler when requesting a surgery date?
    A. Type of procedure
    B. Name of assisting physician
    C. Name of patient
    D. Age of patient
    E. Telephone number of patient

63. The notation *c: Julia Jones, MD* means:
    A. A copy is made for Dr. Jones
    B. A copy of the letter is sent to Dr. Jones
    C. The receiver had been advised that a copy has been sent to Dr. Jones
    D. Dr. Jones will answer the letter
    E. The copy was sent to Dr. Jones by certified mail

64. Under a managed care plan, the physician agrees to:
   A. Set fees within certain ranges provided by the plan
   B. Accept predetermined fees
   C. Charge fees based on community average
   D. Base fees on the national average
   E. Limit the number of patients seen

65. Which type of insurance organization uses the fee-for-service concept?
   A. HMO
   B. Managed care
   C. Independent practice association
   D. PPO
   E. Medicaid

66. On arrival to the medical office, the established patient informs the medical assistant of a change in insurance coverage. Which of the following computer screens should be accessed?
   A. Charge entry screen
   B. Patient ledger screen
   C. Billing screen
   D. The patient record
   E. All of the above

67. When money is placed in an account, which of the following documents is prepared?
   A. Check
   B. Statement
   C. Debit slip
   D. Credit slip
   E. Deposit slip

68. The most common color-coding system color codes the:
   A. Patient's Social Security number
   B. Patient's date of birth
   C. Patient's given name
   D. Patient's surname
   E. Patient's account number

69. When preparing the appointment matrix, the first action is to indicate:
   A. Hospital calls
   B. Times available
   C. Times not available
   D. Facilities available
   E. Staff available

70. The patient must pay a regular monthly premium for:
   A. Medicare Part A
   B. Medicare Part B
   C. Neither Part A nor Part B—the cost is the same for both
   D. Neither Part A nor Part B—there is no cost for either
   E. Both Part A and Part B

71. A major advantage of using a computer for word processing is:
   A. Extensive editing capability
   B. Speed of processing
   C. Spell-check
   D. Column layout
   E. Storage capacity

72. Which is *not* true of certified mail?
   A. Insurance coverage is available
   B. Receipt of delivery can be obtained for a fee
   C. Only first-class mail can be certified
   D. Record of delivery is kept by the post office
   E. Restricted delivery can be obtained for a fee

73. Which of the following information provided by the patient on the patient registration form is considered to be demographic information?
   A. Referring physician
   B. Effective date of insurance
   C. Chief complaint
   D. Place of employment
   E. Patient's height and weight

74. A Medicare claim for a deceased beneficiary may be paid directly to the physician if:
   A. The physician accepts assignment
   B. The spouse assigns benefits to the physician
   C. Social Security verifies Medicare coverage
   D. Charges are paid by the intermediary
   E. The estate is billed

75. All checks received as payment for charges should be endorsed:
   A. Immediately
   B. At the end of the day
   C. When they are deposited
   D. After they are posted
   E. Monthly

76. In an alphabetical file, which is filed first?
   A. R. Stephenson
   B. John Stephenson
   C. George Stephens
   D. Ann Stephenson-Bailey
   E. Andrew Stephen

77. Which is correct for an inside address?
   A. Dr. David Roberts
   B. Dr. David Roberts, M.D.
   C. Mr. David Roberts, M.D.
   D. Roberts, David, M.D.
   E. David Roberts, M.D.

78. The two-letter abbreviation for Nebraska is:
   A. NB
   B. NE
   C. NA
   D. NR
   E. NK

79. Which letter style requires the complimentary closing and typed signature to be placed in line with the left margin of the body of the letter?
   A. Block style
   B. Semiblock style
   C. Full block style
   D. Indented style
   E. Semiindented style

80. Which of the following is *not* included in a memorandum?
   A. Date
   B. Subject
   C. Complimentary close
   D. Writer's name
   E. Reference initials

81. The second page of a two-page letter contains which of the following in the heading?
   A. Name and date
   B. Name and page number
   C. Name, page number, and date
   D. Name, page number, date, and subject
   E. Name, writer's name, subject, and date

82. The complimentary close of a letter is typed how many lines below the last line of the body?
    A. 2
    B. 3
    C. 4
    D. 5
    E. 10

83. A fee profile is derived from:
    A. Insurance payments
    B. Patient's payments
    C. Government payments
    D. Physician charges
    E. Insurance charges

84. Which of the following is demographic information included in a medical record?
    A. Present illness
    B. Date of birth
    C. Laboratory reports
    D. X-ray findings
    E. Complete physical examination

85. Which of the following requires an ICD-10-CM code?
    A. Proctoscopy
    B. Pap smear
    C. Appendectomy
    D. Irritable bowel syndrome
    E. Mastectomy

86. When it is 4:00 PM in New York City, what time is it in Seattle, WA?
    A. 12:00 PM
    B. 1:00 PM
    C. 2:00 PM
    D. 3:00 PM
    E. 4:00 PM

87. Ideally, a telephone should be answered before the:
    A. First ring
    B. Third ring
    C. Fourth ring
    D. Fifth ring
    E. Other line picks up the call

88. After a patient is seen in the medical office, when is the first bill sent to the patient?
    A. Immediately
    B. Within a week after the visit
    C. When the patient requests a bill
    D. The next time bills are prepared
    E. At the next scheduled billing after the insurance has been paid

89. The universal claim form developed by Health Care Financing Administration (HCFA) is:
    A. Form 1904
    B. ICD-9
    C. Form 1040
    D. CMS-1500
    E. HCFA-1999

90. Patients who are always late or who habitually cancel appointments should be scheduled:
    A. First in the morning
    B. Right before lunch
    C. Midafternoon
    D. At the end of the day
    E. On Fridays

91. An error was made in charting the patient's record. The method used to correct the error is to:
    A. Erase the error and write the correction
    B. Reenter the notation on the next line
    C. Draw a single line through the error, write the word "error," make the correction, and date and initial the entry
    D. Cross out the error and make the correction in the margin
    E. Cross out the entry and correct it

92. SOAP is an acronym for:
    A. Child protection services
    B. A medical assistant society
    C. Source-oriented medical records
    D. Problem-oriented progress notes
    E. Traditional medical records

93. A patient refuses to follow medical advice, and the physician decides to terminate the relationship. The letter to the patient should state all of the following *except:*
    A. A referral to another physician
    B. An offer to make records available
    C. That the physician withdraws from the case
    D. A future date after which the physician is not available
    E. That the patient still needs medical care

94. When the medical office works on a fixed appointment schedule and a patient arrives without an appointment requesting to see the physician, the patient:
    A. Should be sent away
    B. Should be referred to another physician
    C. Should be called as soon as a cancellation has been made
    D. Should be told to come back tomorrow
    E. Should be squeezed in for a brief visit so the physician can decide what the next treatment step should be

95. If a patient calls to cancel his or her appointment:
    A. Express regret
    B. Immediately offer a new appointment time
    C. Have the patient speak to the office manager
    D. Discourage cancellations sternly
    E. All of the above

96. A good telephone technique is a:
    A. High-pitched voice
    B. Low-pitched and expressive voice
    C. Monotone voice
    D. Breathless and excited voice
    E. Soft-spoken voice

97. If a patient's account has been turned over to a collection agency and the patient calls about the bill, the patient should be told:
    A. To remit payment to the physician's office
    B. To deal with the collection agency
    C. To talk with the office manager
    D. To disregard further statements
    E. To find another physician

98. The entry, editing, manipulation, and storage of text using the computer is:
    A. Telecommunications
    B. Documentation
    C. Interfacing
    D. Word processing
    E. Formatting

99. When a shipment of supplies is received, the supplies should be checked against the:
A. Advertised prices
B. Enclosed packing slip
C. Invoice
D. Requisition slip
E. Inventory

100. A credit balance on an account occurs when:
A. The patient's check was returned for insufficient funds
B. The insurance company disallows the claim
C. The patient pays in advance
D. A discount is given
E. The patient's account is sent for collection

Pretest 3

Clinical

Directions: Each of the following questions is followed by five possible responses. Select the *best* response.

1. The physician orders an intramuscular injection of meperidine (Demerol) 50 mg for pain relief. On hand is a 30-mL, multiple-dose vial of Demerol that contains 50 mg/mL. The Medical Assistant would administer:
   A. 0.5 mL
   B. 1.0 mL
   C. 1.5 mL
   D. 2.0 mL
   E. None of the above
2. A hemoglobin value of 10 g/dL is approximately equivalent to a hematocrit of:
   A. 10%
   B. 20%
   C. 30%
   D. 40%
   E. 50%
3. This type of microorganism appears as grapelike clusters when stained and viewed microscopically:
   A. Bacilli
   B. Cocci
   C. Staphylococci
   D. Streptococci
   E. Protozoa
4. To cauterize a small lesion on the oral mucosa, the physician might use an applicator with:
   A. Silver nitrate
   B. Alcohol
   C. Formalin
   D. Betadine
   E. Any of the above
5. Which of the following laboratory values might indicate cardiac muscle injury?
   A. Alanine aminotransferase (ALT)
   B. Blood urea nitrogen (BUN)
   C. Creatine kinase (CK)
   D. Bilirubin
   E. Hemoglobin
6. 1 cc is equivalent to:
   A. 1 mL
   B. 5 mL
   C. 10 mL
   D. 20 mL
   E. 0.5 mL
7. A cholecystogram is used to view the:
   A. Urinary bladder
   B. Liver
   C. Gallbladder
   D. Kidneys
   E. All of the above
8. When assisting with a sigmoidoscopy, which of the following would be most appropriate to wear?
   A. Laboratory coat and goggles
   B. Nonsterile gloves and goggles
   C. Nonsterile gloves, laboratory coat, and goggles
   D. Nonsterile gloves, laboratory coat, and mouth barrier
   E. Disposable scrubs
9. A postprandial blood glucose level is measured after:
   A. Drinking water
   B. Exercising
   C. Fasting
   D. Eating
   E. Resting

10. The purpose of pouring off a small amount of a sterile solution from a container with a sterile cap is to:
    A. Rinse contaminants from the lip of the bottle
    B. Avoid staining the label of the bottle
    C. Generate an even flow so the solution does not splash
    D. Expel air bubbles in the solution
    E. None of the above

11. A patient who weighs 45 kg weighs how many pounds?
    A. 45
    B. 99
    C. 105
    D. 145
    E. 150

12. A patient who is 72 inches tall is:
    A. 6 feet, 0 inches
    B. 6 feet, 2 inches
    C. 6 feet, 4 inches
    D. 5 feet, 2 inches
    E. 5 feet, 6 inches

13. During a physical examination, percussion is most commonly used to examine the:
    A. Chest and back
    B. Mouth and throat
    C. Eyes and ears
    D. Breasts
    E. Nose and neck

14. A patient's reaction to stress, use of defense mechanisms, and resources for support would be recorded under:
    A. Chief complaint
    B. Past history
    C. History of present illness
    D. Social history
    E. Family history

15. Subjective information includes:
    A. How the patient feels
    B. Information about the patient's family
    C. Previous pregnancies
    D. All of the above
    E. A and B

16. The temporal artery site can be used to measure temperature in:
    A. Infants
    B. Children
    C. Adults
    D. Elderly
    E. All of the above

17. Visual acuity is:
    A. Pressure in the eyeball
    B. Nearsightedness
    C. Farsightedness
    D. Color vision
    E. Clearness of vision

18. The numeric scale used to grade pain is:
    A. 0–5
    B. 0–10
    C. 1–10
    D. 1–100
    E. None of the above

19. The purpose of a proctoscopy is to examine the:
    A. Prostate gland
    B. Uterus
    C. Rectum
    D. Sigmoid colon
    E. Esophagus

20. A patient in the Sims' position is lying on the:
    A. Right side, with left leg flexed
    B. Left side and chest, with right leg flexed
    C. Back, with both legs bent
    D. Right side, with right leg flexed
    E. Left side, with left leg flexed

21. A patient lying flat on the abdomen is in the:
    A. Dorsal position
    B. Lithotomy position
    C. Supine position
    D. Prone position
    E. Fowler's position

22. The physician uses which of the following to examine the patient's eyes?
    A. Ophthalmoscope
    B. Percussion hammer
    C. Tonometer
    D. Otoscope
    E. Speculum

23. For an obstetric examination, urine is routinely checked for the presence of:
    A. Glucose and protein
    B. Glucose and ketones
    C. Human chorionic gonadotropin (HCG)
    D. Protein and ketones
    E. Blood and glucose

24. A patient should be taught that the best time to perform breast self-examination is approximately:
    A. 1 week after her period
    B. The sixth day of every month
    C. 1 week before her period
    D. 2 weeks after her period
    E. 2 weeks before her period

25. An infection that has a rapid onset, severe symptoms, and subsides in a short period is called:
    A. Acute
    B. Chronic
    C. Local
    D. Systemic
    E. Contagious

26. Sterile-wrapped items that are safely stored are considered sterile for up to:
    A. 7 to 14 days
    B. 14 to 21 days
    C. 21 to 28 days
    D. 28 to 30 days
    E. Indefinitely

27. When removing a pack from the autoclave, you notice that the sterilization indicator has not changed color. You should:
    A. Do nothing
    B. Place the pack back in the autoclave and resterilize
    C. Place a new indicator on the pack and resterilize
    D. Place the pack back in the autoclave but in a different location
    E. Unwrap the pack, rewrap the pack, replace the indicator, and resterilize

28. Patient teaching concerning a minor surgical procedure should include:
    A. Signs of infection
    B. Wound care
    C. Prescriptions
    D. Return appointment
    E. All of the above

29. Scrubbing an item with soap and water before sterilization is referred to as:
    A. Cleaning
    B. Sanitization
    C. Disinfection
    D. Sterilization
    E. Antisepsis

30. The type of immunity that develops from having a disease is:
    A. Natural active
    B. Natural passive
    C. Acquired active
    D. Acquired passive
    E. Congenital

31. Of the following, the finest suture material is:
    A. 0
    B. 00
    C. 000
    D. 4-0
    E. 8-0

32. A type of instrument that is used to grasp or hold tissues or objects is a:
    A. Probe
    B. Scalpel
    C. Scissors
    D. Forceps
    E. Retractor

33. Betadine should not be used on the skin of a patient who is allergic to:
    A. Alcohol
    B. Metal
    C. Iodine
    D. Soap
    E. Latex

34. Wound drainage that contains pus (foul odor, greenish in color) is charted as:
    A. Serous
    B. Normal
    C. Serosanguineous
    D. Sanguineous
    E. Purulent

35. The angle for the insertion of the needle for an intradermal injection is:
    A. 10 to 15 degrees
    B. 20 to 30 degrees
    C. 45 degrees
    D. 90 degrees
    E. Not important

36. A medication that is placed under the tongue is being administered by which technique?
    A. By mouth
    B. Buccal
    C. Sublingual
    D. Instillation
    E. Topical

37. To administer an intramuscular injection in an average-sized adult, which needle would you use?
    A. 1 inch, 25 gauge
    B. 1½ inch, 21 gauge
    C. 1 inch, 18 gauge
    D. ½ inch, 22 gauge
    E. 2 inch, 20 gauge

38. A type of drug that increases urinary output is a(n):
    A. Emetic
    B. Diuretic
    C. Miotic
    D. Cathartic
    E. Antibiotic

39. The physician orders 250 mg amoxicillin intramuscularly. The vial reads "500 mg per 1 mL." How much would be given to the patient?
    A. 0.5 mL
    B. 1 mL
    C. 2 mL
    D. 3 mL
    E. 5 mL

40. Cholesterol levels are influenced by which of the following factors?
    A. Family heritage
    B. Physical activity
    C. Diet
    D. Caloric intake
    E. All of the above

41. Normal specific gravity is generally between:
    A. 1.000 and 1.005
    B. 1.010 and 1.050
    C. 1.025 and 1.500
    D. 1.005 and 1.050
    E. 1.010 and 1.025

42. A complete blood count (CBC) includes:
    A. Platelet count
    B. Hemoglobin and hematocrit
    C. WBC count
    D. All of the above
    E. A and C

43. The instrument used to measure blood glucose is a:
    A. Microscope
    B. Centrifuge
    C. Photometer
    D. Glucometer
    E. Hemocytometer

44. Capillary blood is usually obtained:
    A. From a skin puncture
    B. From a venipuncture
    C. From an arterial puncture
    D. All of the above
    E. B and C

45. A cholecystogram is used to view the:
    A. Urinary bladder
    B. Liver
    C. Gallbladder
    D. Kidneys
    E. Ureters

46. Application of heat:
    A. Dilates blood vessels
    B. Constricts blood vessels
    C. Elevates blood pressure
    D. Decreases respiration
    E. Produces weight loss
47. Which of the following are considered to be physical characteristics of urine?
    A. Specific gravity
    B. Color
    C. Clarity
    D. Odor
    E. All of the above
48. The wave on an electrocardiogram that represents contraction of the atria is:
    A. P
    B. QRS
    C. T
    D. V
    E. R
49. A standard electrocardiogram records how many leads?
    A. 4
    B. 8
    C. 10
    D. 12
    E. 14
50. The standard speed for recording an electrocardiogram is:
    A. 5 mm/s
    B. 10 mm/s
    C. 20 mm/s
    D. 25 mm/s
    E. 50 mm/s
51. The abbreviation used to record the oxygen saturation measured by a pulse oximeter is:
    A. O_2
    B. PCO_2
    C. SaO_2
    D. SpO_2
    E. PO_{22}
52. A common laboratory test that may be ordered for a patient on warfarin (Coumadin) therapy is:
    A. Prothrombin time
    B. ESR
    C. WBC count
    D. Hematocrit
    E. CBC
53. Which one of the following types of suture material is absorbable?
    A. Steel
    B. Cotton
    C. Catgut
    D. Nylon
    E. Silk
54. Which of the following would *not* be included in a well-child visit?
    A. Physical examination
    B. Health maintenance
    C. Strep test
    D. Routine vaccinations
    E. Parent education
55. The purpose of having the patient empty his/her bladder before the physical exam includes all of the following *except*
    A. To obtain a urine specimen for testing
    B. To make the examination easier
    C. To prevent urinary in-continence
    D. To provide for patient comfort
    E. None of the above
56. A hemoglobin of 10 g/dL is approximately equivalent to a hematocrit of:
    A. 10%
    B. 20%
    C. 30%
    D. 36%
    E. 40%
57. Which of the following laboratory results should be called to the attention of the physician?
    A. WBC count: $7200/mm^3$
    B. Red blood cell count: 4.4 million/mm^3
    C. Hemoglobin: 12 g/dL
    D. ESR 30 mm/hr
    E. Total cholesterol: 180 mg
58. The stain used to identify bacteria on a prepared slide is the:
    A. Gram stain
    B. Wright's stain
    C. Giemsa stain
    D. India ink
    E. All of the above
59. After sitting for a long time, a urine sample becomes:
    A. Clear
    B. Alkaline
    C. Acid
    D. Neutral
    E. Darker
60. A blood sample for serum is collected in which of the following tubes?
    A. Blue-stoppered (topped)
    B. Lavender-stoppered (topped)
    C. Green-stoppered (topped)
    D. Red-stoppered (topped) (serum separator tube [SST], tiger)
    E. Black-stoppered (topped)
61. Which of the following should be recorded in a patient's medical record?
    A. Nonprescription medications
    B. Prescription medications
    C. Herbal products
    D. Vitamins
    E. All of the above
62. Which of the following is true of spirometry?
    A. It is noninvasive
    B. It measures exhalation capacity
    C. It monitors chronic conditions
    D. It is considered a screening test
    E. All of the above
63. The first thing that should be done in an emergent situation involving an unconscious person is to:
    A. Assess the victim's airway
    B. Control any bleeding
    C. Apply a tourniquet
    D. Dial 911
    E. Give the patient breaths

64. A tray setup includes examination gloves, lubricant, vaginal speculum, ThinPrep container, cervical spatula, and uterine sponge forceps. This is a setup for which of the following examinations?
    A. Visual acuity
    B. ENT
    C. Rectal
    D. Pelvic
    E. None of the above

65. Most drugs are metabolized in the:
    A. Lungs
    B. Blood
    C. Stomach
    D. Liver
    E. Intestines

66. The Ishihara test:
    A. Tests for visual acuity
    B. Tests for glaucoma
    C. Tests for color blindness
    D. Tests for presbyopia
    E. Tests for nerve deafness

67. Hemostats are a type of:
    A. Forceps
    B. Probe
    C. Applicator
    D. Scissors
    E. Retractors

68. The normal ratio for respiration to pulse is:
    A. 1: 6
    B. 1: 2
    C. 1: 4
    D. 2: 4
    E. 4: 1

69. Symptoms of insulin shock include:
    A. Restlessness and confusion
    B. Cold, clammy skin
    C. Profuse sweating
    D. Rapid, weak pulse
    E. All of the above

70. The drug fluoxetine (Prozac) is an example of an:
    A. Antihistamine
    B. Antidiuretic
    C. Antidepressant
    D. Antifungal
    E. Antibiotic

71. The two most important factors in performing effective hand washing are:
    A. Temperature of water and soap
    B. Friction and running water
    C. Position of hands and hot water
    D. Length of time and soap
    E. Friction and soap

72. At which age is the first mumps, measles, and rubella (MMR) vaccination recommended?
    A. Birth
    B. 2 months
    C. 4 months
    D. 12 months
    E. 5 years

73. If a patient describes an aura before the onset of a severe headache, this is often a sign of:
    A. Cerebrovascular accident
    B. Migraine
    C. Hay fever
    D. Brain tumor
    E. Seizure

74. Aspirin:
    A. Has antipyretic properties
    B. Has analgesic properties
    C. Has antiinflammatory properties
    D. Has anticoagulant properties
    E. All of the above

75. A quality assurance program in the laboratory:
    A. Ensures the accuracy of results
    B. Requires less paperwork
    C. Eliminates outside laboratory tests
    D. Increases convenience
    E. Provides quick results

76. The reaction of the purified protein derivative (PPD) test is read:
    A. 12 to 24 hours after it has been placed
    B. 48 to 72 hours after it has been placed
    C. Immediately after it has been placed
    D. 24 to 36 hours after it has been placed
    E. 4 to 8 hours after it has been placed

77. Malignant melanomas are often identified by the:
    A. 1234 rule
    B. Rule of nines
    C. ABCDE rule
    D. Pain index
    E. None of the above

78. The blood type known as the universal donor is:
    A. A
    B. B
    C. AB
    D. O
    E. All of the above

79. A lower gastrointestinal (GI) series is performed to outline the:
    A. Esophagus
    B. Stomach
    C. Ileum
    D. Duodenum
    E. Colon

80. A technique that provides three-dimensional images of soft tissues is:
    A. Ultrasound
    B. Computed tomography (CT) scan
    C. Myelography
    D. Tomography
    E. Intravenous pyelogram (IVP)

81. Massive and prolonged exposure to radiation can result in:
    A. Cancer
    B. Anemia
    C. Leukocytosis
    D. Arthritis
    E. Death

82. Which is the first group of leads to be recorded on an electrocardiogram?
    A. Augmented leads
    B. Leads I, II, and III
    C. aVR, aVL, and aVF
    D. Leads V_1 through V_3
    E. Leads V_1 through V_6

83. Streptococci are arranged in:
    A. Clusters
    B. Chains
    C. Circles
    D. Pairs
    E. Fours

84. Pulse rate may be increased in all of the following *except:*
    A. Fear
    B. Anger
    C. Anxiety
    D. Increasing age
    E. Exercise

85. The electrode that is used for grounding in an electrocardiogram is placed on the:
    A. LA
    B. RA
    C. LL
    D. RL
    E. C

86. Which federal agency oversees the safety of health facilities?
    A. OSHA
    B. CLIA '88
    C. CDC
    D. DEA
    E. COLA

87. A laboratory test profile is
    A. A laboratory test required by state law
    B. A substance to be identified by testing
    C. An array of tests for identifying a disease
    D. A quantitative laboratory test
    E. The source of the specimen

88. Ibuprofen has analgesic and antipyretic properties and is used to treat:
    A. Pain
    B. Arthritis
    C. Headache
    D. Dysmenorrhea
    E. All of the above

89. Which of the following patient instructions is critical for a successful Holter monitor recording interpretation?
    A. Avoid stress
    B. Refrain from exercise
    C. Keep a written record of all daily activities
    D. Wear the monitor for 5 days
    E. Do not take any medications

90. The first dose of diphtheria tetanus acellular pertussis (DTaP) vaccine should be administered at:
    A. 2 months
    B. 4 months
    C. 12 months
    D. 5 years
    E. 12 years

91. Which of the following antecubital veins is considered the best site for venipuncture?
    A. Basilica
    B. Cephalic
    C. Brachial
    D. Femoral
    E. Median cubital

92. Which of the following would be *least* likely to contaminate the sterile field?
    A. Talking over the field
    B. Hair not pulled back
    C. A nonsterile person entering the room
    D. A sterile instrument touching the edge of the field
    E. Moisture on the sterile field

93. Massage therapy is considered to be:
    A. Alternative medicine
    B. Conventional medicine
    C. Integrative medicine
    D. Complementary medicine
    E. Diagnostic medicine

94. An antihistamine that may be used to treat an allergic reaction is:
    A. Bactrim
    B. Motrin
    C. Benadryl
    D. Inderal
    E. Indocin

95. Each of the following abbreviations is correctly defined *except:*
    A. bid—twice a day
    B. tid—three times a day
    C. OD—right eye
    D. qod—every day
    E. ac—before meals

96. Surgical asepsis should be maintained when performing which of the following?
    A. Dipstick urinalysis
    B. Pelvic examination
    C. Snellen test
    D. Needle biopsy
    E. Blood pressure

97. How often should quality control tests be performed in the laboratory?
    A. Daily
    B. Weekly
    C. Monthly
    D. When necessary
    E. Before each test

98. A decrease in bone density may indicate:
   A. Osteolysis
   B. Osteoclasis
   C. Osteoporosis
   D. Crepitus
   E. Osteomyelitis

99. A disorder of accommodation usually associated with aging is known as:
   A. Myopia
   B. Hyperopia
   C. Astigmatism
   D. Presbyopia
   E. Macular degeneration

100. An infection of the middle ear may be charted as:
   A. Otitis media
   B. Tinnitus
   C. Conjunctivitis
   D. Mastoiditis
   E. Tympanitis

Medical Terminology

I. General

A. Language of Medicine

B. Mostly Latin and Greek Origins

C. Made Up of Word Parts

1. Root word
   a. Core of the word
   b. Tells the fundamental meaning of the word
   c. More than one root word may exist in a medical term
2. Suffix
   a. Word part attached to the end of a root word
   b. Changes or modifies the meaning of the medical word but not the root word
   c. Can be:
      - Symptomatic: describes evidence of illness
      - Diagnostic: names a medical condition
      - Operative: describes a surgical treatment
      - General: general applications
3. Prefix
   a. Word part attached to the beginning of a root word
   b. Changes or modifies the meaning of the medical word but not the root word
4. Combining vowel or form
   a. Used between two root words or between a root word and a suffix to make pronunciation easier
   b. Not used between a prefix and the root word
   c. Usually an *o*
   d. Combining form is a root word with the combining vowel attached

D. To Analyze a Medical Term

- Divide the word into word parts
- Divide the word by slashes, and label each word part

Example: arthroscopy

arthr/o/scopy

rw / cv / s

rw = root word
cv = combining vowel
s = suffix

E. To Define a Medical Term

- Give each word part a meaning
- Begin by defining the suffix, then the prefix, then the root word

F. To Build a Medical Term, Use the Same Procedure as Previously Described

II. Medical Word Parts

A. General Body Combining Forms

1.	acr/o	extremities; top
2.	anter/o	before; front
3.	axil/o	armpit
4.	bol/o	cast; throw
5.	brachi/o	arm
6.	caud/o	lower part of the body; tail
7.	crypt/o	hidden
8.	cyt/o	cell
9.	dist/o	far

10. dors/o — back of the body
11. epitheli/o — epithelium
12. faci/o — face
13. hist/o — tissue
14. inguin/o — groin
15. kary/o — nucleus
16. later/o — side
17. lei/o — smooth
18. lip/o — fat
19. medi/o — middle
20. nucle/o — nucleus
21. organ/o — organ
22. plant/o — sole of the foot
23. poster/o — toward the back; behind
24. proxim/o — near
25. sarc/o — flesh; connective tissue
26. somat/o — body
27. super/o — above; excessive; higher than
28. system/o — system
29. thel/o — nipple
30. ventr/o — in front; belly side of the body
31. viscer/o — internal organs; viscera

B. Integumentary System Combining Forms

1. cutane/o, derm/o, dermat/o — skin
2. diaphor/o — sweat
3. hidr/o — sweat
4. ichthy/o — dry; scaly
5. myc/o — fungus
6. onych/o, ungu/o — nail
7. pachy/o — thick
8. rhytid/o — wrinkle
9. seb/o — sebum (oil)
10. trich/o, pil/o — hair
11. xer/o — dry

C. Musculoskeletal System Combining Forms

1. acetabul/o — acetabulum
2. ankyl/o — stiff
3. aponeur/o — aponeurosis
4. arthr/o, articul/o — joint
5. burs/o — bursa
6. calcane/o — calcaneus (heel bone)
7. carp/o — carpals
8. cervic/o — neck
9. chondr/o — cartilage
10. clavic/o, clavicul/o — clavicle
11. cost/o — rib
12. crani/o — skull
13. disk/o — intervertebral disk
14. fasci/o — fascia
15. femor/o — femur
16. fibul/o, perone/o — fibula
17. humer/o — humerus
18. ili/o — ilium
19. ischi/o — ischium
20. ligament/o — ligament
21. kinesi/o — movement
22. kyph/o — hump
23. lamin/o — thin, flat layer
24. lord/o — bent forward; abnormal convexity of the spine
25. lumb/o — lower back; loin
26. malleol/o — malleolus

27. mandibul/o — mandible
28. maxill/o — maxilla
29. menisc/o — meniscus
30. metacarp/o — metacarpal
31. metatarsal/o — metatarsal
32. myel/o, myelon/o — bone marrow; spinal cord
33. my/o, myos/o — muscle
34. olecran/o — olecranon (elbow)
35. orth/o — straight
36. oste/o — bone
37. patell/o — patella
38. pelv/i, pelv/o — pelvic bone; hip
39. phalang/o — phalanges
40. pub/o — pubis
41. radi/o — radius
42. sacr/o — sacrum
43. scapul/o — scapula
44. scoli/o — bent; curved
45. spin/o — spine; backbone
46. stern/o — sternum
47. synovi/o — synovial fluid; synovial membrane
48. tars/o — tarsals
49. ten/o, tend/o, tendin/o — tendon
50. tibi/o — tibia
51. uln/o — ulna
52. vertebr/o, rachi/o, spondyl/o — vertebrae; vertebral column

D. Nervous System Combining Forms

1. cerebell/o — cerebellum
2. cerebr/o — cerebrum
3. dur/o — dura mater
4. encephal/o — brain
5. esthesi/o — feeling; sensation; sensitivity
6. gangli/o, ganglion/o — ganglion
7. gli/o — glue; supportive tissue of the nervous system
8. meningi/o, mening/o — meninges
9. myel/o — spinal cord
10. neur/o — nerve
11. osm/o — sense of smell
12. phas/o — speech
13. pont/o — pons
14. psych/o, ment/o, phren/o — mind
15. radicul/o — nerve root
16. somn/o — sleep
17. thalam/o — thalamus
18. thec/o — sheath
19. vag/o — vagus nerve

E. Sensory System Combining Forms

1. acous/o, audi/o, audit/o — hearing
2. aur/o, aur/i, auricul/o, ot/o — ear
3. blephar/o, palpebr/o — eyelid
4. cochle/o — cochlea
5. conjunctiv/o — conjunctiva
6. cor/o, corne/o, kerat/o — cornea
7. cycl/o — ciliary body; cycle
8. dacry/o, lacrim/o — tear
9. ir/o, irid/o, iri/o — iris
10. mastoid/o — mastoid process
11. myring/o, tympan/o — tympanic membrane
12. ocul/o, ophthalm/o — eye
13. opt/o, optic/o — vision
14. ossicul/o — ossicle

15. phac/o, phak/o — lens of the eye
16. pupill/o — pupil (of the eye)
17. retin/o — retina
18. salping/o — eustachian tube
19. scler/o — sclera
20. staped/o — stapes
21. uve/o — iris (of the eye)
22. vestibul/o — vestibule (of the ear)
23. vitr/o — vitreous body (of the eye)

F. Cardiovascular, Blood, and Lymphatic Systems Combining Forms

1. angi/o, vas/o, vascul/o — vessel
2. aort/o — aorta
3. arteri/o, arter/o — artery
4. ather/o — fatty deposit
5. atri/o — atrium
6. cardi/o, coron/o — heart
7. coagul/o — coagulation (clotting)
8. hem/o, hemat/o — blood
9. immun/o — immune; protection
10. lymph/o — lymph
11. lymphaden/o — lymph gland (node)
12. pericard/o — pericardium
13. phleb/o, ven/o, ven/i — vein
14. plasm/o — plasma
15. sphygm/o — pulse
16. therm/o — heat
17. thromb/o — clot
18. valv/o, valvul/o — valve
19. ventricul/o — ventricle

G. Respiratory System Combining Forms

1. adenoid/o — adenoid
2. alveol/o — alveolus
3. atel/o — incomplete; imperfect
4. bronchi/o, bronch/o — bronchus
5. bronchiol/o — bronchiole
6. diaphragm/o, diaphramat/o, phren/o — diaphragm
7. epiglott/o — epiglottis
8. laryng/o — larynx
9. lob/o — lobe
10. mediastin/o — mediastinum
11. nas/o, rhin/o — nose
12. pector/o — chest
13. pharyng/o — pharynx
14. pleur/o — pleura
15. pneum/o, pneumat/o, pneumon/o — lung; air
16. pulmon/o — lung
17. sept/o — septum; wall off
18. sinus/o, sin/o — sinus
19. spir/o — breathe; breathing
20. thorac/o — thorax; chest
21. tonsill/o — tonsil
22. trache/o — trachea

H. Digestive System Combining Forms

1. an/o — anus
2. appendic/o, append/o — appendix
3. bucc/o — cheek
4. cec/o — cecum
5. cheil/o, labi/o — lip

6. chol/e, bil/i — bile; gall
7. cholecyst/o — gallbladder
8. cholangi/o — bile duct
9. choledoch/o — common bile duct
10. col/o, colon/o — colon, large intestine
11. dent/i, odont/o — tooth
12. diverticul/o — diverticulum; blind pouch extending from an organ
13. duoden/o — duodenum
14. enter/o — small intestines
15. esophag/o — esophagus
16. gastr/o — stomach
17. gingiv/o — gum
18. gloss/o, lingu/o — tongue
19. hepat/o — liver
20. herni/o — hernia
21. ile/o — ileum
22. jejun/o — jejunum
23. lapar/o, abdomin/o, celi/o — abdomen
24. palat/o — palate
25. pancreat/o — pancreas
26. peritone/o — peritoneum
27. proct/o, rect/o — rectum
28. polyp/o — polyp; small growth on a stalk
29. pylor/o — pylorus; pyloric sphincter
30. sial/o — saliva
31. sialaden/o — salivary gland
32. sigmoid/o — sigmoid colon
33. stomat/o, or/o — mouth
34. uvul/o — uvula

I. Urinary System Combining Forms

1. cyst/o, vesic/o — bladder; sac
2. glomerul/o — glomerulus
3. meat/o — meatus; opening
4. nephr/o, ren/o — kidney
5. olig/o — scanty; few
6. pyel/o — renal pelvis
7. ureter/o — ureter
8. urethr/o — urethra
9. urin/o, ur/o — urine; urinary tract

J. Endocrine System Combining Forms

1. adeno/o — gland
2. adren/o, adrenal/o — adrenal glands
3. cortic/o — cortex
4. crin/o — secrete
5. endocrin/o — endocrine
6. gonad/o — sex gland
7. hormon/o — hormone
8. pancreat/o — pancreas
9. parathyroid/o — parathyroid glands
10. pituitary/o — pituitary gland
11. thyroid/o, thyr/o — thyroid gland

K. Male Reproductive System Combining Forms

1. andr/o — male; man
2. balan/o — glans penis
3. epididym/o — epididymis
4. orchid/o, orchi/o, orch/o, test/o — testicle; testes
5. pen/i, phall/o — penis

6. prostat/o — prostate gland
7. scrot/o — scrotum
8. semin/i — semen; seed; sperm
9. sperm/o, spermat/o — sperm
10. vas/o — vessel; duct
11. vesicul/o — seminal vesicles

L. Female Reproductive System Combining Forms

1. arche/o — beginning; first
2. amni/o — amnion
3. cervic/o — cervix
4. chorion/o, chor/i — chorion
5. colp/o, vagin/o — vagina
6. culd/o — cul-de-sac
7. gynec/o, gyn/o, estr/o — female; woman
8. episi/o — vulva
9. hymen/o — hymen
10. hyster/o, metr/o, metri/o, uter/o — uterus
11. lact/o, galact/o — milk
12. mamm/o, mast/o — breast
13. men/o — menstruation
14. nat/i — birth
15. obstetr/o — obstetrics; midwife
16. oophor/o, ovari/o — ovary
17. ov/o, ov/i, o/o — egg; ovum
18. perine/o — perineum
19. salping/o — fallopian tubes
20. toc/o — labor; birth
21. vulv/o, episi/o — vulva

M. Combining Forms Indicating Colors

1. albin/o, leuk/o — white
2. anthrac/o, melan/o — black
3. chlor/o — green
4. cirrh/o — yellow
5. cyan/o — blue
6. eosin/o — rosy
7. erythr/o — red
8. jaund/o — yellow
9. lute/o — yellow
10. melan/o — black
11. poli/o — gray
12. purpur/a — purple
13. xanth/o — yellow

N. Body Substances Combining Forms

1. adip/o, steat/o — fat
2. albumin/o — albumin (protein)
3. amyl/o — starch
4. azot/o — urea; nitrogen
5. bilirubin/o — bilirubin
6. calc/o, calci/o — calcium
7. capn/o — carbon dioxide
8. chlorhydr/o — hydrochloric acid
9. cholesterol/o — cholesterol
10. coni/o — dust
11. gluc/o, glyc/o — glucose; sugar
12. glycogen/o — glycogen; animal starch
13. hidr/o — sweat
14. hydr/o — water

15. kal/i — potassium
16. ket/o, keton/o — ketones; acetone
17. lact/o, galact/o — milk
18. lith/o — stone; calculus
19. muc/o, myx/o — mucus
20. natr/o — sodium
21. ox/o, ox/i — oxygen
22. prote/o — protein
23. py/o, purul/o — pus
24. seb/o, sebace/o — sebum
25. sial/o — saliva
26. sider/o — iron
27. tox/o, toxic/o — poison

O. Pathology Combining Forms

1. bacteri/o — bacteria
2. carcin/o, cancer/o — cancer; cancerous
3. eti/o — cause
4. fung/i, myc/o — fungus
5. onc/o — tumor
6. path/o — disease
7. staphyl/o — clusters; staphylococcus
8. strept/o — twisted chains; streptococcus
9. vir/o — virus

P. Miscellaneous Combining Forms

1. aque/o — water
2. aut/o — self; own
3. bar/o — weight
4. bi/o — life
5. caus/o — burn; burning
6. cauter/o — heat; burn
7. cid/o — killing
8. chem/o — chemical; drug
9. chrom/o — color
10. cry/o — cold
11. crypt/o — hidden
12. dips/o — thirst
13. ech/o — sound
14. electro — electricity; electric
15. fibr/o — fiber
16. ger/o — old age
17. gno/o — knowledge
18. heter/o — other
19. hom/o, home/o — same
20. iatr/o — physician; medicine
21. is/o — equal
22. isch/o — blockage; deficiency
23. kerat/o — hard; horny
24. lept/o — thin; slender
25. lex/o — word
26. log/o — study of
27. morph/o — shape
28. neo — new
29. necr/o — death
30. neutr/o — neutral; neither
31. noct/o, noct/i — night
32. orth/o — straight
33. ped/o — child; foot
34. pod/o — foot
35. phon/o — voice; sound
36. poikil/o — irregular
37. psych/o — mind

38.	pyr/o, pyret/o, pyrex/o	fever
39.	rhabd/o	rod-shaped
40.	radi/o	x-rays
41.	sect/o	to cut
42.	son/o	sound
43.	spher/o	round
44.	squam/o	scale
45.	tax/o	coordination; order
46.	terat/o	monster
47.	therm/o	heat
48.	voc/o	voice

Q. Suffixes Used to Indicate Pathological Conditions

1.	-acusis	hearing
2.	-agra	excessive pain
3.	-algia, -dynia	pain
4.	-asthenia	loss of strength
5.	-ation	a process
6.	-cele	hernia
7.	-capnia	carbon dioxide
8.	-chalasis	relaxation; thickening
9.	-constriction	constriction; narrowing
10.	-cytosis	abnormal increase in cells
11.	-derma	skin
12.	-ectasis, -ectasia	dilation; swelling
13.	-edema	swelling
14.	-emesis	vomiting
15.	-emia	blood condition
16.	-esis	condition; state of
17.	-esthesia	feeling; sensation
18.	-ia	state of; condition
19.	-iasis	abnormal condition
20.	-ism	condition
21.	-itis	inflammation
22.	-lapse	to fall; to sag
23.	-lepsy	seizure
24.	-lith	stone; calculus
25.	-lithiasis	condition of stones
26.	-lysis	destruction; separation; breakdown
27.	-lytic	to destroy; to reduce
28.	-malacia	softening
29.	-mania	obsessive preoccupation
30.	-megaly	enlargement
31.	-oma	tumor; mass
32.	-osis	abnormal increase; abnormal condition
33.	-otia	ear condition
34.	-paresis	weakness
35.	-pareunia	sexual intercourse
36.	-pathy	disease process
37.	-penia	decrease; deficiency
38.	-phobia	irrational fear
39.	-plegia	paralysis
40.	-ptosis	drooping; sagging; prolapse
41.	-ptysis	spitting
42.	-rrhage, -rrhagia	bursting forth
43.	-rrhea	flow; discharge
44.	-rrhexis	rupture
45.	-sclerosis	hardening
46.	-spasm	involuntary contraction
47.	-stenosis	narrowing
48.	-y	process; state; condition

R. Suffixes Used to Indicate Diagnostic and Surgical Procedures

1.	-apheresis	removal
2.	-centesis	surgical puncture to remove fluid
3.	-clasis	to break
4.	-clysis	irrigation
5.	-desis	surgical binding; surgical fusion
6.	-ectasia, -ectasis	dilation
7.	-ectomy	excision; surgical removal
8.	-gram	record; writing
9.	-graph	instrument used to record
10.	-graphy	process of recording; producing images
11.	-lithotomy	incision for removal of a stone
12.	-meter	instrument used to measure
13.	-metry	to measure; measurement
14.	-opsy	to view
15.	-pexy	surgical fixation
16.	-plasty	surgical repair; surgical reconstruction
17.	-rrhaphy	suture; sew
18.	-scope	instrument used to examine visually
19.	-scopy	process of visually examining
20.	-stasis	stoppage; stopping; controlling
21.	-stomy	new opening
22.	-tension	pressure
23.	-therapy	treatment
24.	-tome	instrument used to cut
25.	-tomy	process of cutting; incision into
26.	-tripsy	surgical crushing

S. General Suffixes

1.	-ac, -al, -an, -ar, -ary, -eal, -iac, -ic, -ical, -ine, -ior, -ose, -ous, -ical	pertaining to
2.	-agon	assemble; gather together
3.	-agra	excessive pain
4.	-arche	beginning
5.	-ase	enzyme
6.	-ation	process; condition
7.	-blast	immature form
8.	-chezia	defecation
9.	-cide, -cidal	killing
10.	-cyesis	pregnancy
11.	-clast	breaking down
12.	-crine	secrete; separate
13.	-cusis, -acusis	hearing
14.	-cyte	cell
15.	-derma	skin
16.	-dipsia	thirst
17.	-dote	to give
18.	-e, -or, -ician, -logist, -ist	specialist; one who specializes
19.	-esthesia	nervous sensation
20.	-form	resembling; in the shape of
21.	-fusion	to come together
22.	-genesis	producing; forming
23.	-genic, -genous	produced by or in
24.	-globin, -globulin	protein
25.	-gravida	pregnant
26.	-in; -ine	substance
27.	-ion	process

28.	-ium	membrane; structure; tissue
29.	-kinesis, -kinetic, -kinesia	movement
30.	-lexia	word
31.	-logy	study of
32.	-lucent	to shine
33.	-mortem	death
34.	-motor	movement
35.	-oid	derived from; like; resembling
36.	-ole, -ule	small
37.	-one	hormone
38.	-opia, -opsia	vision
39.	-orexia	appetite
40.	-ose	sugar; full of; pertaining to
41.	-osmia	smell
42.	-para	labor; delivery
43.	-paresis	slight paralysis
44.	-pareunia	sexual intercourse
45.	-parous	bearing; bringing forth
46.	-partum	birth; labor
47.	-pepsia	digestion
48.	-phagia, -phage	to eat; swallow
49.	-phasia	speech
50.	-philia	attraction for
51.	-phobia	fear
52.	-phonia	voice; sound
53.	-physis	to grow
54.	-plasia	formation; development
55.	-pnea	breathing
56.	-poiesis	production; formation
57.	-porosis	pore; passage
58.	-prandial	meal
59.	-ptysis	spitting
60.	-sis	state of; condition
61.	-somnia	sleep
62.	-sphyxia	pulse
63.	-tension	pressure
64.	-therapy	treat
65.	-thorax	chest
66.	-tion	process of
67.	-tocia	labor; birth
68.	-tresia	opening
69.	-trophy	development; growth
70.	-tropia	turn
71.	-tropin	stimulate the formation of
72.	-uria	urine

T. Prefixes Used to Indicate Direction and Position

1.	ab-	away from
2.	ad-, af-	toward
3.	ante-	before
4.	cata-	down
5.	circum-	around
6.	dia-	complete; through
7.	ecto-, ec-	outside
8.	endo-, en-	within
9.	e-, ex-, exo-, extra-	out; outward; outside
10.	em-	in
11.	epi-	upon; on; above
12.	eso-	inward; within
13.	hyper-	above; excessive
14.	hypo-	below; under; deficient
15.	in-	in; into; not
16.	infra-	below; beneath
17.	inter-	between
18.	intra-	within

19.	ipsi-	same
20.	meso-	middle
21.	meta-	beyond; change
22.	para-	beside; near
23.	per-	through
24.	peri-	around
25.	post-	after
26.	pre-	before; in front of
27.	pro-	before
28.	re-	back; backward; again
29.	retro-	back; behind
30.	sub-	under; below
31.	supra-	above
32.	trans-	across; through

U. Prefixes Referring to Number or Measurement

1.	amphi-	both
2.	bi-, di-	two
3.	hemi-, semi-	half
4.	mono-, uni-	one
5.	multi-, poly-	many
6.	nulli-	none
7.	primi-	first
8.	quadri-, tetra-	four
9.	tri-	three

V. Miscellaneous Prefixes

1.	a-, an-	no; not; lack of; without
2.	acu-	sharp
3.	ana-	apart; up
4.	anti-	against
5.	apo-	separate; away
6.	auto-	self
7.	brachy-	short
8.	brady-	slow
9.	con-	together; with
10.	contra-	against
11.	de-	lack of; removal
12.	dis-	apart from
13.	dys-	bad; abnormal; difficult; painful
14.	echo-	sound
15.	eu-	good; well; normal; easy
16.	in-, ir-, im-	not
17.	macro-	large
18.	mal-	bad
19.	micro-	small
20.	neo-	new
21.	non-	without
22.	pan-	all
23.	par-	other than; abnormal
24.	pseudo-	false
25.	syn-, sym-	together; joined; with
26.	tachy-	fast; rapid
27.	ultra-	beyond; excessive

III. Plurals

To form a plural, change the:

a as in bur**sa**	→	**ae** as in burs**ae**
ax as in thor**ax**	→	**aces** as in thor**aces**

en as in foram**en**	→	**ina** as in foram**ina**
is as in cris**is**	→	**es** as in cris**es**
is as in ir**is**	→	**ides** as in ir**ides**
is as in femor**is**	→	**a** as in femor**a**
ix as in append**ix**	→	**ices** as in append**ices**
nx as in phala**nx**	→	**ges** as in phala**nges**
on as in spermatozo**on**	→	**a** as in spermatozo**a**
um as in ov**um**	→	**a** as in ov**a**
us as in nucle**us**	→	**i** as in nucle**i**
y as in arter**y**	→	**ies** as in arter**ies**

IV. Abbreviations

Follow the institution's policies for use of abbreviations. Some institutions do not use abbreviations because of the increased chance of errors. Abbreviations can be written with or without periods.

A. Charting Terms

abd	abdomen
AB, ab	abortion
ABCDE	asymmetry, border, color, diameter, elevation (melanoma scale)
abx	antibiotic
ACL	anterior cruciate ligament
ACLS	advanced cardiac life support
ADL	activities of daily living
AED	automated external defibrillator
A & P	auscultation and percussion
approx	approximately
ASAP	as soon as possible
ax	axillary
BCP	birth control pills
BE	barium enema
bil	bilateral
BM	bowel movement
BMI	body mass index
BP, B/P	blood pressure
BPM	beats per minute; breaths per minute
BRAT	bananas, rice, applesauce, toast (BRAT diet)
BS	bowel sounds; breath sounds
BSE	breast self-examination
bx	biopsy
C1, C2	first cervical vertebra, second cervical vertebra (and so forth)
CABG	coronary artery bypass graft
CAM	complementary and alternative medicine
cath	catheterization; catheter
CC	chief complaint
CHEDDAR	chief complaint, history, examination, details of problems, drugs and dosages, assessment, return visit if applicable
chemo	chemotherapy
c̄ gl	with glasses
c/o	complains of
CSF	cerebrospinal fluid
CPAP	continuous positive airway pressure
CPR	cardiopulmonary resuscitation
C-section	cesarean section
Cx	cervix
D&C	dilatation (dilation) and curettage
disc, d/c, dc	discontinue
DOB	date of birth
DOD	date of death

DNR	do not resuscitate
Dr.	doctor
DRE	digital rectal examination
DRG	diagnosis-related group
drsg, dsg	dressing
DTP	diphtheria, tetanus, pertussis (vaccine)
DTaP	diphtheria, tetanus, acellular pertussis (vaccine)
DTR	deep tendon reflex
dx	diagnosis
ECG, EKG	electrocardiogram
ECHO	echocardiography
ECP	emergency contraceptive pill
EDC, EDD	estimated date of confinement (due date); estimated date of delivery
ED, ER	emergency department, emergency room
EEG	electroencephalogram
EENT	eyes, ears, nose, throat
EHR	electronic health record
EMR	electronic medical record
ENT	ear, nose, and throat
ERT	estrogen replacement therapy
ETOH	ethyl alcohol (liquor)
FB	foreign body
FH	family history
FHR	fetal heart rate
FROM	full range of motion
FU, F/U	follow-up
FUO	fever of unknown origin
Fx	fracture
GB	gallbladder
GI	gastrointestinal
GIFT	gamete intrafallopian transfer
GP	general practitioner
G/TPAL	no. of pregnancies, no. of term births, no. of premature births, no. of abortions (spontaneous or induced), no. of living children
grav, gravida	pregnancy
GU	genitourinary
GYN	gynecology
HAART	highly reactive antiretroviral therapy (for AIDS)
H&P	history and physical
HEENT	head, eye, ear, nose, throat
Hib	*Haemophilus influenzae* type b vaccine
H/O	history of
HRT	hormone replacement therapy
ht	height
hx	history
I&D	incision and drainage
IPV	inactivated polio vaccine
IUD	intrauterine device
IVF	in vitro fertilization
Ⓛ	left
L1, L2	first lumbar vertebra, second lumbar vertebra (and so forth)
lac	laceration
LLQ	left lower quadrant
LMP	last menstrual period
LUQ	left upper quadrant
MCV4	meningococcal vaccine
med(s)	medication(s)
mets	metastasis
MMR	mumps, measles, and rubella (vaccine)
MRI	magnetic resonance imaging
N&V	nausea and vomiting
NKA	no known allergies
NKDA	no known drug allergies
NPO	nothing by mouth
NVD	nausea, vomiting, diarrhea

OB	obstetrics
OB/GYN	obstetrics and gynecology
OC	oral contraceptives
OCP	oral contraceptive pill
O/E	on examination
OR	operating room
os	opening
P	pulse
P&A	percussion and auscultation
para	live birth
PCV	pneumococcal vaccine
PE, px	physical examination
Peds	pediatrics
PERLA	pupils equally reactive to light and accommodation
PERRLA	pupils equal, round, react to light and accommodation
PH	past history
postop	postoperative
PPD	purified protein derivative (TB testing)
preop	preoperative
prep	prepare for
pt	patient
R	respiration
	right
RICE	rest, ice, compression, elevation
RLQ	right lower quadrant
r/o	rule out
ROM	range of motion
ROS	review of systems
RRR	regular rate and rhythm (heart)
Rota	rotavirus vaccine
RUQ	right upper quadrant
S1, S2	first sacral vertebra, second sacral vertebra (and so forth)
s̄ gl	without glasses
SOAP	subjective, objective, assessment, plan
SOAPER	subjective, objective, assessment, plan, response
stat	immediately
sx	symptoms
T	temperature
T1, T2	first thoracic vertebra, second thoracic vertebra (and so forth)
T&A	tonsilloadenoidectomy (tonsils and adenoids)
TAB	therapeutic abortion
TLC	tender loving care
TM	tympanic membrane
TMJ	temporomandibular joint
TPR	temperature, pulse, respiration
TSE	testicular self-examination
tx	treatment, therapy
UCHD	usual childhood diseases
vo	verbal order
VS	vital signs
WDWN	well-developed, well-nourished
WNL	within normal limits
wt	weight
y/o	year old

B. Diagnostic Terms

AD	Alzheimer disease
ADD	attention-deficit disorder
ADHD	attention-deficit/hyperactivity disorder
Afib	atrial fibrillation
AIDS	acquired immunodeficiency syndrome
ALL	acute lymphoblastic leukemia
ALS	amyotrophic lateral sclerosis (Lou Gehrig disease)

AMI	acute myocardial infarction
AML	acute myelogenous leukemia
ARMD	age-related macular degeneration
ARDS	acute respiratory distress syndrome
ASHD	arteriosclerotic heart disease
BPH	benign prostatic hyperplasia/hypertrophy
CA, Ca	cancer
CAD	coronary artery disease
CF	cystic fibrosis
CHD	coronary heart disease
CHF	congestive heart failure
CIN	cervical intraepithelial neoplasia
CIS	carcinoma in situ
CKD	chronic kidney disease
CLD	chronic liver disease
CLL	chronic lymphocytic leukemia
CML	chronic myelogenous leukemia
CMV	cytomegalovirus
COLD	chronic obstructive lung disease
COPD	chronic obstructive pulmonary disease
CP	cerebral palsy
CTS	carpal tunnel syndrome
CVA	cerebrovascular accident
DCIS	ductal carcinoma in situ
DJD	degenerative joint disease
DLE	discoid lupus erythematosus
DT	delirium tremens
DVT	deep vein thrombosis
ED	erectile dysfunction
ESRD	end-stage renal disease
FTT	failure to thrive
GAD	generalized anxiety disorder
Gc	gonococcus
GERD	gastroesophageal reflux disease
HAV	hepatitis A virus
HBV	hepatitis B virus
HCV	hepatitis C virus
HIB	haemophilus influenza type B
HIV	human immunodeficiency virus
HPV	human papillomavirus
HSV-1	herpes simplex virus 1
HSV-2	herpes simplex virus 2; herpes genitalis
HTN	hypertension
IBD	inflammatory bowel disease (Crohn disease and ulcerative colitis)
IBS	irritable bowel syndrome
IDDM	insulin-dependent diabetes mellitus
LE	lupus erythematosus
MG	myasthenia gravis
MI	myocardial infarction
mono	mononucleosis
MRSA	methicillin-resistant *Staphylococcus aureus*
MS	multiple sclerosis
NIDDM	non–insulin-dependent diabetes mellitus
OA	osteoarthritis
OCD	obsessive-compulsive disorder
OM	otitis media
PAC	premature atrial contraction
PAD	peripheral artery disease
PID	pelvic inflammatory disease
PIH	pregnancy-induced hypertension
PKU	phenylketonuria
POCS	polycystic ovary syndrome
PMDD	premenstrual dysphoric disorder
PMS	premenstrual syndrome
PTSD	posttraumatic stress disorder
PVC	premature ventricular contraction
RA	rheumatoid arthritis

RAD	reactive airways disease
RDS	respiratory distress syndrome
RSV	respiratory syncytial virus
SAD	seasonal affective disorder
SARS	severe acute respiratory syndrome
SIDS	sudden infant death syndrome
SLE	systemic lupus erythematosus
SOB	shortness of breath
STD	sexually transmitted disease
STI	sexually transmitted infection
TMJ	temporomandibular joint
TB	tuberculosis
TIA	transient ischemic attack
URI	upper respiratory infection
UTI	urinary tract infection
VSD	ventricular septal defect

C. Medication Orders and Administration Terms

aa	of each
$\bar{a}$	before
ac	before meals
AD	right ear
ad lib	as desired
AM, am	morning
amp	ampule
amt	amount
APAP	acetyl-para-aminophenol (acetaminophen)
aq	water
AS	left ear
ASA	aspirin
ASAP	as soon as possible
AU	both ears
bid	twice daily; two times a day
$\bar{c}$	with
cap	capsule
d	day
elix	elixir
et	and
h, hr	hour
hs, HS	bedtime; hour of sleep
ID	intradermal
IM	intramuscular
inj	by injection
IV	intravenous
MDI	metered dose inhaler
noct	night
NSAIDs	nonsteroidal antiinflammatory drugs
OTC	over-the-counter (drug)
OD	right eye; overdose
os	mouth
OS	left eye
OU	both eyes
$\bar{p}$	after
pc	after meals
per	by means of
po	by mouth
PM, pm	afternoon
prn	as needed
$\bar{q}$	every
qd	every day
qh	every hour
qid	four times daily; four times a day
qod	every other day
qoh	every other hour

Rx	take; prescription
$\bar{s}$	without
SC; subq; subcu; subcut	subcutaneous
SL	sublingual
SSRI	selective serotonin reuptake inhibitor (antidepressant)
$\overline{\overline{ss}}$	half
supp	suppository
tab	tablet
tid	three times daily; three times a day
top	topically
vag	vaginal

D. Laboratory and Diagnostic Testing Terms

ABG	arterial blood gas
ABO	main blood grouping system
ANA	antinuclear antibody
AP	anterior/posterior (x-ray)
ASCUS	atypical squamous cells of undetermined significance
AST	aspartate aminotransferase
bands	immature white blood cells
BaS	barium swallow
baso	basophils
BRCA1, BRCA2	breast cancer 1, breast cancer 2 (genetic markers for risk)
BS	blood sugar
BUN	blood urea nitrogen
CBC	complete blood count
C&S	culture and sensitivity
chol	cholesterol
crit	hematocrit
CSF	cerebrospinal fluid
C-spine	cervical spine (x-ray)
CT	computed tomography (scan)
CVS	chorionic villus sampling
CXR	chest x-ray
cysto	cystoscopy
DEXA	dual-energy x-ray absorptiometry
Diff	differential white blood cell count
E. coli	*Escherichia coli*
EBV	Epstein-Barr virus
ECT	electroconvulsive therapy
ELISA	enzyme-linked immunosorbent assay (used in AIDS diagnosis)
EPCA-2	early prostate cancer antigen 2
ESR	erythrocyte sedimentation rate; sed rate
ESWL	extracorporeal shock-wave lithotripsy
FBS	fasting blood sugar
FOBT	fecal occult blood test
GTT	glucose tolerance test
H&H	hemoglobin and hematocrit
hct	hematocrit
hgb	hemoglobin
HbA1c	glycosylated hemoglobin (A1c)
hCG	human chorionic gonadotropin
HDL	high-density lipoprotein
INR	international normalized ratio
IVP	intravenous pyelogram
KUB	kidney, ureter, bladder
Lap	laparoscopy
LASIK	laser-assisted in situ keratomileusis
Lat	lateral (x-ray)
LEEP	loop electrocautery excision procedure
LP	lumbar puncture

LFT	liver function tests
lpf	low-power field (microscope)
LDL	low-density lipoprotein
NST	nonstress test
O&P	ova and parasites
obl	oblique (x-ray)
Pap	Pap smear
PET	positron emission tomography (scan)
pH	degree of acidity or alkalinity
PKU	phenylketonuria
PSA	prostate-specific antigen
PT	prothrombin time; pro-time
PTT	partial thromboplastin time
qns	quantity not sufficient
RBC	red blood cell
RPR	rapid plasma reagin test (for syphilis)
segs	segmented neutrophil
SMAC	sequential multiple analyzer computer (automated blood testing)
staph	staphylococcus
strep	streptococcus
T_3	triiodothyronine
T_4	thyroxine
TENS	transcutaneous electrical nerve stimulation
TFT	thyroid function tests
TNM	tumor-node-metastasis (tumor staging)
TURP; TUR	transurethral resection of the prostate
UA	urinalysis
US	ultrasound
VBAC	vaginal birth after cesarean section
VDRL	Venereal Disease Research Laboratory (test for syphilis)
WBC	white blood cell

E. Measures

C	centigrade
cc	cubic centimeter
cm	centimeter
dr	dram
F	Fahrenheit
g, gm	gram
gr	grain
gtt(s)	drop(s)
kg	kilogram
L	liter
lb, #	pound
mcg, μg	microgram
mg	milligram
mL	milliliter
mn	minum
oz	ounce
pt	pint
qt	quart
tbsp, T	tablespoon
tsp, t	teaspoon
U	unit

F. Compounds and Chemicals

Ag	silver
AgNO3	silver nitrate
Au	gold
Ba	barium
C	carbon
Ca	calcium

Cl	chloride
CO	carbon monoxide
CO_2	carbon dioxide
Cu	copper
Fe	iron
H	hydrogen
H_2O	water
HCl	hydrochloric acid
HCO_3	bicarbonate
Hg	mercury
K	potassium
KOH	potassium hydrochloride
Na	sodium
NaCl	sodium chloride
O_2	oxygen
Pb	lead

G. Symbols

♂	male
♀	female
>	greater than
<	less than
↑	increase, above
↓	decrease, below
×	times (multiply by)
%	percent
=	equal
≠	does not equal
+	plus
−	minus
:	ratio
::	proportion
#	pound
±	plus or minus; negative or positive
⊕	positive
⊖	negative
@	at
°	degree; hour
⯗	standing
⯗	sitting
⯗	lying down
Δ	change

H. Professional

AAMA	American Association of Medical Assistants
AAPC	American Academy of Professional Coders
ADA	American Diabetes Association; Americans with Disabilities Act
AHIMA	American Health Information Management Association
AMA	American Medical Association
AMT	American Medical Technologists
BC/BS	Blue Cross/Blue Shield
CCMA (NHA)	Certified Clinical Medical Assistant
CCS	Certified Coding Specialist
CDC	Centers for Disease Control and Prevention
CHAMPVA	Civilian Health and Medical Program of the Department of Veterans Affairs
CLIA	Clinical Laboratory Improvement Amendments
CMA	Certified Medical Assistant (AAMA)
CMAA	Certified Medical Administrative Assistant (NHA)
CMAC	Clinical Medical Assistant Certification (AMCA)

CMAS	Certified Medical Administrative Specialist (AMT)	HCPCS	Healthcare Common Procedure Coding System
CMS	Centers for Medicare and Medicaid Services	HIPAA	Health Insurance Portability and Accountability Act
CMT	Certified Medical Transcriptionist	MD	Doctor of Medicine
CPC	Certified Professional Coder	MFS	Medicare Fee Schedule
DC	Doctor of Chiropractic	MT	Medical Technologist; Medical Transcriptionist
DEA	US Drug Enforcement Agency	NHA	National Healthcare Association
DHHS	US Department of Health and Human Services	NP	Nurse Practitioner
DO	Doctor of Osteopathic Medicine	OD	Doctor of Optometry
DPM	Doctor of Podiatric Medicine	OSHA	US Occupational Safety and Health Administration
FACP	Fellow of the American College of Physicians	PCP	Primary Care Physician
FACS	Fellow of the American College of Surgeons	PharmD	Doctor of Pharmacy
FDA	US Food and Drug Administration	RN	Registered Nurse
GP	General Practitioner	RMA	Registered Medical Assistant (AMT)

2

Anatomy and Physiology

I. Introduction to the Body

A. General

1. Anatomy: the study of body structures
2. Physiology: the study of body functions

B. Levels of Organization

1. Arranged from smallest to largest
2. Chemical: includes atoms and molecules
3. Cell: basic unit of all life
4. Tissue: group of cells with similar structure and function
5. Organ: group of tissues that work together to perform a function
6. System: group of organs working together to accomplish a set of functions
7. Organism: made up of systems that work together to maintain life

C. Organ Systems

1. Each system has a specific function, yet all systems work together
2. Integumentary system
   a. Made up of skin and accessory organs
   b. Provides protection, temperature regulation, chemical synthesis, water balance, and sensory reception
3. Skeletal system
   a. Made up of bones, joints, tendons, and ligaments
   b. Provides protection, provides a framework for the body, assists with movement, stores minerals, and responsible for hematopoiesis/hemopoiesis
4. Muscular system
   a. Made up of muscles
   b. Provides movement, body heat, and storage of energy
5. Nervous system
   a. Made up of the brain, spinal cord, and nerves
   b. Coordinates all body activities and detects changes in the outside environment
6. Endocrine system
   a. Made up of glands that secrete chemical messengers (hormones)
   b. Coordinates and balances body activities and regulates reproductive systems
7. Cardiovascular system
   a. Made up of the heart and blood vessels
   b. Transports substances to tissues and removes waste products from tissues
8. Lymphatic system
   a. Made up of the lymph, lymph vessels, lymph nodes, and lymphoid organs
   b. Removes excess fluid and helps protect the body against diseases
9. Digestive system
   a. Made up of the mouth, esophagus, stomach, intestines, rectum, liver, gallbladder, and pancreas
   b. Takes in food and processes it into molecules that can be used by the body; eliminates solid waste products
10. Urinary system
    a. Made up of the kidneys, ureters, bladder, and urethra
    b. Removes liquid nitrogenous waste products and helps regulate water balance
11. Respiratory system
    a. Made up of the nose, pharynx, larynx, trachea, bronchi, and lungs
    b. Brings oxygen (O_2) into the lungs and removes carbon dioxide (CO_2) from the body
12. Reproductive system
    a. Made up of gonads (ovaries and testes), duct systems, accessory glands, and support structures
    b. Produces new individuals

D. Life Processes

1. Characteristics that distinguish a living organism from a nonliving organism
2. Organization: each part has a function and cooperates with all other parts
3. Metabolism: all chemical reactions in the body
4. Responsiveness: ability to detect changes in the internal and external environment and respond to them
5. Movement: all activities accomplished by the muscular system
6. Reproduction: formation of new cells; formation of a new individual
7. Growth: increase in size by an increase in the number of cells
8. Respiration: exchange of O_2 and CO_2
9. Digestion: ability to break down complex foodstuffs into simpler molecules the body can use
10. Excretion: process of removing waste products from the body
11. Maintaining boundaries: keeping the inside environment separate from the outside
12. Differentiation: developmental process by which unspecialized cells change into specialized cells

E. Survival Needs

1. Requirements of an organism to sustain life
2. Physical factors that come from the environment
3. Water
   a. Probably more necessary than food
   b. Provides a medium for all chemical reactions
   c. Provides a fluid base for body secretions and excretions
   d. Makes up approximately 60% of body weight
4. Oxygen: necessary for metabolic reactions
5. Nutrients
   a. Taken in from diet
   b. Provide raw materials necessary for growth, replacement, and repair
   c. Provide energy for body processes
6. Temperature
   a. Necessary for chemical reactions to occur
   b. Optimum is 98.6°F (37.0°C)
7. Pressure
   a. Application of a force
   b. Necessary for breathing and blood pressure

F. Homeostasis

1. Body's ability to maintain a constant internal environment, regardless of the external environment
2. When the body is healthy, the internal environment remains stable within limited normal ranges
3. Lack of homeostasis can lead to disease and eventually death

G. Anatomical Terms

1. Universal language
2. Used to describe directions and regions of the body
3. Anatomical position
   a. Beginning position for point of reference
   b. Body is standing erect, face forward, arms at sides with palms facing forward, and toes pointing forward
4. Directions in the body (Fig. 2.1): used to describe relative position of one part to another
   a. Superior: part above another part; toward the head
   b. Inferior: part below another part; toward the feet
   c. Anterior (ventral): toward the front
   d. Posterior (dorsal): toward the back
   e. Medial: toward or near the midline of the body
   f. Lateral: toward or near the side of the body; away from the midline
   g. Proximal: closer to the point of attachment
   h. Distal: farther away from the point of attachment
   i. Superficial: on or near the surface
   j. Deep: away from the surface
5. Planes and sections of the body (see Fig. 2.1): used to visualize spatial relationships of body parts
   a. Sagittal plane: divides the body into left and right parts
   b. Midsagittal plane: divides the body into equal right and left halves
   c. Transverse plane: divides the body into upper and lower parts; cross section
   d. Frontal (coronal) plane: divides the body into front and back parts
6. Body cavities (Fig. 2.2): hollow body spaces that contain internal organs
   a. Dorsal cavity: made up of two cavities along the back of the body
      1) Cranial cavity: contains the brain
      2) Spinal cavity: contains the spinal cord
   b. Ventral cavity: made up of two cavities along the front of the body
      1) Thoracic cavity: contains the heart, lungs, esophagus, and trachea
      2) Abdominopelvic cavity: contains organs below the diaphragm
   c. Diaphragm: separates thoracic and abdominopelvic cavities
7. Abdominal regions (Fig. 2.3): two methods used to describe locations of body organs or pain
   a. Quadrants: divide abdomen into four regions
      1) Right upper quadrant (RUQ)
      2) Left upper quadrant (LUQ)
      3) Right lower quadrant (RLQ)
      4) Left lower quadrant (LLQ)
   b. Nine regions: more specific
      1) Epigastric
      2) Umbilical
      3) Hypogastric
      4) Right hypochondriac
      5) Left hypochondriac
      6) Right lumbar
      7) Left lumbar
      8) Right iliac
      9) Left iliac
8. Body areas
   a. Abdominal: portion of trunk below diaphragm; between the thorax and pelvis
   b. Antebrachial: forearm; region between the elbow and wrist

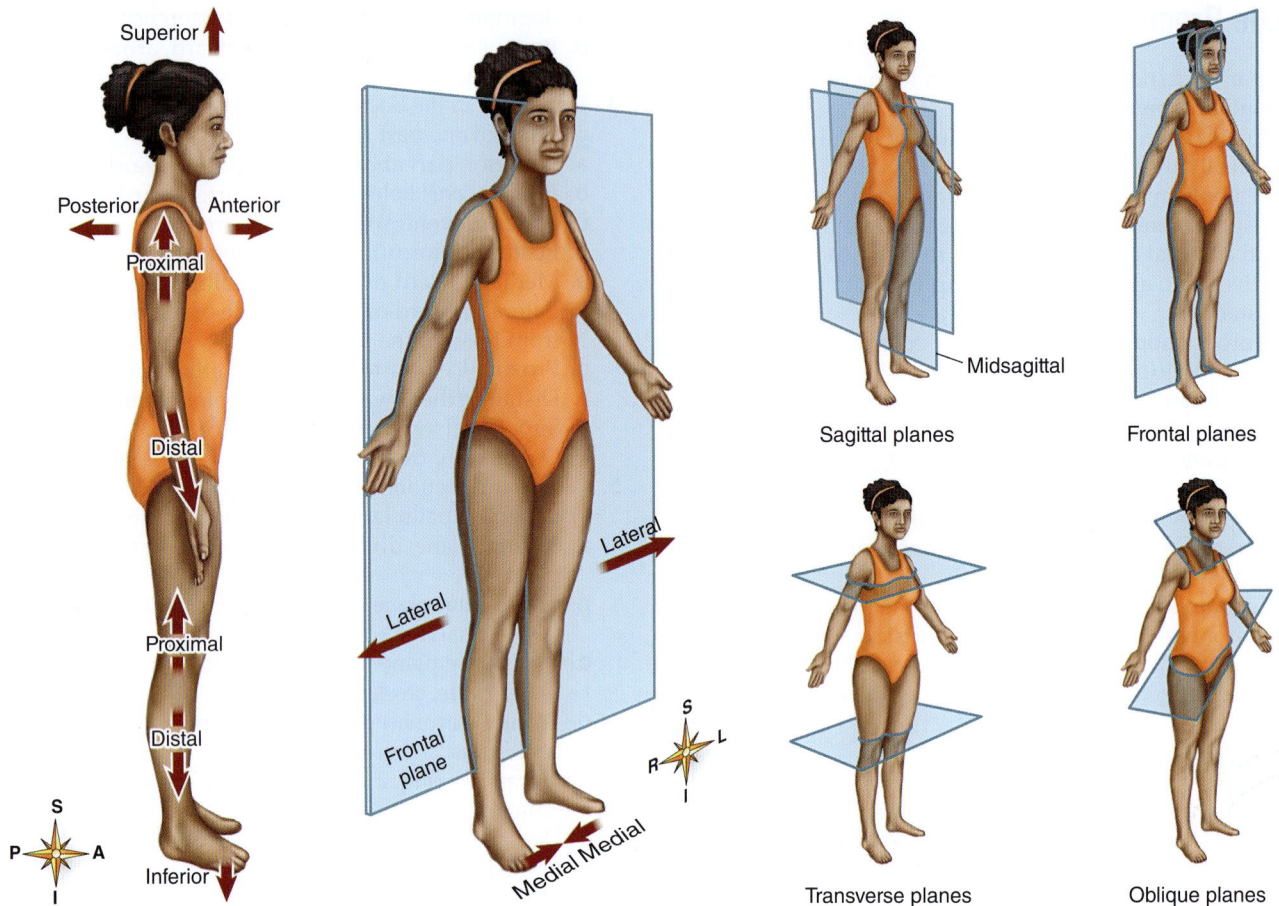

Fig. 2.1 Directions and planes of the body. (Modified from Musculino JE: *Know the body: muscle, bone, and palpation essentials*, 2012, Mosby.)

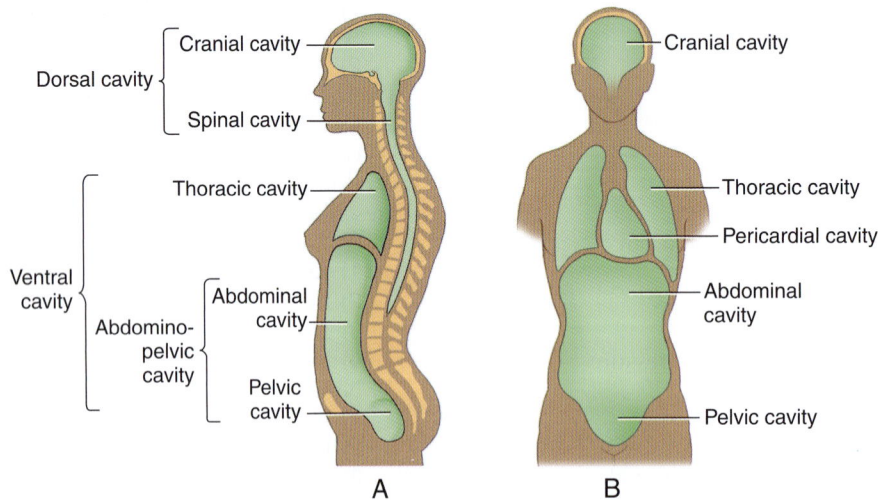

Fig. 2.2 Major body cavities. (From Shiland, BJ: *Mastering healthcare terminology*, ed 5, 2016, Mosby.)

c. Antecubital: space in front of the elbow
d. Axillary: armpit area
e. Brachial: arm; region between the elbow and shoulder
f. Buccal: cheek area
g. Carpal: wrist area
h. Celiac: abdomen
i. Cephalic: head

j. Cervical: neck area; cervix
k. Costal: ribs
l. Cranial: skull
m. Crural: region between the knee and foot; leg
n. Cubital: region between the elbow and wrist; forearm
o. Cutaneous: skin
p. Femoral: thigh area; region between the hip and knee

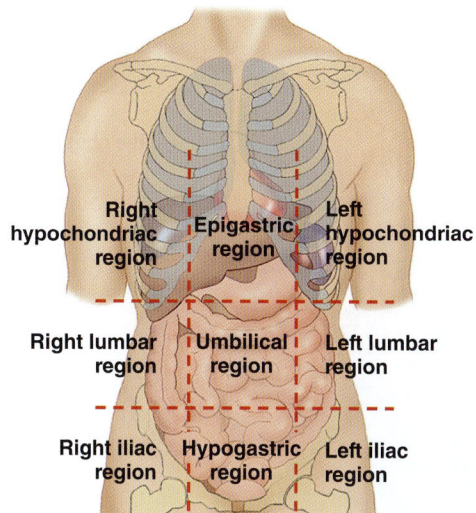

Fig. 2.3 Areas of the abdomen. (From Shiland, BJ: *Mastering healthcare terminology*, ed 5, 2016, Mosby.)

q. Frontal: forehead
r. Gluteal: buttock area
s. Inguinal: groin
t. Lumbar: lower back area between ribs and pelvis
u. Mammary: breast
v. Occipital: lower portion of back of head
w. Ophthalmic: eyes
x. Oral: mouth
y. Otic: ears
z. Palmar: palm of the hand
aa. Pectoral: chest area
ab. Pedal: foot
ac. Pelvic: inferior region of abdominal cavity
ad. Perineal: region between the anus and pubic symphysis; includes region of external reproductive organs
ae. Plantar: sole of the foot
af. Popliteal: area behind the knee
ag. Sacral: posterior region between hipbones
ah. Sternal: anterior midline of the thorax
ai. Tarsal: ankle area
aj. Thoracic: chest
ak. Umbilical: navel
al. Vertebral: backbone

II. Cell

A. General

1. Basic structural and functional unit of the body
2. Vary in size, shape, and function
3. Well organized in structure
4. Homeostasis depends on the interaction between the cell and its environment

B. Structure (Fig. 2.4)

1. Cell (plasma) membrane
   a. Thin, flexible, outermost barrier of the cell
   b. Made up of a double layer of phospholipids
   c. Allows water and chemicals to pass in and out
   d. Permeable and selective
2. Cytoplasm
   a. Cytosol
   b. Thick, semisolid substance that contains mostly water
   c. Site of cellular activity
   d. Holds organelles in place
3. Nuclear membrane
   a. Encloses the membrane
   b. Double layered
   c. Has pores that allow passage of material as necessary
4. Nucleus
   a. Controls center of the cell
   b. Contains genetic material (deoxyribonucleic acid [DNA])
5. Nucleolus
   a. Small, dense structure located in the nucleus
   b. Important in the synthesis of ribosomes
6. Centrioles
   a. Hollow, rod-shaped structures found in the cytoplasm near the nucleus
   b. Play an important role in cell division
7. Endoplasmic reticulum
   a. Complex network of tubular channels
   b. "Transportation system" of the cell
   c. Allows molecules to move from one part of the cell to another
   d. Two types
      1) Rough: ribosomes attached; transports proteins
      2) Smooth: without ribosomes; manufactures lipids and hormones
8. Golgi apparatus
   a. Stack of flattened sacs
   b. Located near the nucleus
   c. Processes and packages proteins
9. Lysosomes
   a. Sacs of various sizes and shapes
   b. Contain strong chemicals that digest various substances that enter the cytoplasm
10. Mitochondria
    a. Sausage-shaped sacs
    b. Inner layer arranged in folds
    c. "Powerhouse" of the cell
    d. Source of energy for cells and tissues
11. Microtubules
    a. Extremely small, hollow tubes
    b. Crisscross cytoplasm to form a "skeleton"
    c. Give cells strength and shape
12. Peroxisomes
    a. Membranous sacs that resemble lysosomes
    b. Contain enzymes that detoxify harmful substances
13. Ribosomes
    a. Composed of ribonucleic acid (RNA) and protein
    b. Form amino acids into new protein molecules
    c. Some are free-floating in the cytoplasm; some are attached to the endoplasmic reticulum
14. Vacuoles
    a. Membrane-bound sacs that appear in the cytoplasm when the cell membrane folds inward on itself
    b. Contain fluid or solid substances
    c. Lysosomes can empty their enzymes into the sac
    d. Aid in the metabolic activity of the cell

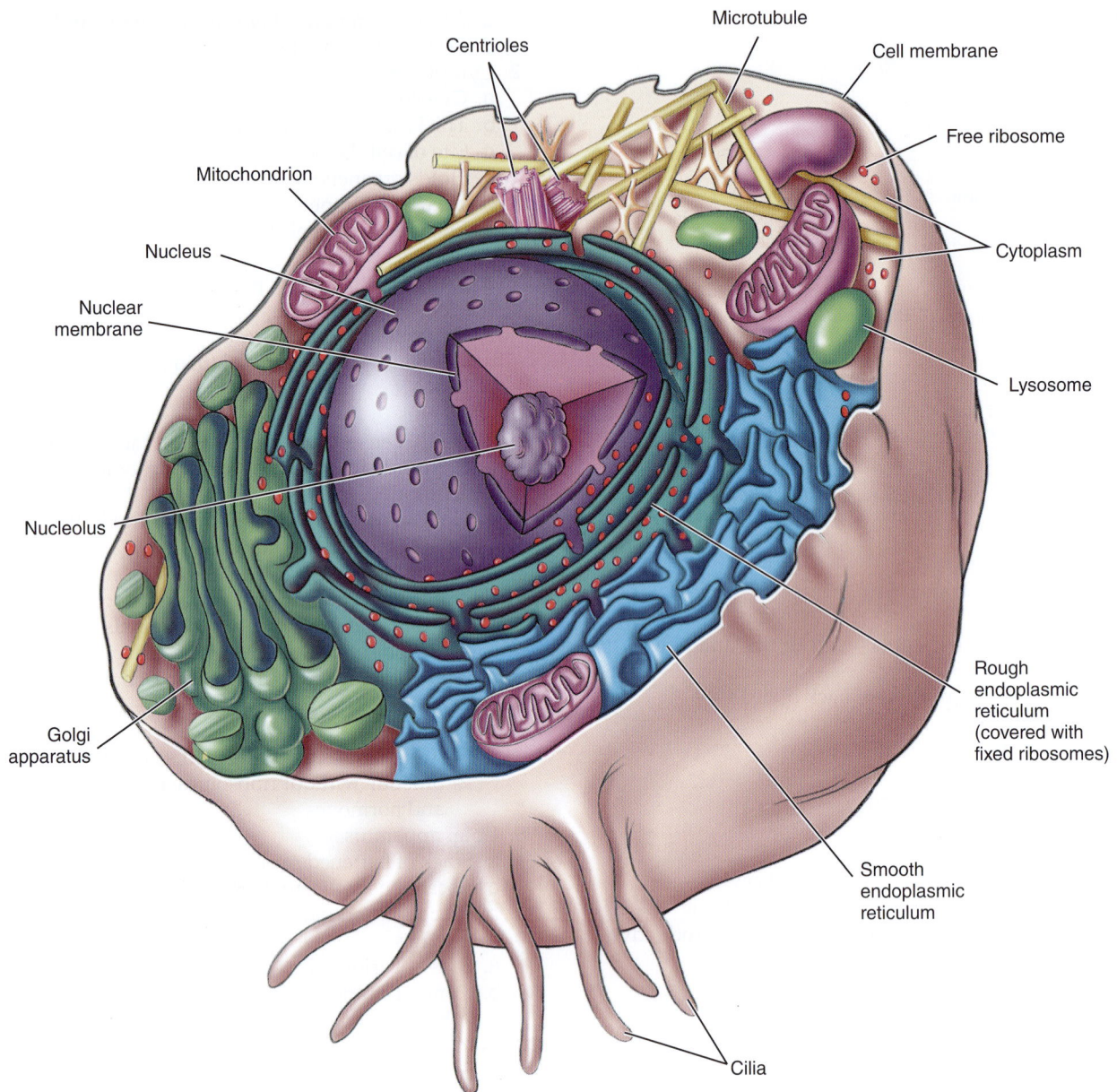

Fig. 2.4 A typical cell. (From Herlihy B: *The human body in health and illness*, ed 6, 2018, Saunders.)

15. Microvilli
    a. Tiny fingerlike extensions that project from the surface of certain cells
    b. Increase absorptive surface of the cell
16. Cilia
    a. Hairlike projections on the surface of the cell
    b. Move substances along the cell surface
17. Flagella
    a. Hairlike projection from the surface of the cell
    b. Provides movement

C. Types of Movement Across the Cell Membrane

1. Ability of the cell to carry out its function depends on the movement or exchange of fluids, particles, and molecules
2. Movement controlled and facilitated by cell membrane

a. Diffusion
    1) Movement of solids from an area of higher concentration to an area of lower concentration
    2) Does not require cellular energy
b. Filtration
    1) Movement of a fluid by hydrostatic pressure
    2) Does not require cellular energy
c. Osmosis
    1) Movement of water from an area of higher concentration to an area of lower concentration
    2) Does not require cellular energy
d. Phagocytosis
    1) "Cell eating"; cell engulfs particles
    2) Requires cellular energy
e. Pinocytosis
    1) "Cell drinking"; cell engulfs fluid
    2) Requires cellular energy

f. Active transport
  1) Movement of substances from an area of lower concentration to an area of higher concentration
  2) Requires cellular energy
g. Passive transport
  1) Movement of small molecules across the cell membrane by diffusion
  2) Does not require cellular energy

D. Cell Division

1. Mitosis
2. Continuous process
3. Results in two identical daughter cells
4. Consists of two separate operations
   a. Division of the nucleus (karyokinesis)
   b. Division of cytoplasm (cytokinesis)
5. Entire process has several phases
   a. Interphase: period of growth and development; chromosomes double
   b. Prophase: centrioles move to opposite ends of the cell, trailing a thin, threadlike substance that forms a structure resembling a spindle
   c. Metaphase: chromosomes line up across the spindles
   d. Anaphase: spindle fibers pull chromosomes toward opposite ends
   e. Telophase: nuclear area becomes pinched in the middle until two regions have formed; similar change happens in the cell membrane; the cell eventually splits in two
6. Meiosis: division of gametes producing half the number of chromosomes (23) as in mitosis when fertilization occurs; nuclei of sperm and egg come together to produce a zygote with the full number of chromosomes (46)

III. Tissues and Membranes

A. General

1. Group of cells similar in structure and function
2. Histology: microscopic study of tissues
3. Organized into four general types

B. Types of Tissues

1. Connective tissue
   a. Variety of forms throughout the body
   b. Serves as a framework for other tissues
   c. Combines to form more complex tissues (organs)
   d. Provides support and protection
   e. Serves as storage sites
   f. Fills in spaces between body structures
   g. Most have good blood supply; some do not
   h. Types include:
     1) Loose (areolar)
       a) Attaches skin to underlying tissues
       b) Surrounds blood and lymph vessels
       c) Fills spaces around muscles and other organs
     2) Dense fibrous
       a) Provides great strength
       b) Makes up tendons and ligaments
     3) Elastic
       a) Capable of stretching
     4) Adipose
       a) Stores fat
       b) Serves to insulate the body and as an energy reserve
     5) Blood
       a) Liquid matrix (plasma) with cells suspended in it
     6) Cartilage
       a) Rigid connective tissue
       b) Forms sliding surface for joints
       c) Contains no blood vessels
       d) Three types
         (1) Hyaline cartilage
         (2) Elastic cartilage
         (3) Fibrocartilage
     7) Bone (osseous)
       a) Compact and rigid
       b) Calcium deposits in fibers give it hardness and strength
2. Epithelial tissue
   a. Epithelium
   b. Found throughout the body
   c. Provides covering and lining for surfaces, body cavities, and hollow organs
   d. Major tissue of glands
   e. Functions include protection, absorption, secretion, excretion, and sensory reception
   f. Classified according to number of cells, arrangement of cells, location of tissue, and shape of cells at the surface of the tissue
3. Muscle tissue
   a. Makes up muscles
   b. Has ability to contract (shorten)
   c. Basis of and provides for movement
   d. Three types
     1) Skeletal muscle tissue
       a) Attaches to bone and produces movement
       b) Voluntary (under conscious control)
     2) Smooth muscle
       a) Found in internal organs
       b) Involuntary (not under conscious control)
     3) Cardiac muscle tissue
       a) Found only in the heart
       b) Complex network of cells
       c) Involuntary
4. Nervous tissue
   a. Composed of cells that can respond to surroundings
   b. Found in the brain, spinal cord, and nerves
   c. Cells called neurons: supported and nourished by neuroglial cells
   d. Regulates all activities and functions of the body

C. Inflammation and Tissue Repair

1. Inflammation: nonspecific defense mechanism; attempts to localize tissue injury and prepare area for healing; characterized by redness, swelling, heat, and pain
2. Tissue repair: type that occurs depends on the tissue and the severity of damage
3. Two types

a. Regeneration: replacement of destroyed tissue by reproducing identical cells; occurs only in tissues that have mitotic capabilities
b. Fibrosis: replacement of destroyed tissue by generation of fibrous connective tissue (scar)

D. Membranes (Fig. 2.5)

1. Thin sheet of tissue
2. Can cover a surface, serve as a partition, line organs and cavities, or anchor an organ
   a. Serous membrane
      1) Serosa
      2) Lines the walls of body cavities that do not open to the outside
      3) Has two layers
         a) Parietal layer: layer attached to the wall of the cavity or sac
         b) Visceral layer: layer attached to the internal organs
      4) Three main serous membranes
         a) Pleura: lines the thoracic cavity and covers the lungs
         b) Pericardium: sac that encloses the heart
         c) Peritoneum: largest serous membrane; lines the wall of the abdominal cavity and covers the abdominal organs
   b. Mucous membrane
      1) Mucosa
      2) Lines the walls of body cavities that open to the outside
      3) Produces a thick, sticky substance (mucus)
   c. Cutaneous membrane: the skin

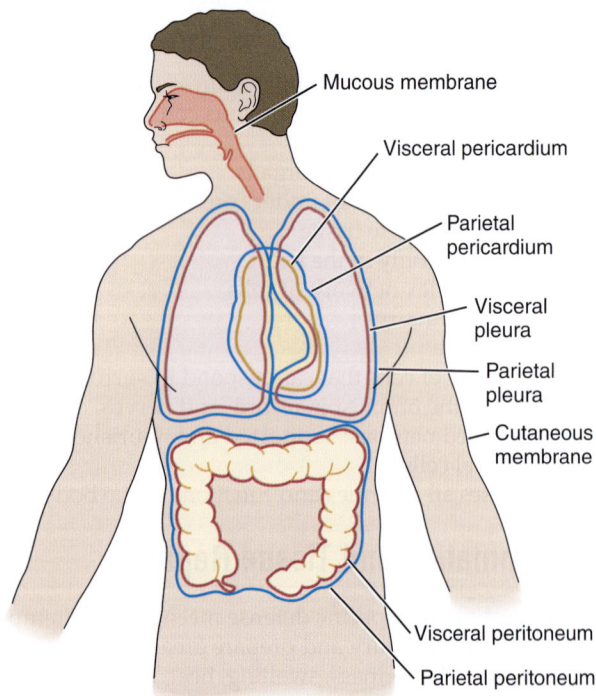

Fig. 2.5 Epithelial membranes: cutaneous membrane (skin), mucous membranes, and serous membranes (pleura, pericardium, and peritoneum). (From Herlihy B: *The human body in health and illness*, ed 6, 2018, Saunders.)

d. Synovial membrane
   1) Lines joint cavities
   2) Secretes a lubricating fluid that reduces friction

IV. Integumentary System

A. General

1. Considered to be the largest system and organ of the body
2. Made up of skin and its appendages (hair, glands, nails)
3. Forms outer boundary of the body

B. Functions

1. Protection from radiation, water loss, drying, and invasion of microorganisms
2. Control of body temperature
3. Detection of sensation
4. Secretion of waste products
5. Production of vitamin D

C. Structure (Fig. 2.6)

1. Two main layers
   a. Epidermis
      1) Outer layer
      2) Made up of four to five sublayers (strata)
      3) Innermost layer continuously supplies cells that move up to the next strata
      4) Cells continue to pick up keratin as they pass through the strata
      5) Outermost layer contains lifeless, keratin-filled cells that continually slough off
      6) Contains melanocytes that produce pigment (melanin), which gives skin color
      7) Contains no blood supply
   b. Dermis
      1) Corium; "true skin"
      2) Innermost layer
      3) Contains nerve and blood supply
      4) Also contains appendages of the skin
      5) Provides strength to the skin
      6) Stores water and electrolytes
2. Appendages: special structures that perform various functions
   a. Sudoriferous glands
      1) Sweat glands
      2) Coiled, tubelike structures in the dermis
      3) Produce and transport sweat to the skin surface
      4) Sweat evaporates and cools the body
   b. Ceruminous glands
      1) Modified sweat glands found in the ear
      2) Secrete cerumen (earwax)
   c. Sebaceous glands
      1) Oil glands
      2) Connected to the hair follicle
      3) Secrete sebum that oils the hair and lubricates the skin
   d. Hair
      1) Covers most of the body

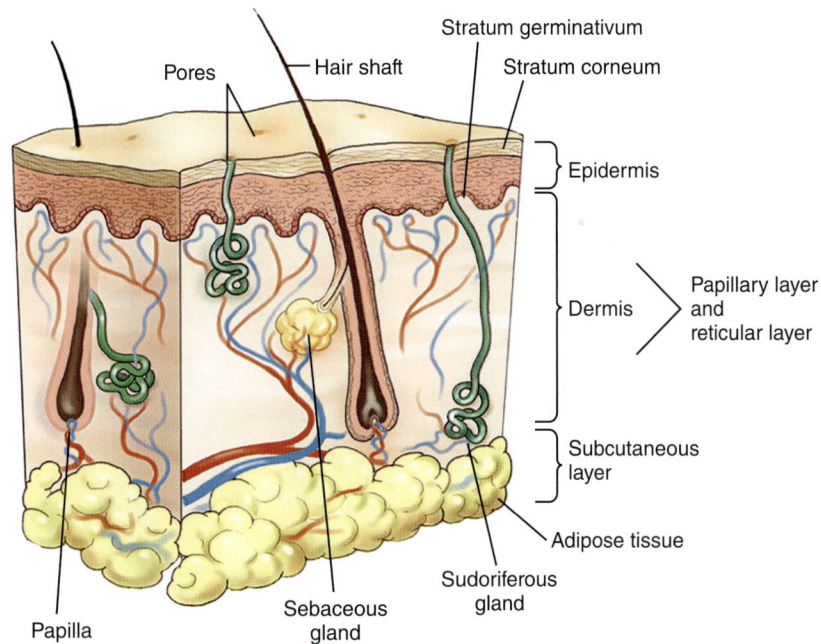

Fig. 2.6 Normal skin. (From Shiland, BJ: *Mastering healthcare terminology*, ed 5, 2016, Mosby.)

2) Made up of dead, keratinized tissue
3) Root is below the surface of the skin; shaft extends beyond epidermis
4) Connected to small muscles (erector pili)
   e. Nails
      1) Hard, keratinized structures found on the fingertips and tips of toes
      2) Protective function
3. Subcutaneous tissue
   a. Layer of tissue below the dermis
   b. Connects dermis to the surface of muscles
   c. Made up of adipose tissue, elastic fibers, and fibers
   d. Injection site

V. Skeletal System

A. General (Fig. 2.7)

1. Composed of bones, cartilage, tendons, and ligaments
2. Adult skeleton composed of 206 bones

B. Functions

1. Provides a framework for the body: shape and support for other structures
2. Provides for movement: places for muscles to attach
3. Provides protection: surrounds body cavities
4. Provides hematopoiesis: blood cell formation in marrow
5. Provides storage: inorganic minerals (calcium [Ca], phosphorus [P], magnesium [Mg], potassium [K], sodium [Na]) stored in matrix and released into circulation as needed

C. Bone Tissue

1. Two types
   a. Compact: cells packed tightly together
   b. Spongy: less dense than compact
2. Made up of three types of cells
   a. Osteoblasts: bone-forming cells
   b. Osteoclasts: break down and resorb bone
   c. Osteocytes: mature bone cells

D. Anatomy of Long Bone

1. Diaphysis: shaft of the long bone; made up of compact and cancellous bone
2. Epiphysis: ends of the long bone
3. Epiphyseal cartilage (plate): "growth plate"; layer of cartilage between the diaphysis and epiphysis where the growth in length occurs
4. Articular cartilage: thin sheet of cartilage that covers the end of the epiphysis; provides a cushion and lubrication for joint
5. Periosteum: tough, vascular covering of the bone; made up of fibrous connective tissue; does not cover the epiphysis
6. Endosteum: lining of the medullary cavity
7. Medullary cavity: cavity in the center of long bones; contains marrow
   a. Red marrow: produces red blood cells
   b. Yellow marrow: made up of fat
8. Process: bony projection on the surface of a bone
9. Foramen: an opening in a bone
10. Sinus: bony cavity in a bone

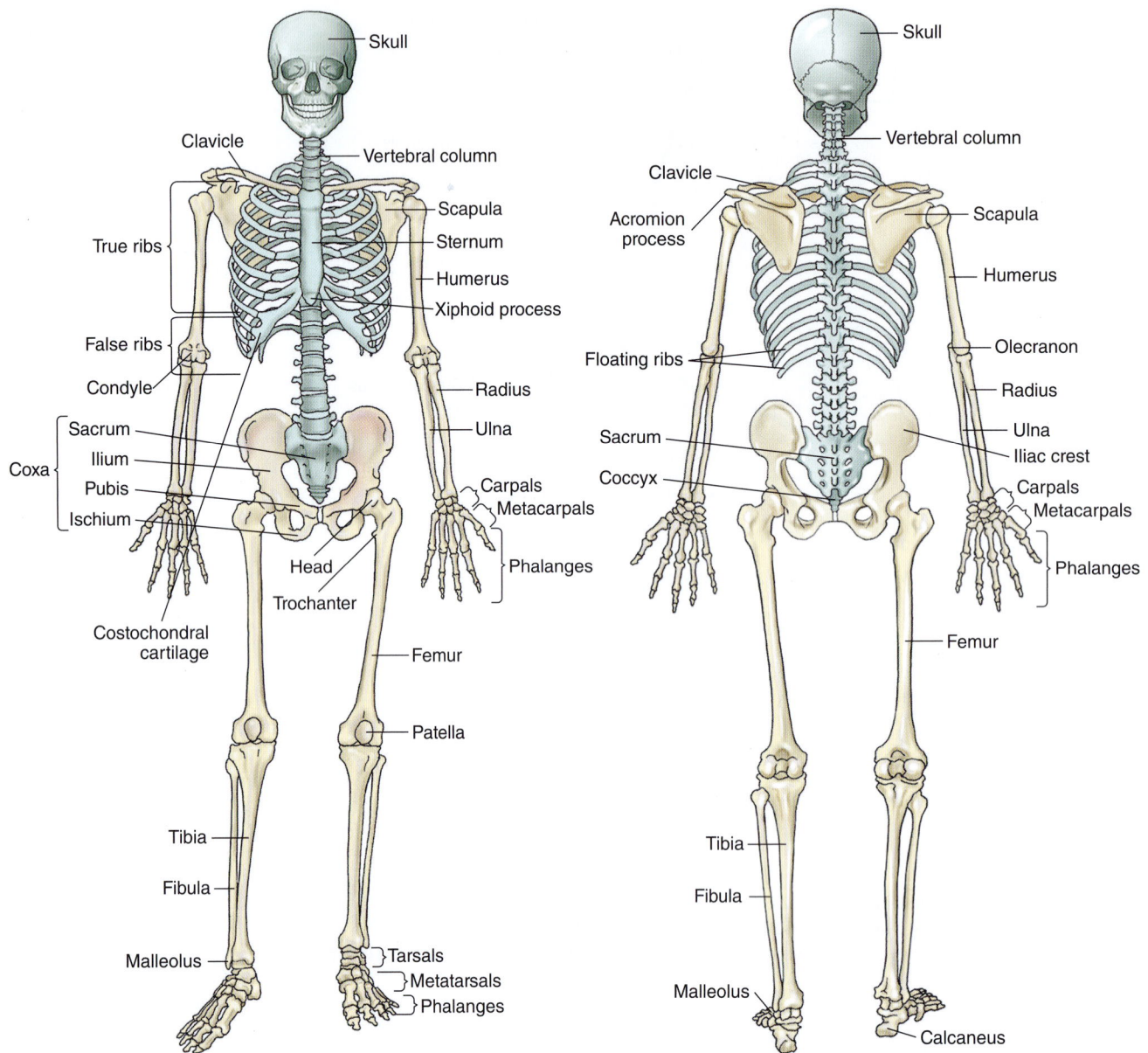

Fig. 2.7 Normal skeletal. (A) Anterior view; (B) posterior view. (From Shiland, BJ: *Mastering healthcare terminology*, ed 5, 2016, Mosby.)

E. Bone Classifications

1. Long: length exceeds width
2. Short: smaller than long bone with expanded ends
3. Flat: thin, sheetlike
4. Sesamoid: rounded bones embedded in tendons; round bones
5. Irregular: various shapes

F. Organization of the Skeleton

1. Axial skeleton: consists of bones of the skull, spine, and chest
   a. Cranium (skull): bones that enclose the brain (Fig. 2.8)
      1) Frontal: forms forehead
      2) Parietal: forms sides and top

3) Temporal: forms lower sides and floor; contains ossicles (bones of middle ear—malleus, incus, and stapes) and external auditory meatus (opening into middle ear)
4) Mastoid process: projection located on the temporal bone
5) Styloid process: sharp projection inferior to the external auditory meatus
6) Zygomatic process: projects anteriorly to form prominence of cheek
7) Occipital: single bone forming the posterior of the cranium; contains foramen magnum, where the spinal cord exits the skull
8) Sphenoid: butterfly-shaped bone that bridges the temporal regions to form the floor of the cranium; contains sella turcica, where the pituitary gland sits

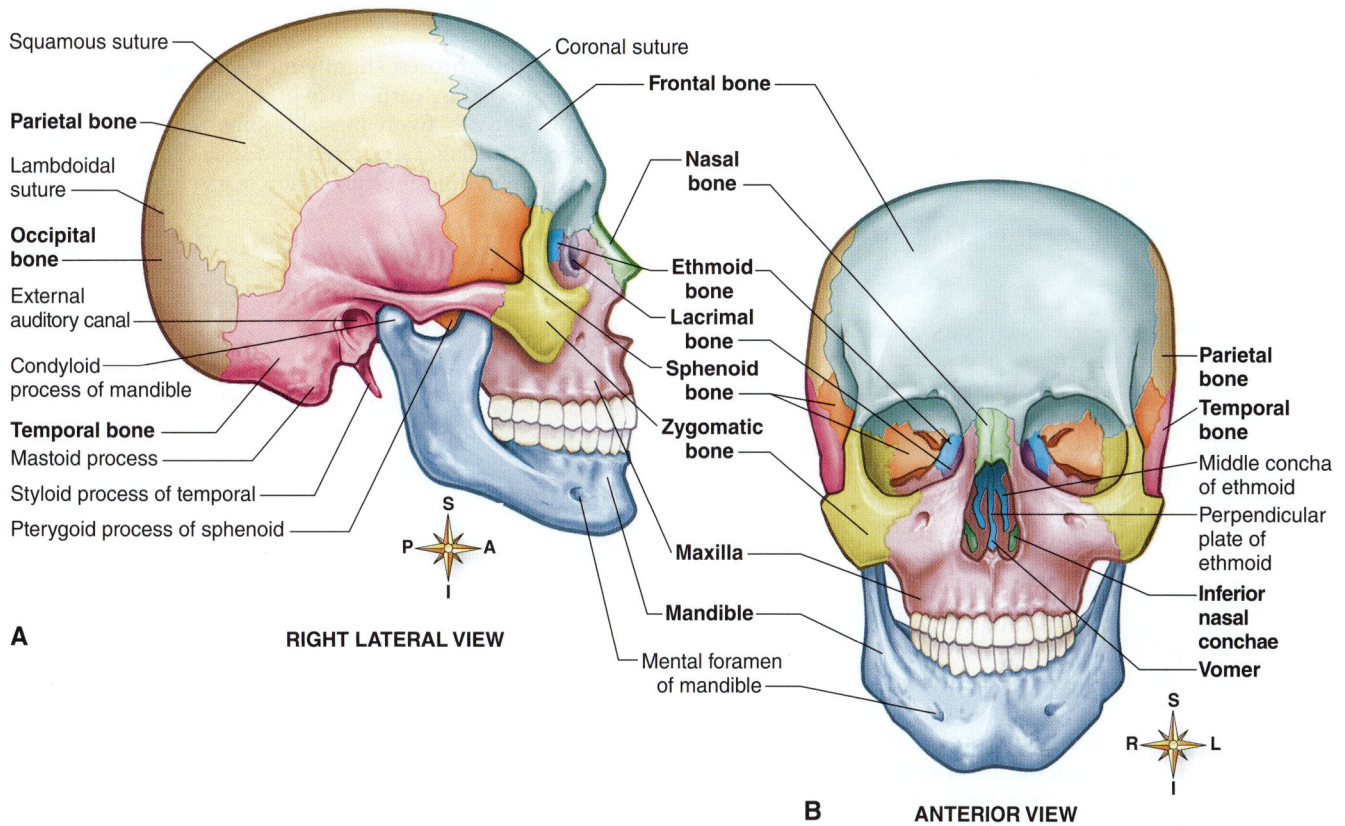

Fig. 2.8 Bones of the skull. (A) Right side; (B) front. (From Patton KT, Thibodeau GA: *The human body in health and disease*, ed 7, 2020, Mosby.)

9) Ethmoid: single bone that forms most of bony area between the nasal cavity and orbits

b. Facial: forms the basic framework for the face

1) Nasal: two bones forming the bridge of the nose
2) Vomer: thin bone that forms the inferior nasal septum
3) Lacrimal: located in the medial walls of the orbits; contains the lacrimal glands
4) Zygomatic: forms the arch of the cheekbone
5) Palatine: forms the posterior of the hard palate
6) Mandible: lower jawbone (only movable bone in the face)
7) Hyoid: U-shaped bone that supports the tongue; only bone that does not articulate with another

c. Vertebral (spinal) column: composed of 26 vertebrae separated by pads of cartilage (intervertebral disks); houses the spinal cord; four distinct curves; common structural pattern (Fig. 2.9)

1) Cervical vertebrae: first seven, C1 through C7; forms the neck
   a) C1: atlas; supports the skull
   b) C2: axis; allows for rotation of the skull
2) Thoracic vertebrae: next 12, T1 through T12; articulate with the ribs
3) Lumbar vertebrae: next five, L1 through L5; forms the small of the back
4) Sacrum: triangle-shaped bone; forms the posterior wall of the pelvic cavity
5) Coccyx: tailbone

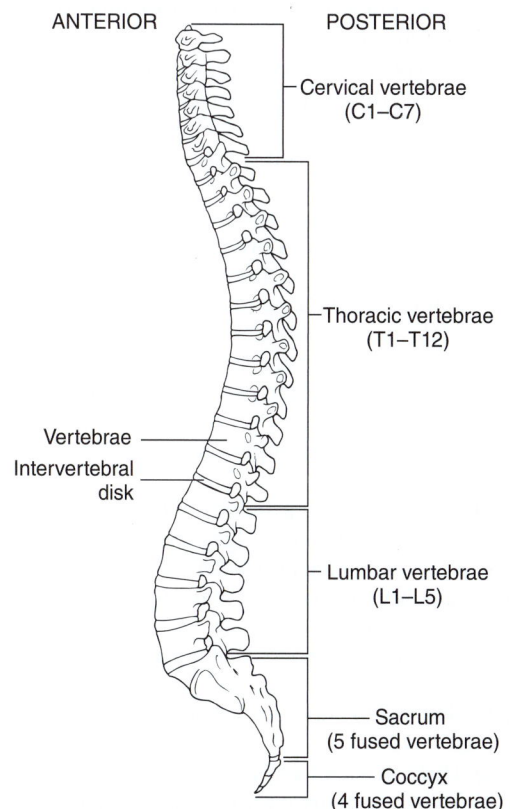

Fig. 2.9 The vertebral column. (From Frazier MS, Drzymkowski JW: *Essentials of human diseases and conditions*, ed 6, St. Louis, 2016, Elsevier.)

d. Thorax: thoracic cage; protects heart, lungs, and great vessels
   1) Sternum: breastbone; three parts
      a) Manubrium: superior, triangular part
      b) Body: middle, slender part
      c) Xiphoid process: projection at end of the body; landmark for cardiopulmonary resuscitation
   2) Ribs
      a) Curved, flat bones that form the lateral sides of thorax
      b) 12 pairs
         (1) True ribs: first seven pairs; articulate with the sternum by means of costal cartilage
         (2) False ribs: next three pairs; articulate with the seventh rib by means of costal cartilage
         (3) Floating ribs: last two pairs; do not articulate with the sternum
2. Appendicular skeleton: made up of bones of upper and lower extremities and girdles that are anchored to the axial skeleton
   a. Pectoral (shoulder) girdle
      1) Clavicle: collarbone; forms a bridge between shoulder blades and breastbone
      2) Scapula: shoulder blade
      3) Humerus: bone of the upper arm
      4) Radius: lateral bone of the forearm (thumb side)
      5) Ulna: medial bone of the forearm (little finger side)
      6) Carpals: two rows of four bones tightly bound by ligaments; make up the wrist
      7) Metacarpals: five bones that make up the hand
      8) Phalanges
         a) Three bones in each finger (proximal, medial, and distal)
         b) Two bones in each thumb (proximal and distal)
   b. Pelvic (hip) girdle: attaches lower extremities to axial skeleton
      1) Pelvis: os coxae; basin-shaped bones on floor of trunk; three parts
         a) Ilium: superior, wing-shaped bones of hips
         b) Ischium: inferior portion; "sit-down" bone
         c) Pubis: anterior portion; right and left sides join at symphysis pubis (pad of cartilage)
         d) Male and female pelvis differ; female pelvis shaped to accommodate childbirth
      2) Femur: thighbone; largest, longest, and strongest bone in the body
      3) Patella: kneecap; triangle shaped, enclosed in tendon
      4) Tibia: shinbone
         a) Lateral malleolus: bulge on the outside of the ankle
         b) Medial malleolus: bulge on the inside of the ankle
      5) Fibula: smaller leg bone lateral to the tibia
      6) Tarsals: seven bones that make up the ankle; largest is calcaneus (heel bone)
      7) Metatarsals: five bones that make up the instep of the foot
      8) Phalanges: 14 bones in each foot that make up the toes
         a) Three in each toe (proximal, medial, and distal)
         b) Two in each great toe (proximal and distal)
   c. Articulations: joints; where two bones come together; classified by the amount of movement allowed (Fig. 2.10)
      1) Synarthroses: immovable joints (e.g., sutures in the skull)
      2) Amphiarthroses: slightly movable joints; bones are connected by cartilage (e.g., symphysis pubis)
      3) Diarthroses: freely movable joints; ends covered with cartilage; separated by a space containing synovial fluid for lubrication (e.g., elbow)

VI. Muscular System

A. General

1. Approximately 650 muscles in the body
2. Accounts for approximately 40% of body weight

B. Functions

1. Movement: contractions (shortening) allow movement of bone
2. Protection: sheets of muscle protect the internal organs
3. Posture: provides position and alignment of body parts
4. Heat production: movement produces heat
5. Shape: muscles plus bones give the body shape

C. Types of Muscle Tissue (Fig. 2.11)

1. Skeletal: under conscious control (voluntary); appears striated (striped); provides movement of the body
2. Smooth: involuntary (operates automatically); appears nonstriated; helps with metabolic functions
3. Cardiac: found only in the heart; involuntary; causes contraction of heart muscle to maintain blood flow

D. Characteristics of Muscle

1. Excitability: ability to receive and respond to a stimulus
2. Contractility: ability to shorten (contract), which produces movement
3. Extensibility: ability to stretch
4. Elasticity: ability to return to original shape and length

E. Skeletal Muscle Structure

1. Composed of bundles of fibers held together by fibrous connective tissue
   a. Fiber: skeletal muscle cell
   b. Endomysium: connective tissue membrane that covers a muscle fiber
   c. Fasciculus: bundle of muscle fibers
   d. Perimysium: connective tissue membrane that surrounds the fasciculus
   e. Epimysium: tough tissue membrane that covers the entire muscle
   f. Fascia: connective tissue outside of the epimysium; surrounds and separates the muscles
   g. Tendon: strong, cordlike structure that attaches muscles to bones
   h. Aponeurosis: sheetlike tendon that attaches muscle to muscle

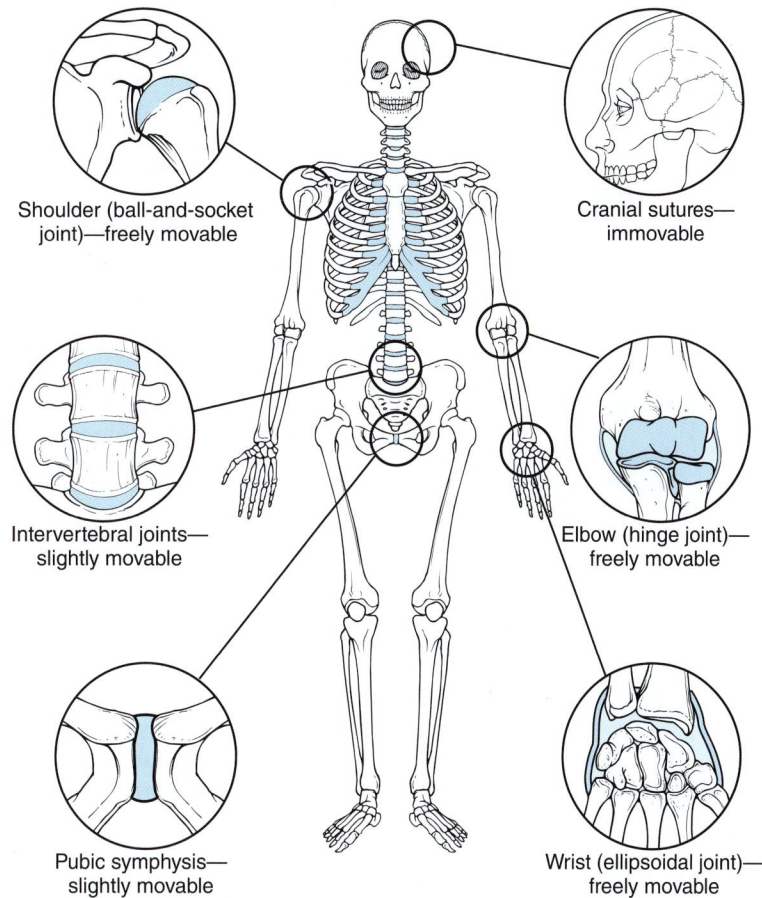

Fig. 2.10 Examples of types of joints. (From Frazier MS, Drzymkowski JW: *Essentials of human diseases and conditions*, ed 6, 2016, Elsevier.)

F. Naming of Muscles

1. May be named according to the following
   a. Size: maximus, medius, longus
   b. Shape: deltoid, latus
   c. Fiber direction: rectus, oblique
   d. Location: pectoralis, gluteus
   e. Points of attachment
      1) Origin: point of attachment that does not move on contraction
      2) Insertion: point of attachment that moves on contraction
   f. Number of attachments: biceps, quadriceps
   g. Action of muscle: adductor, flexor, levator

G. Muscle Actions

1. Prime mover: provides movement
2. Antagonist: opposes prime mover; can cause opposite movement or provide more control and precision to prime mover
3. Synergist: helps prime mover work more efficiently and effectively
4. Fixator: stabilizes the origin of the prime mover

H. Movement

1. Caused by contraction (shortening) of muscle
2. Complex series of events based on chemical reactions at cellular level
3. Begins with stimulation by the nerve cell and ends when muscle is relaxed
4. Requires adenosine triphosphate as an energy source

I. Types of Movements (Fig. 2.12)

1. Flexion: to bend; brings two bones closer together and decreases the angle between them
2. Extension: to straighten; opposite of flexion; increases the angle between bones
3. Hyperextension: extension beyond the anatomic position; joint angle greater than 180 degrees
4. Abduction: to take away; movement of a bone or limb away from the midline of the body
5. Adduction: to bring together; opposite of abduction; movement of a bone or limb toward the midline of the body
6. Circumduction: circular motion of a body part or segment; the proximal end is stationary, whereas the distal end outlines a large circle

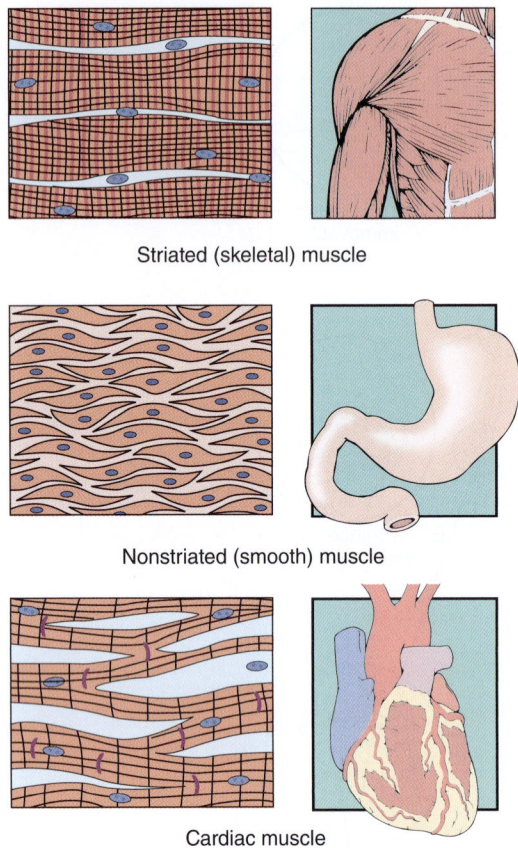

Striated (skeletal) muscle

Nonstriated (smooth) muscle

Cardiac muscle

Fig. 2.11 Three types of muscle: skeletal, smooth, and cardiac. (From Frazier MS, Drzymkowski JW: *Essentials of human diseases and conditions*, ed 6, 2016, Elsevier.)

7. Rotation: movement of a bone around its own axis
8. Inversion: turning a body part inward
9. Eversion: opposite of inversion; turning a body part outward
10. Supination: movement of a body part to face upward
11. Pronation: opposite of supination; movement of a body part to face downward

J. Major Skeletal Muscles (Fig. 2.13)

1. Muscles of facial expression
   a. Frontalis: over the frontal bone; raises eyebrows and wrinkles forehead
   b. Orbicularis oris: circular muscle that surrounds the mouth; closes the mouth, forms words, puckers lips
   c. Orbicularis oculi: circular muscle that surrounds the eye; helps in winking, blinking, and squinting
   d. Buccinator: principal muscle of the cheek; helps in whistling, sucking, and blowing out air
   e. Zygomaticus: extends from the zygomatic arch to corner of mouth; raises the corners of the mouth when smiling
2. Muscles of mastication (chewing)
   a. Temporalis: largest muscle; inserts in mandible; responsible for chewing
   b. Masseter: inserts in mandible; used for chewing

3. Neck muscles
   a. Sternocleidomastoid: runs across front of neck from the sternum to clavicle to mastoid process; flexes neck
   b. Trapezius: extends from occipital bone to end of thoracic vertebrae; extends head
4. Vertebral column muscles
   a. Erector spinae: group of muscles on each side of vertebral column from sacrum to skull; keeps vertebral column erect
   b. Quadratus lumborum (deep back muscles): short muscles between vertebrae; responsible for movement of vertebral column
5. Thoracic wall muscles
   a. Intercostal muscles (internal and external): located between ribs; help with breathing
   b. Diaphragm: dome-shaped muscle located between thorax and abdomen; muscle of respiration
6. Abdominal wall muscles
   a. External oblique: fibers run medially and inferiorly
   b. Internal oblique: fibers run opposite to the external obliques
   c. Transversus abdominis: fibers run horizontally
   d. Rectus abdominis: fibers run vertically
7. Muscles that move the shoulder and arm
   a. Trapezius: large, triangular muscle of the back; used to shrug shoulders
   b. Serratus anterior: located on side of chest; used in pushing
   c. Pectoralis major: superficial muscle on anterior chest; adductor; moves arm medially across chest
   d. Latissimus dorsi: large superficial muscle of lower back
   e. Deltoid: large triangular muscle that covers the shoulder; used to abduct arm; injection site
   f. Rotator cuff muscles: infraspinatus, supraspinatus, subscapularis, teres minor; assist with movement of the humerus; form cuff over proximal humerus
8. Muscles that move the forearm and hand
   a. Triceps brachii: posterior of arm; extends the forearm
   b. Biceps brachii: flexes the forearm
   c. Brachialis: flexes the forearm
   d. Brachioradialis: lateral side of forearm; flexes the forearm
9. Muscles that move the thigh
   a. Gluteus maximus: forms the buttocks; extends and straightens the thigh at the hip
   b. Gluteus medius: deep to the gluteus maximus; common injection site; abducts the thigh
   c. Gluteus minimus: deepest of gluteal group; abducts the thigh
   d. Iliopsoas: anterior muscle; flexes the thigh
   e. Adductor longus: medial muscle; adducts the thigh
   f. Adductor brevis: medial muscle; adducts the thigh
   g. Adductor magnus: medial muscle; adducts the thigh
   h. Gracilis: medial muscle; adducts the thigh
10. Muscles that move the leg
    a. Quadriceps femoris: group of muscles located on anterior and lateral sides of the thigh; extends and straightens leg at the knee

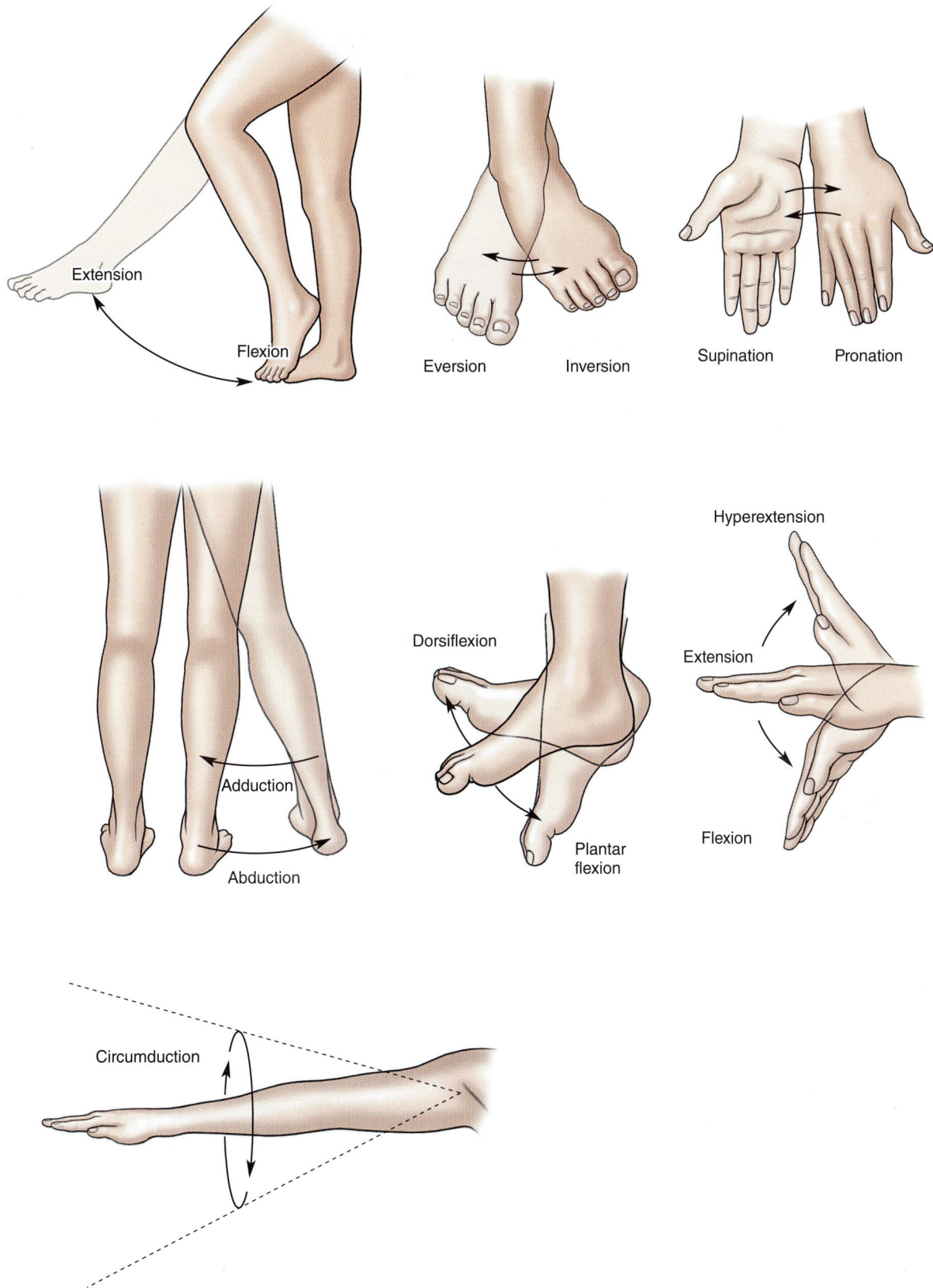

Fig. 2.12 Types of movements at joints. (From Herlihy B: *The human body in health and illness*, ed 6, 2018, Saunders.)

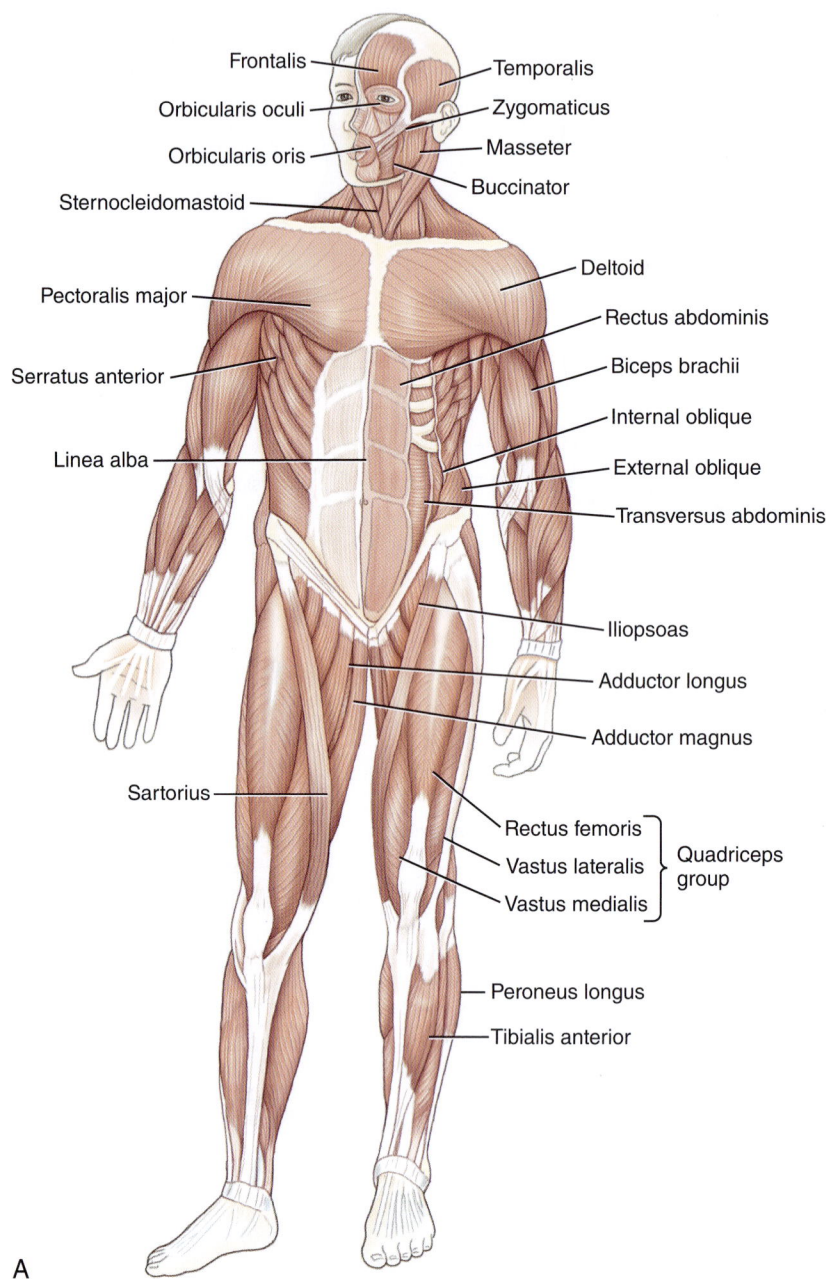

Fig. 2.13 Major muscles of the body. (A) Anterior view;

1) Vastus lateralis: injection site for infants and children; extends leg and supports knee joint
2) Vastus intermedius: extends leg
3) Vastus medialis: extends leg
4) Rectus femoris: extends leg
b. Sartorius: longest muscle in the body; runs obliquely over the quad group; flexes and medially rotates the legs (to sit cross legged)
c. Hamstrings: posterior to the thigh; flexes the leg at the knee; strong tendons; includes the following:
    1) Biceps femoris

2) Semitendinosus
3) Semimembranosus
11. Muscles that move the ankle and foot
    a. Tibialis anterior: primary muscle of anterior group; dorsiflexion of foot
    b. Peroneus longus: lateral to the leg; everts the foot
    c. Gastrocnemius: posterior to leg (calf); plantar flexion ("toe-dancer's" muscles)
    d. Soleus: posterior to the leg (calf)
    e. Achilles tendon: common tendon for gastrocnemius and soleus; connects muscles to calcaneus; largest tendon in the body

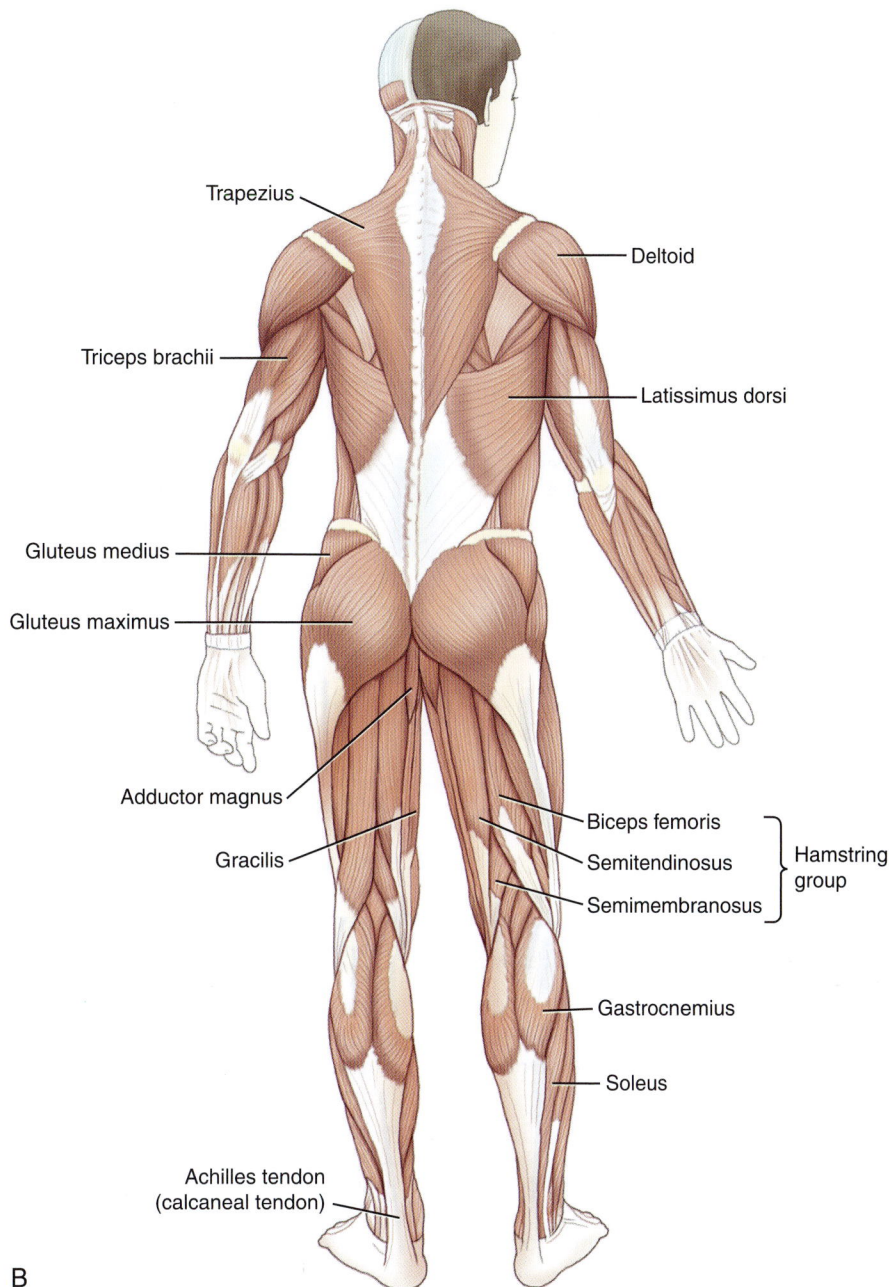

Fig. 2.13, cont'd (B) posterior view. (From Shiland, BJ: *Mastering healthcare terminology*, ed 5, 2016, Mosby.)

VII. Nervous System

A. General

1. Major controlling, regulating, and communicating system of the body
2. Works with the endocrine system to regulate and maintain homeostasis

B. Functions

1. Control: regulates internal body functions and processes
2. Communication: directs processes among body systems

3. Mental processes: generates thoughts, feelings, perceptions, sensations, and emotions

C. Organization (Fig. 2.14)

1. Central nervous system (CNS): made up of the brain and spinal cord
2. Peripheral nervous system (PNS): made up of nerves and ganglia; includes the following:
   a. Twelve pairs of cranial nerves originating in the brain
   b. Thirty-one pairs of spinal nerves originating from the spinal cord
   c. Afferent (sensory) division: transmits information to the brain

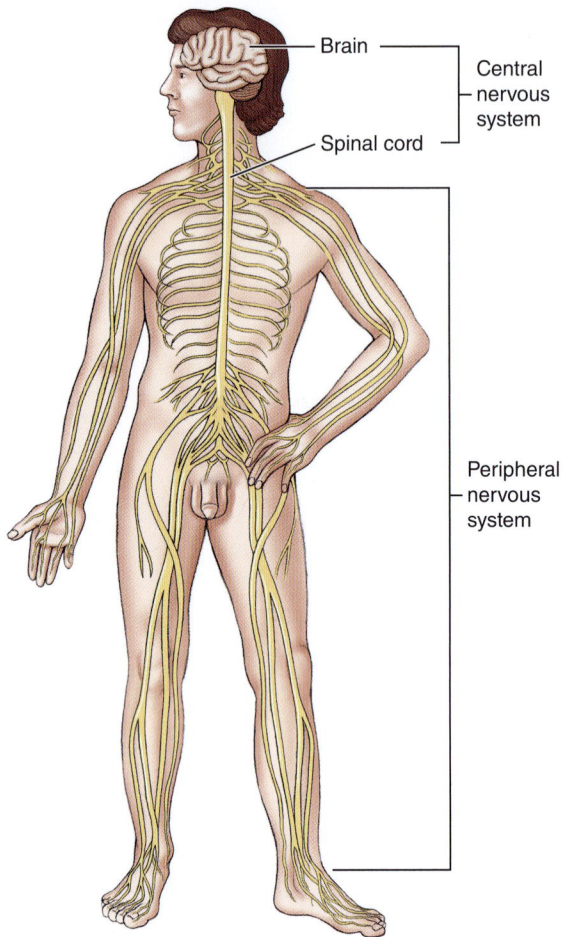

Fig. 2.14 Divisions of the nervous system: central and peripheral. (From Herlihy B: *The human body in health and illness*, ed 6, 2018, Saunders.)

d. Efferent (motor) division: transmits information from the brain to organs and body parts
e. Somatic nervous system: transmits impulses to voluntary muscles
f. Autonomic nervous system: transmits impulses to involuntary muscles and glands
g. Sympathetic nervous system: prepares the body for stressful conditions
h. Parasympathetic nervous system: coordinates normal resting activities

D. Organs of the Nervous System

1. Neuron (Fig. 2.15): nerve cell; structural and functional unit of nerve tissue; highly specialized; if destroyed, cannot be replaced (does not go through mitosis)
   a. Cell body: contains nucleus and organelles
   b. Dendrites: one or more branching extensions; receive signals from other neurons and bring them to the cell body
   c. Axon: single extension from the cell body; carries impulses away from the cell body
   d. Myelin sheath: white, segmented, fatty substance that surrounds axons; produced by Schwann cells that cover the axons; serves as an insulator and to speed up the conduction of nerve impulses; gives white appearance to fibers (white matter)

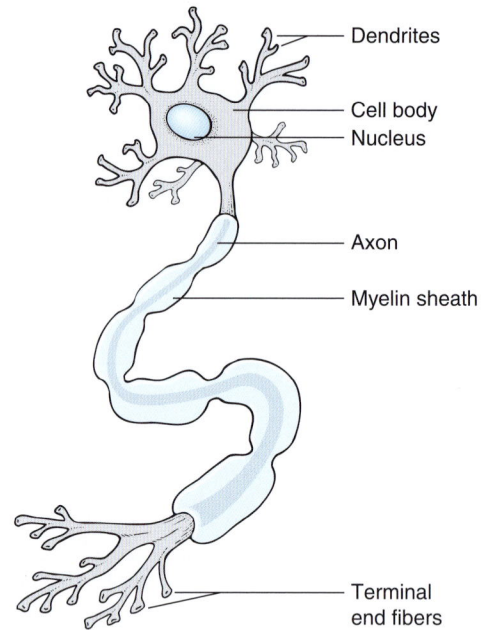

Fig. 2.15 Structure of a neuron. (From Frazier MS, Drzymkowski JW: *Essentials of human diseases and conditions*, ed 6, 2016, Elsevier.)

   e. Neurilemma: outer membrane of the axon
   f. Nodes of Ranvier: gaps in the myelin sheath
   g. Neurotransmitter: chemical substance that allows neurons to communicate with each other
2. Neuroglia: "nerve glue"; nonconductive cells of nerve tissue; provides support system (nourishment and protection) for neurons; more numerous than neurons; different types with specialized functions; capable of mitosis
3. Nerves: collection of nerve fibers held together by layers of connective tissue
   a. Afferent (sensory): carry impulses from PNS to CNS
   b. Efferent (motor): carry impulses from CNS to PNS
4. Brain (see Fig. 2.15)
   a. Cerebrum (see Fig. 2.15): largest superior portion; consists of thin layer of gray matter (cerebral cortex) and white matter (bulk of cerebrum)
      1) Cortex: makes us "human"; concerned with memory, language, reasoning, intelligence, personality, and other factors associated with human life
      2) Divided into two halves (hemispheres) by longitudinal fissure
         a) Right hemisphere: controls the left side of the body; responsible for auditory perception, tactile perception, and interpretation of spatial relationships
         b) Left hemisphere: controls the right side of the body; responsible for language and hand movements
      3) Each hemisphere is divided into five lobes named for bones that cover them (except for the insula)
         a) Frontal lobe: controls voluntary muscle movements and speech
         b) Parietal lobe: receives and integrates sensory output
         c) Temporal lobe: interprets sound; involved with personality, emotion, memory, and behavior
         d) Occipital lobe: interprets sight
         e) Insula: visceral effects

      4) Ventricles: cavities within each hemisphere that make and store cerebrospinal fluid (CSF)

b. Diencephalon: centrally located; surrounded by cerebral hemispheres

      1) Thalamus: relay station for all sensory input; associated with pain, temperature, and touch sensations; located between cerebrum and midbrain

      2) Hypothalamus: located below thalamus; important role in regulating heart rate, blood pressure, body temperature, water balance, hunger, sleep, and wakefulness

c. Brainstem (see Fig. 2.15)

      1) Medulla oblongata: lowest portion of brain, connects to spinal cord; contains vital centers for control of heartbeat, respiration, and blood pressure

      2) Pons: bulge at the base of the brain; links the cerebellum to the rest of the nervous system; nerve fibers cross here; one side of the brain controls the other side of the body

      3) Midbrain: upper portion of the brainstem; correlates information about muscle tone and posture; relay center for certain eye and ear reflexes

d. Cerebellum (see Fig. 2.15): second largest portion of the brain, located below the cerebrum; responsible for coordination of voluntary movement, posture, and balance

e. Spinal cord (see Fig. 2.15): extends from the brainstem through the foramen magnum into the vertebral column to the second lumbar vertebra; approximately 17 inches long; conducts nerve impulses to and from brain; center for spinal reflexes; 31 pairs of spinal nerves connected to cord

f. Meninges: protective membrane covering the brain and spinal cord; three layers:

      1) Dura mater: strong, fibrous outer layer

      2) Arachnoid: middle, delicate weblike layer that allows for movement of CSF

      3) Pia mater: thin inner layer; contains blood vessels to supply the brain

g. Meningeal spaces

      1) Epidural space: located between dura mater and bone (skull or vertebra); acts as a cushion

      2) Subdural space: located between dura mater and arachnoid; contains serous fluid for lubrication

      3) Subarachnoid space: located between arachnoid and pia mater; contains CSF

h. Cerebrospinal fluid: clear, colorless, watery fluid found in subarachnoid space and in the ventricles of the brain; constantly circulates; provides protective cushion for the brain; can detect physiologic changes in the body

VIII. Sensory System

A. General

1. Variety of receptors located in various structures
2. Stimulation of a receptor by an appropriate stimulus results in an impulse, which is sent to the CNS, where it is processed
3. Allow the individual to be aware of the world around him or her

4. Depend on sensory receptors classified as
   a. General (widely distributed)
   b. Special (localized in a specific area)

B. General Senses (Fig. 2.16)

1. Somatic senses: found throughout the body
2. Touch and pressure
   a. Mechanoreceptor (responds to a bending, or a change in the shape, of a cell)
   b. Widely distributed in the skin
   c. Includes free nerve endings, Meissner corpuscle (touch), Pacinian corpuscles (pressure)
3. Position and orientation: proprioceptors
4. Temperature
   a. Thermoreceptor (detects change in temperature)
   b. Found immediately under the skin
   c. Ten times more cold receptors than heat receptors
5. Pain
   a. Nociceptors (respond to tissue damage)
   b. Widely distributed in the skin and tissues of internal organs
   c. Protective function

C. Special Senses

1. Located within special organs
2. Gustatory sense
   a. Sense of taste
   b. Organs of taste (taste buds) localized on the surface of tongue
   c. Chemoreceptors (sensitive to chemicals in food)
   d. Includes receptors for sensations of salty, sweet, sour, and bitter
3. Olfactory sense
   a. Sense of smell
   b. Receptors found in the upper nose
   c. Chemoreceptors
   d. Closely related to sense of taste
4. Visual sense (Fig. 2.17)
   a. Receptors located in the eye
   b. Photoreceptors (detect light)
      1) Eye
         a) Found in protective bony socket (orbit)
         b) Three layers (tunics)
           (1) Sclera
             (a) Outer layer; white of the eye
             (b) Made of tough fibrous tissue
             (c) Anterior portion covered by cornea, which focuses light rays
           (2) Choroid
             (a) Middle layer
             (b) Highly vascular
             (c) Ciliary body; changes shape of the lens
             (d) Suspensory ligament: connects the ciliary body to lens
             (e) Iris: colored portion of the eye
               (i) Doughnut-shaped muscle with a hole in the middle (pupil)
               (ii) Continually contracts and relaxes to regulate the amount of light entering the eye

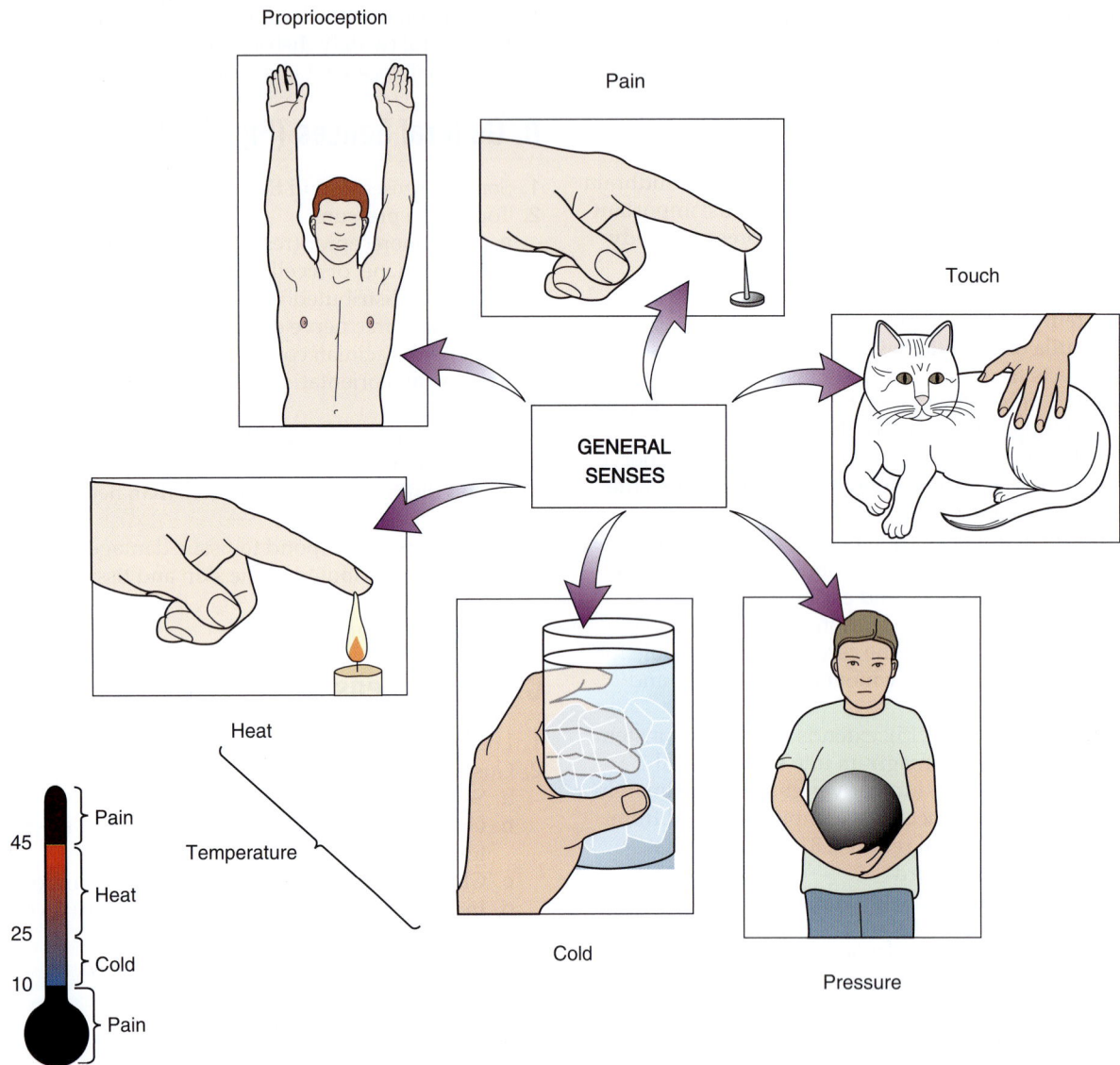

Fig. 2.16 The general senses. (From Herlihy B: *The human body in health and illness*, ed 6, 2018, Saunders.)

(3) Retina
  (a) Innermost layer
  (b) Posterior portion of the eye
  (c) Contains
    (i) Rods: receptors sensitive to shades of gray
    (ii) Cones: receptors sensitive to color
  (d) Fovea centralis: area of closely packed cones that function as the area of sharpest vision
  (e) Optic disk: area on the retina where the optic nerve exits the eye; the "blind spot"
2) Cavities
  a) Anterior cavity: anterior space between the lens and the cornea; filled with aqueous humor (maintains shape and internal pressure)
  b) Posterior cavity: between lens and retina; filled with gel-like substance (vitreous humor); keeps retina against the wall of the eye, supports parts of the eye, and helps maintain shape
3) Accessory structures

  a) Eyebrows and eyelashes: protect against foreign objects
  b) Eyelids: open and close eyes to keep foreign objects out and to keep eyes moist
  c) Lacrimal apparatus: lacrimal glands make tears to lubricate, moisten, and cleanse the eye; nasolacrimal duct drains tears into the nasal cavity
  d) Conjunctiva: mucous membrane that lines the inner eyelids and anterior eyeball
4) Muscles of the eye
  a) Extrinsic muscles: skeletal muscles attached to the orbital bones and outer eye
  b) Intrinsic muscles: smooth muscles located in the eye
5) Visual pathway: light ray → cornea → aqueous humor → pupil → lens → vitreous humor → retina (rods and cones) → optic nerve fibers → optic chiasma → thalamus → cerebral cortex
5. Auditory sense: receptors located in the ears; mechanoreceptors (Fig. 2.18)
  a. Ears: found on both sides of the head

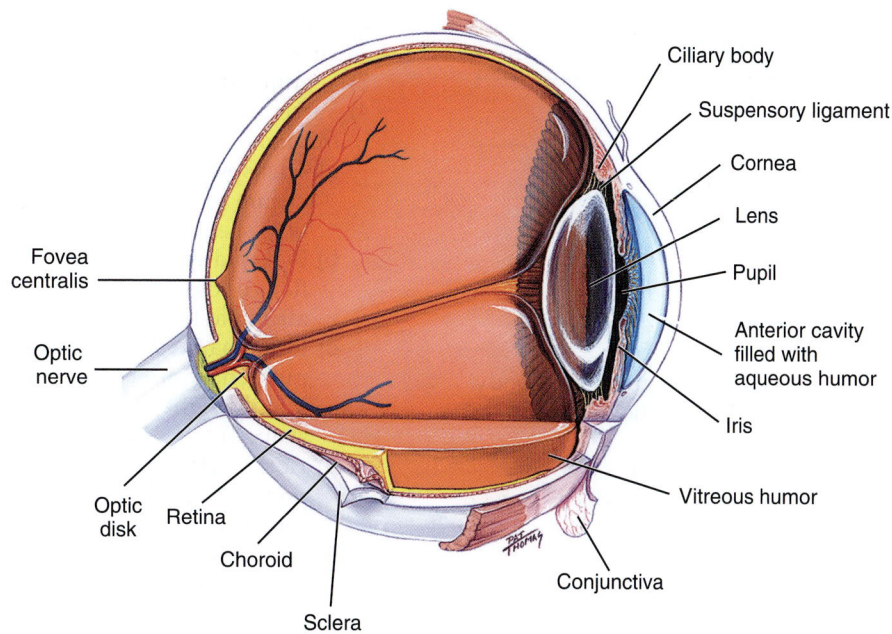

Fig. 2.17 Structure of the eyeball. (From Applegate E: *The anatomy and physiology learning system*, ed 4, 2011, Saunders.)

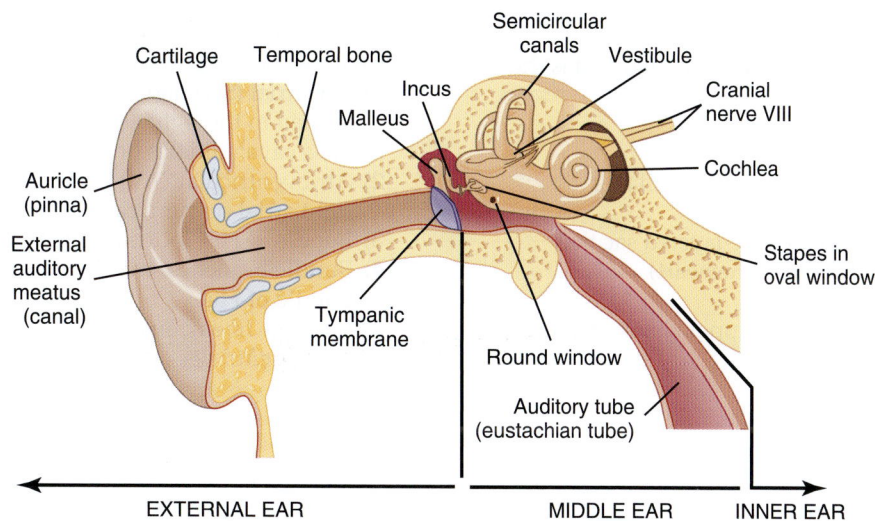

Fig. 2.18 Structure of the ear. (From Applegate E: *The anatomy and physiology learning system*, ed 4, 2011, Saunders.)

1) External ear
   a) Auricle (pinna): fleshy part visible on sides of head; collects sound waves and directs them toward the auditory meatus
   b) External auditory meatus: short tube that extends from the auricle to the tympanic membrane; lined with glands that produce cerumen (earwax) to protect and lubricate
2) Middle ear: found in the temporal bone
   a) Tympanic membrane: eardrum
   b) Auditory tube: eustachian tube; extends from the middle ear to the throat; equalizes pressure between the outside air and the middle ear cavity
   c) Ossicles: three tiny bones of the middle ear
      (1) Malleus: attached to the tympanic membrane
      (2) Incus: connects the malleus to the stapes
      (3) Stapes: attached to the incus and oval window
   d) Oval window: membrane covering the opening into the vestibule

3) Inner ear
   a) Bony labyrinth: series of interconnecting chambers in the temporal bone
   b) Contains membranous labyrinth filled with fluid (endolymph)
   c) Space between the bony and membranous labyrinth; filled with fluid (perilymph)
   d) Divided into three sections
      (1) Vestibule: involved with balance
      (2) Semicircular canals: involved in equilibrium
      (3) Cochlea: snail-shaped structure involved with hearing; contains the organ of Corti, which contains receptors for sound
4) Auditory pathway: sound wave → pinna → external auditory meatus → tympanic membrane → malleus → incus → stapes → oval window → cochlea → perilymph → auditory nerve fibers → cerebral cortex

IX. Cardiovascular System

A. General

1. Closed, sterile system
2. Consists of heart and blood vessels

B. Functions

1. Transportation: carries important elements throughout the body
2. Temperature regulation: helps with the regulation of body temperature through dilation and constriction of blood vessels
3. Waste removal: assists lungs, kidneys, and liver
4. Fluid balance: maintains balance between fluid loss and fluid retention

C. Organs

1. Heart (Fig. 2.19)
   a. Hollow, muscular, cone-shaped organ about the size of a fist; located slightly to the left of midline in the mediastinum; protected by the sternum and ribs; upper end is the base; lower end is pointed and is the apex (apical pulse)
   b. Made up of three layers
      1) Epicardium: outer layer
      2) Myocardium: thick, middle muscular layer
      3) Endocardium: inner layer
   c. Covered by pericardium (double-layered sac that decreases friction and protects the heart)
   d. Contains four chambers
      1) Atria (singular *atrium*): two upper chambers; receive blood from veins
      2) Ventricles: two lower chambers; receive blood from atria and pump it into the body
      3) Septum: divides chambers into right and left
      4) Valves: structures that allow one-way flow of blood throughout the heart
         a) Tricuspid valve: permits blood to flow from right atrium to right ventricle; composed of three flaps of tissue
         b) Bicuspid valve (mitral valve): made up of two flaps of tissue; permits blood to flow from left atrium to left ventricle
         c) Pulmonary valve: located at the entrance of the pulmonary artery; prevents backflow of blood into the right ventricle; semilunar (half-moon shaped)
         d) Aortic valve: located at the entrance of the aorta; prevents backflow of blood into the left ventricle; semilunar
         e) Blood enters right atrium → right ventricle → pulmonary artery → pulmonary capillaries (exchange of gases) → pulmonary vein → left atrium → left ventricle → aorta → capillaries in body tissues (exchange of gases) → superior vena cava and inferior vena cava → right atrium
   e. Electrical conduction system: initiates and maintains rhythmic heart contractions (Fig. 2.20)
      1) Sinoatrial (SA) node: pacemaker of the heart; located in the right atrial wall near the superior vena cava; initiates heartbeat and sets its pace
      2) Atrioventricular (AV) node: located in the lower right atrial septum; causes the atria to contract
      3) Bundle of His: located in ventricular septum
      4) Bundle branches: two branches extending from bundle of His
      5) Purkinje fibers: extend from the bundle branches; cause ventricles to contract

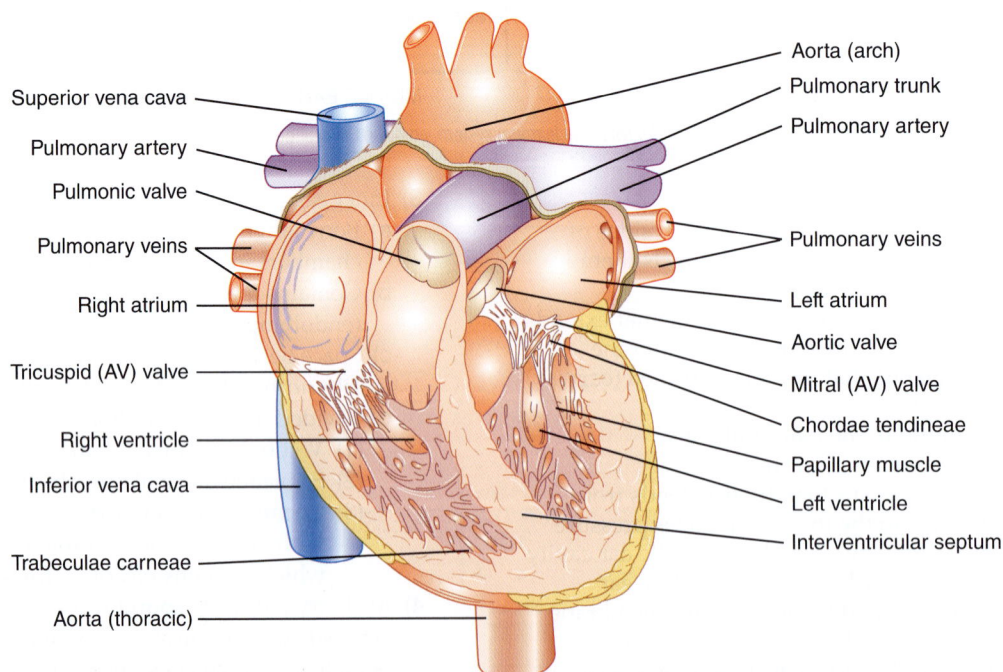

Fig. 2.19 Chambers of the heart and the large vessels; blood flow through the heart. *AV,* Atrioventricular. (From Applegate E: *The anatomy and physiology learning system,* ed 4, 2011, Saunders.)

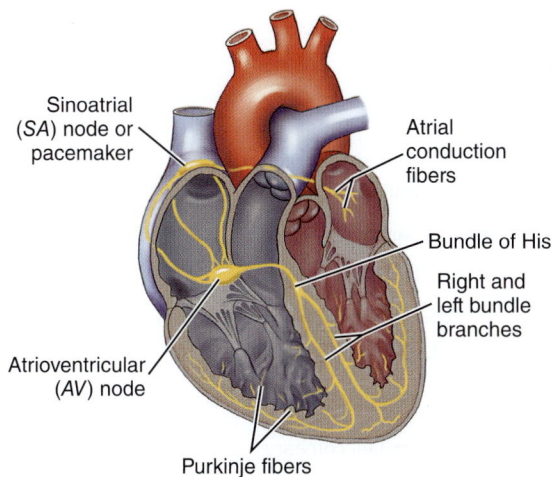

Sinoatrial (SA) node or pacemaker

Atrial conduction fibers

Bundle of His

Right and left bundle branches

Atrioventricular (AV) node

Purkinje fibers

Fig. 2.20 Conduction system of the heart. (From Shiland, BJ: *Mastering healthcare terminology*, ed 5, 2016, Mosby.)

f. Cardiac cycle: complete heartbeat; consists of contraction (systole) and relaxation (diastole) of both atria and ventricles; complete cycle lasts for 0.8 seconds (75 beats per minute [bpm]); sounds associated with heartbeat described as *lubb-dupp*

2. Vessels
   a. Arteries: vessels that carry blood away from the heart
      1) Composed of three layers
         a) Tunica adventitia: outermost layer of tough fibrous connective tissue
         b) Tunica media: middle layer of smooth muscle tissue; allows for contraction and dilation
         c) Tunica intima: innermost layer
      2) Arterioles: small arteries
   b. Veins: vessels that carry blood toward the heart
      1) Same layers as arteries, except tunica adventitia is thicker, and the tunica intima has valves to prevent backflow
      2) Venules: small veins
   c. Capillaries: microscopic vessels, one-cell layer thick
      1) Connect arterioles and venules
      2) Exchange of substances takes place here (as in the capillaries)

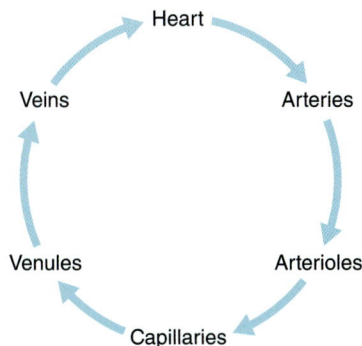

Heart

Veins

Arteries

Venules

Arterioles

Capillaries

3. Major arteries (Fig. 2.21A)
   a. Pulmonary: comes from the right ventricle; transports deoxygenated blood to the lungs
   b. Aorta: largest artery in the body; comes from the heart; divided into ascending aorta, aortic arch, descending aorta, and abdominal aorta

c. Coronary: right and left branches off the ascending aorta; supplies the heart with blood
d. Brachiocephalic: one of three major branches off the aortic arch; supplies blood to the neck, head, axilla, and upper arm
e. Subclavian: supplies arms and vertebrae
   1) Left subclavian branches from aortic arch
   2) Right subclavian branches from brachiocephalic
f. Carotid: supplies neck and head
   1) Left carotid branches from aortic arch
   2) Right carotid branches from brachiocephalic
g. Facial: branch of carotid; supplies the face and cranium
h. Occipital: branch of carotid; supplies the neck and cranium
i. Axillary: extension of subclavian; supplies the axilla
j. Brachial: extension of axillary; supplies the upper arm
k. Radial: branch of brachial; supplies the forearm, wrist, and hand
l. Ulnar: branch of brachial on little finger side; supplies the forearm, wrist, and hand
m. Celiac: branch of abdominal aorta; supplies the upper abdomen and organs
n. Splenic: functions similarly to celiac
o. Renal: branch of abdominal aorta; supplies the kidneys, ureters, and adrenal glands
p. Mesenteric: branch of abdominal aorta; supplies intestines, colon, and rectum
q. Iliac: extension of abdominal aorta; branches and supplies abdominal and pelvic regions and lower limbs
r. Femoral: extension of iliac; supplies abdominal wall, genitalia, and upper leg
s. Popliteal: extension of femoral; supplies the knee and calf
t. Tibial: extension of popliteal
   1) Anterior supplies lower leg, ankle, and foot
   2) Posterior supplies lower leg, foot, and heel
u. Dorsalis pedis: extension of anterior tibial; supplies the foot

4. Major veins (Fig. 2.21B)
   a. Pulmonary: transports blood from the lungs to the left atrium
   b. Coronary: drains blood from the right atrium
   c. Vena cava: largest vein in the body; leads from the body into the right atrium
      1) Superior vena cava: drains upper body
      2) Inferior vena cava: drains lower body
   d. Brachiocephalic: left and right branches go into the superior vena cava; drains the head, neck, and upper extremities
   e. Jugular: branches go into the brachiocephalic; drains the head and neck
   f. Facial: branches go into the jugular; drains the face and cranium
   g. Occipital: branches go into the jugular; drains the cranium
   h. Axillary: branches go into the brachiocephalic; drains the axillary area and the upper arm
   i. Subclavian: branches go into the axillary; drains the upper arm
   j. Cephalic: goes into the axillary; drains the upper and lower arm
   k. Radial: goes into the axillary; drains the thumb side of the forearm and wrist
   l. Basilic: goes into axillary on the little finger side; drains the upper and lower arm
   m. Ulnar: goes into the axillary; drains the little finger side of the forearm and wrist

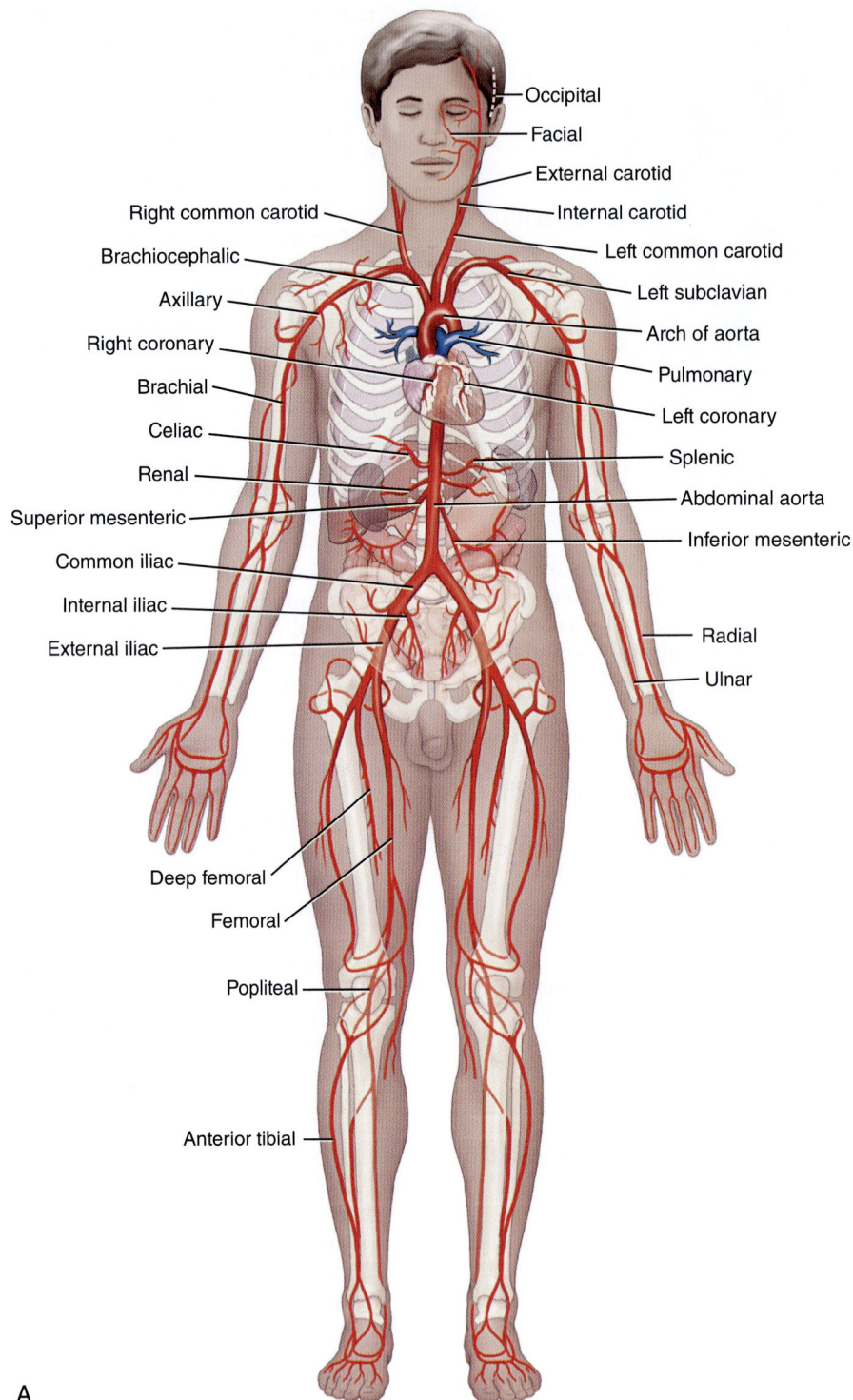

Fig. 2.21 (A) Major arteries of the body.

n. Gastric, cholecystic, and splenic: goes into portal hepatic vein; drains the stomach, gallbladder, and spleen

o. Mesenteric: goes into the hepatic portal vein; drains the intestines, colon, and rectum

p. Hepatic: goes into the inferior vena cava; drains the liver

q. Renal: goes into the inferior vena cava; drains the kidneys and gonads

r. Iliac: extension of the inferior vena cava; drains the abdominal, pelvic, and lower limb regions

s. Femoral: extension of right and left iliac; drains the upper leg

t. Popliteal: extension of femoral; drains the knee and calf

u. Saphenous: longest vein in the body
   1) Great saphenous goes into femoral; drains the medial leg
   2) Small saphenous goes into popliteal; drains the lower leg

v. Tibial: goes into the popliteal; drains the lower leg

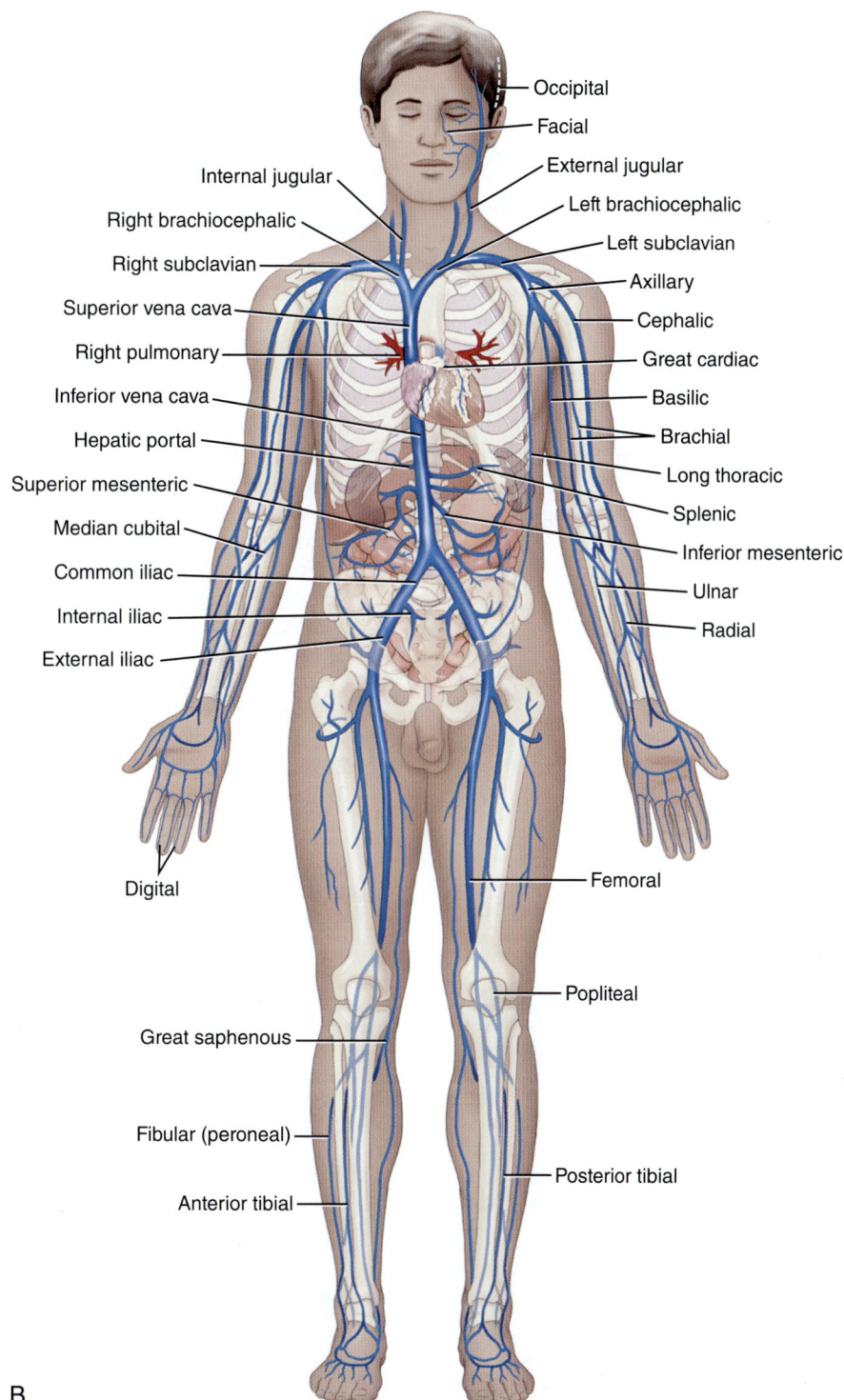

Fig. 2.21, cont'd (B) Major veins of the body. (From Shiland, BJ: *Mastering healthcare terminology*, ed 5, 2016, Mosby.)

Labels on figure:
Occipital
Facial
External jugular
Internal jugular
Left brachiocephalic
Right brachiocephalic
Left subclavian
Right subclavian
Axillary
Superior vena cava
Cephalic
Right pulmonary
Great cardiac
Inferior vena cava
Basilic
Hepatic portal
Brachial
Superior mesenteric
Long thoracic
Median cubital
Splenic
Common iliac
Inferior mesenteric
Internal iliac
Ulnar
External iliac
Radial
Digital
Femoral
Popliteal
Great saphenous
Fibular (peroneal)
Posterior tibial
Anterior tibial

B

D. Circulatory Pathways

1. Pulmonary circuit
   a. Takes blood from the right side of the heart to the lungs and back to the left side of the heart
2. Systemic circuit
   a. Provides blood supply to all body tissues
   b. Blood carries O_2 and nutrients from the left ventricle through arteries to capillaries in tissues to the cells; picks up CO_2 and waste products and returns these through the veins to the right atrium of the heart

X. Blood

A. General

1. Primary transport medium of the body
2. Pumped by the heart through a closed system of vessels
3. Classified as connective tissue (cells and matrix)
4. Approximately 5–6 L in adults
5. 8% of body weight

B. Functions

1. Transportation
   a. Carries O_2 and nutrients to cells
   b. Carries CO_2 and wastes from the tissues to the lungs and kidneys for removal
   c. Carries hormones from the endocrine glands to other parts of the body
2. Regulation
   a. Regulates body temperature by removing heat from active areas and transporting that heat to the skin for dissipation
   b. Helps regulate fluid and electrolyte balance
   c. Regulates pH through buffers
3. Protection
   a. Provides clotting mechanism to prevent fluid loss when vessels are damaged
   b. White blood cells engulf and destroy invading microorganisms
   c. Antibodies react with offending agents

C. Composition of Blood (Fig. 2.22)

1. Plasma
   a. Liquid portion of circulating blood
   b. 55% of the total blood volume
   c. 90% water
   d. Continuously changing because of dissolved solutes
   e. Contains plasma proteins
      1) Albumin: maintains osmotic pressure
      2) Globulin: functions in lipid transport and immune reaction
      3) Fibrinogen: formation of blood clots
   f. Also contains amino acids, urea, uric acids, nutrients, hormones, O_2, CO_2, antibodies, and electrolytes
2. Formed elements: produced by hematopoiesis (red blood cells [RBCs] in red bone marrow; white blood cells [WBCs] in lymphoid tissue); all types develop from stem cell (hematocytoblast)
   a. Erythrocytes (RBCs)
      1) Most numerous of formed elements
      2) Normal range: 4.5–6 million/mm^3 blood
      3) Biconcave disks (thin in the middle and thick around the edge)
      4) Mature cells have no nucleus
      5) Primary function: to carry O_2 to all body cells; O_2 combines with hemoglobin and is transported
      6) Formation regulated by hormone erythropoietin
      7) Iron, vitamin B_{12}, and folic acid are essential to RBC production
      8) Live approximately 120 days; destroyed by the spleen and liver
   b. Leukocytes (WBCs)
      1) Larger in size than RBCs but fewer in number
      2) Normal range: 5000–10,000/mm^3 blood
      3) Each contains a nucleus

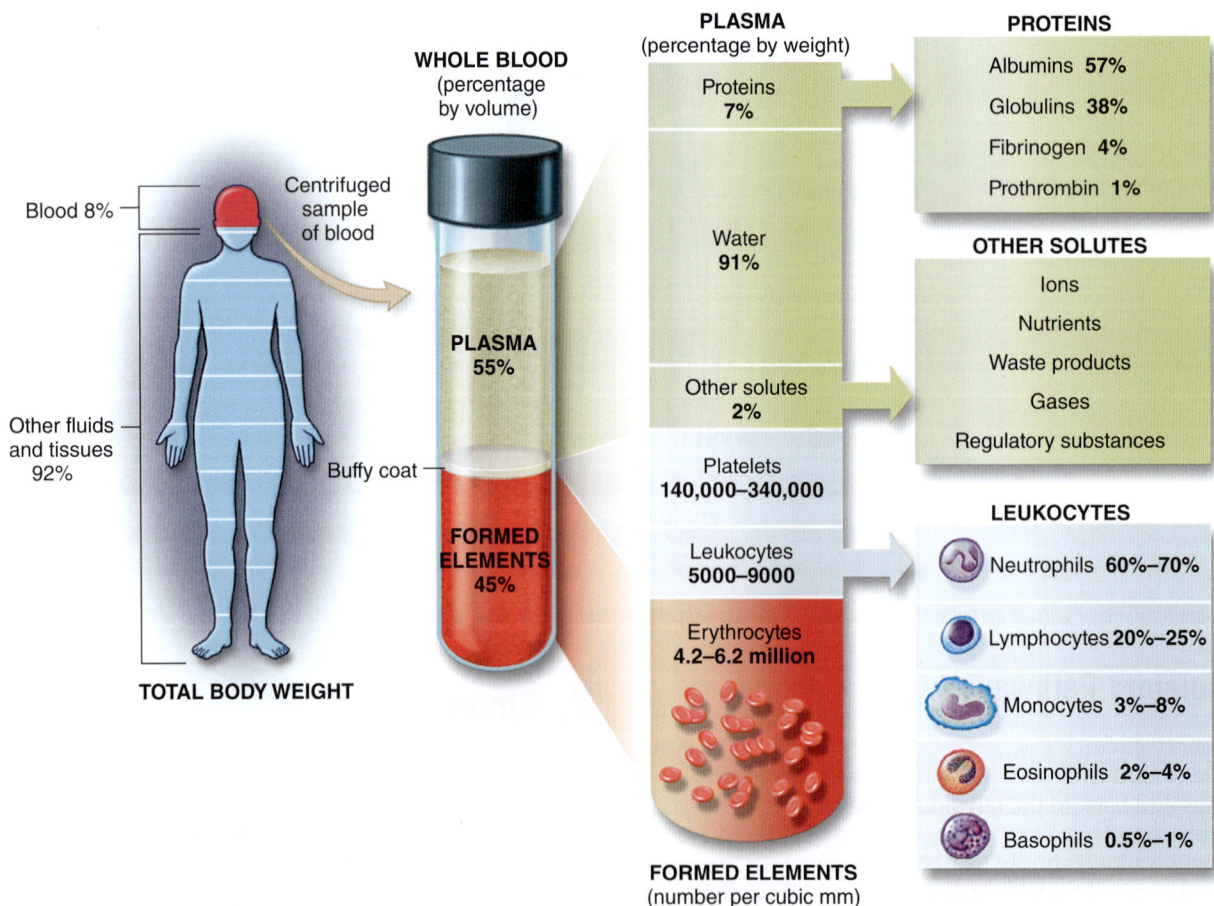

WHOLE BLOOD (percentage by volume)

Blood 8%
Centrifuged sample of blood
Other fluids and tissues 92%
Buffy coat

PLASMA 55%
FORMED ELEMENTS 45%

TOTAL BODY WEIGHT

PLASMA (percentage by weight)

Proteins 7%
Water 91%
Other solutes 2%

PROTEINS

Albumins 57%
Globulins 38%
Fibrinogen 4%
Prothrombin 1%

OTHER SOLUTES

Ions
Nutrients
Waste products
Gases
Regulatory substances

Platelets 140,000–340,000
Leukocytes 5000–9000
Erythrocytes 4.2–6.2 million

LEUKOCYTES

Neutrophils 60%–70%
Lymphocytes 20%–25%
Monocytes 3%–8%
Eosinophils 2%–4%
Basophils 0.5%–1%

FORMED ELEMENTS (number per cubic mm)

Fig. 2.22 Components of blood. (Courtesy Barbara Cousins.)

4) Able to move through capillary walls into the tissue

5) Primary function: to provide defense against invading microorganisms and to promote or inhibit inflammatory response

6) Types

a) Granulocytes: contains granules in the cytoplasm

(1) Neutrophil: most common; has multilobed nucleus; responds first to tissue damage; number increases in acute infection

(2) Eosinophil: two-lobed nucleus; large granules in cytoplasm; neutralizes histamine; numbers increase during allergic reaction and parasitic infections

(3) Basophil: least numerous of WBCs; has large U-shaped nucleus; can leave blood and enter tissue, where they release histamine and heparin

b) Agranulocytes: granules absent in cytoplasm

(1) Lymphocytes: large round nucleus surrounded by small amount of cytoplasm; role in the body's defense system

(a) T lymphocytes: directly attack microorganisms

(b) B lymphocytes: produce antibodies

(2) Monocytes: largest in size of all WBCs; can enter the tissue (macrophage); finish the cleanup process of the neutrophils

c. Thrombocytes (platelets): small fragments of very large cells (megakaryocytes)

1) Normal range: 250,000–500,000/mm^3 blood

2) Initiates formation of blood clots

D. Hemostasis

1. Stoppage of bleeding
2. Can be caused by either an injured vessel or stasis of blood flow
3. Includes three processes (Fig. 2.23)

a. Vascular constriction: reduces flow of blood through torn vessel

b. Platelet plug formation: platelets become sticky and adhere to each other

c. Coagulation: complex series of steps that results in clot formation; requires calcium and vitamin K

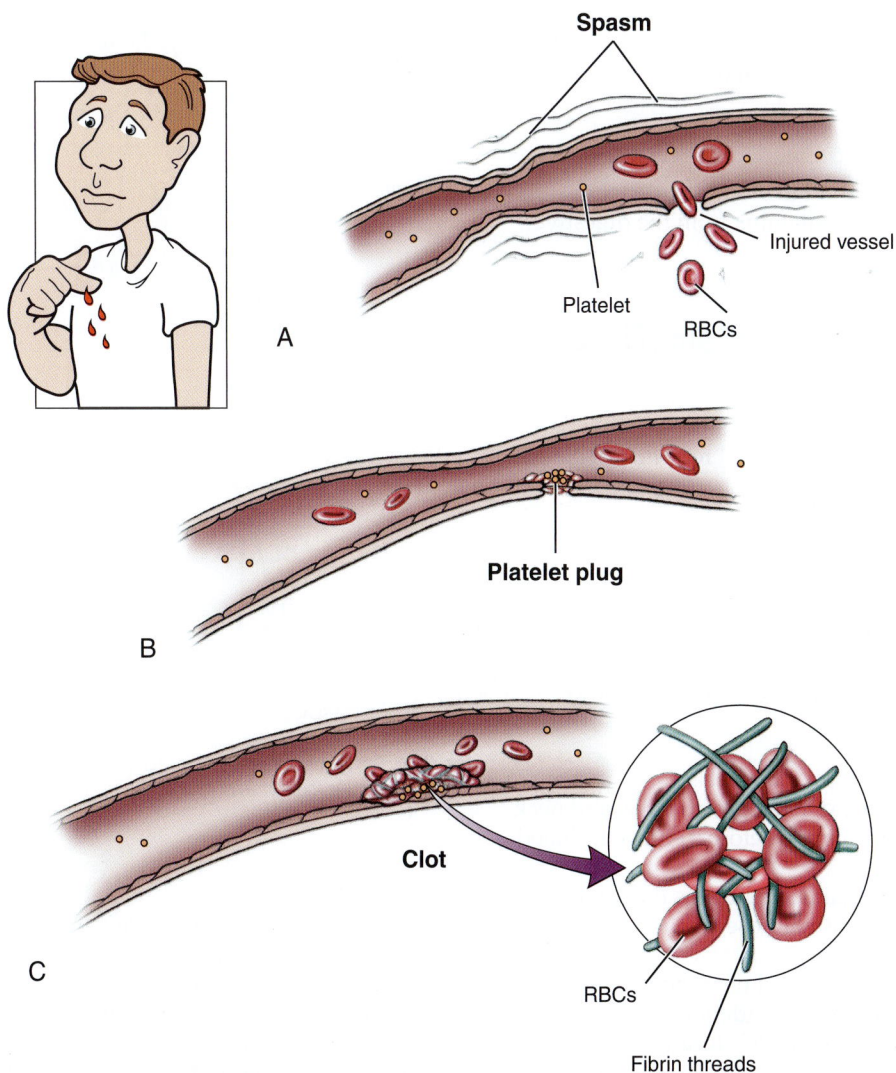

Fig. 2.23 Steps of hemostasis. (A) Vascular constriction; (B) formation of the platelet plug; (C) blood clotting (coagulation). *RBCs*, Red blood cells. (From Herlihy B: *The human body in health and illness*, ed 6, 2018, Saunders.)

E. Blood Typing

1. Based on specific antigens and antibodies related to RBCs; blood type antigens are found on RBCs; antibodies in plasma
2. Main blood groups, ABO blood groups; blood types *must* match in transfusions
   a. Type A: has A antigens on RBCs; has anti-B antibodies
   b. Type B: has B antigens on RBCs; has anti-A antibodies
   c. Type AB: has both A and B antigens on RBCs; has no antibodies
   d. Type O: has neither A nor B antigens on RBCs; has both anti-A and anti-B antibodies
3. Rh factor: Rh-positive individual has Rh antigen on RBCs; Rh-negative individual has no antigens; neither has anti-Rh in plasma; hemolytic disease of the newborn may develop when Rh-negative mother has Rh-positive fetus

XI. Lymphatic System

A. General

1. Part of the circulatory system
2. Transports a fluid (lymph) through lymphatic vessels and empties it into the venous blood
3. Major role in the body's defense system

B. Functions

1. Returns excess interstitial fluid to blood
2. Absorbs fats and fat-soluble vitamins from the digestive system
3. Provides defense against disease

C. Organs of the Lymphatic System (Fig. 2.24)

1. Lymph
   a. Similar in composition to blood plasma
   b. Picked up from interstitial fluid and returned to blood plasma
2. Lymphatic vessels
   a. Found in tissue spaces
   b. Carry fluid away from the tissues
   c. Vessels empty into the lymphatic ducts
      1) Right lymphatic duct: drains the lymph from the RUQ of the body
      2) Thoracic duct: drains the remainder of the body
3. Lymphatic organs
   a. Lymph nodes
      1) Located along the lymphatic vessels
      2) Superficial nodes found in the groin, axilla, and neck
      3) Filter and cleanse the lymph before it enters the blood
   b. Tonsils
      1) Provide protection against pathogens that may enter through the mouth or nose
      2) Three groups
         a) Pharyngeal tonsils: located near the opening of the nose into the pharynx; adenoids
         b) Palatine tonsils: "the tonsils"; located near the opening of the oral cavity into the pharynx
         c) Lingual tonsils: posterior surface of the tongue

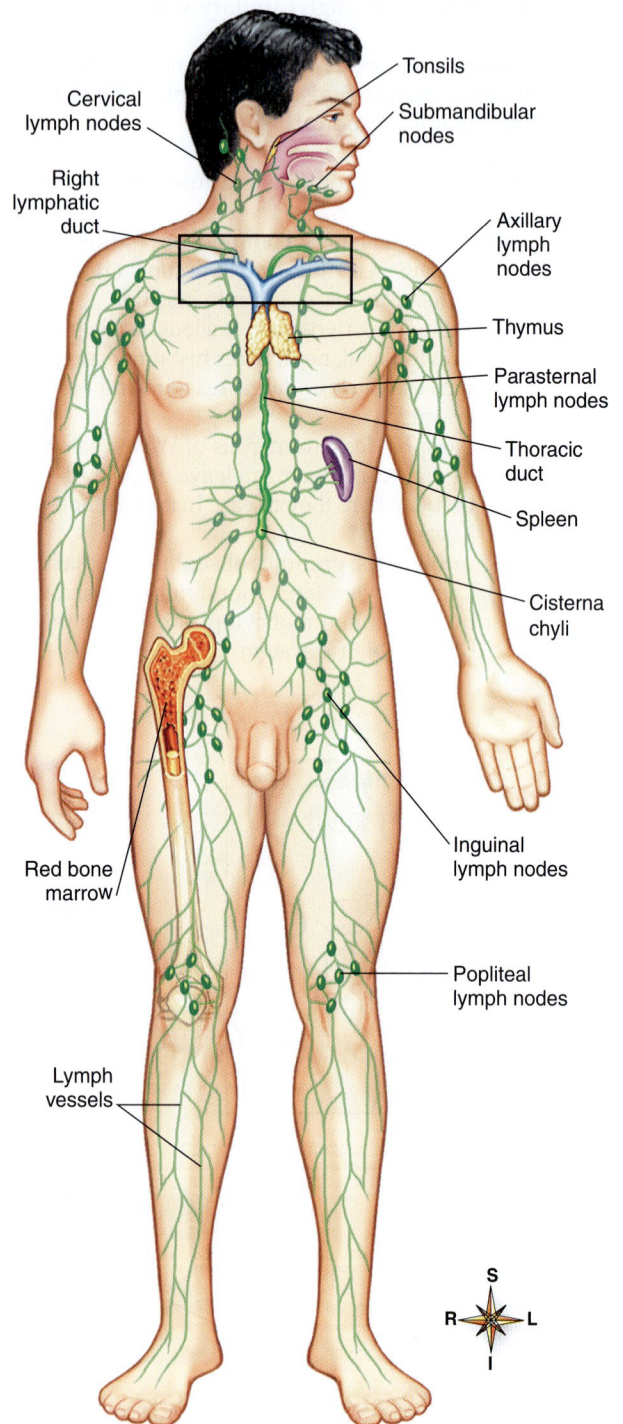

Fig. 2.24 The lymphatic system. Principal organs and lymph drainage. (From Patton KT, Thibodeau GA: *The human body in health and disease*, ed 7, 2020, Mosby.)

4. Spleen: located in the upper left abdomen beneath the diaphragm, posterior to the stomach; filters blood; acts as a reservoir for the blood
5. Thymus: located posterior to the sternum; large in infants, atrophies after puberty; produces thymosin (stimulates the maturation of lymphocytes in the lymphatic organs)

D. Resistance to Disease

1. Resistance: the body's ability to counteract pathogens
2. Susceptibility: the lack of resistance
3. Resistance accomplished through defense mechanisms
   a. Nonspecific defense mechanisms: directed against all pathogens and foreign substances; provides first line of defense against invasion (Fig. 2.25)
      1) Barriers
         a) Mechanical (e.g., skin)
         b) Chemical (e.g., hydrochloric acid in stomach)
      2) Chemical action
         a) Complement: promotes phagocytosis and inflammation
         b) Interferon: produced by virus-infected cells to provide protection for neighboring cells
      3) Phagocytosis: neutrophils and macrophages
      4) Inflammation: characterized by redness, warmth, swelling, and pain
   b. Specific defense mechanisms: programmed to be selective (specificity); ability to remember invading agent (memory); invading agent called antigen; B lymphocytes produce antibodies that react with the antigen (Fig. 2.26)

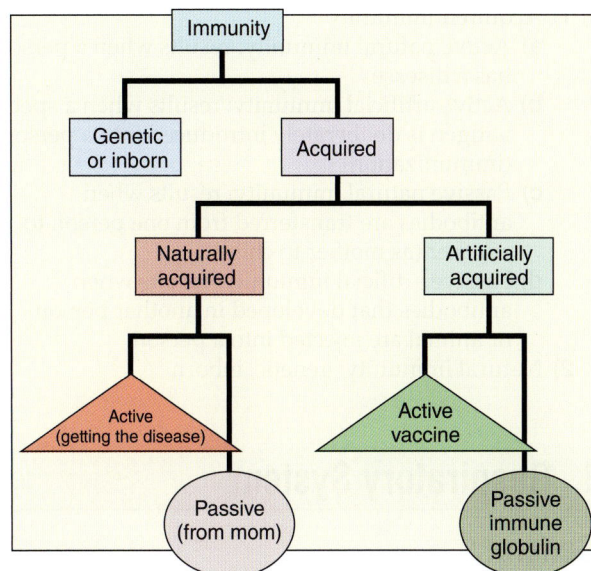

Fig. 2.26 Immunity is either genetic or acquired. Immunity is acquired either naturally or artificially. Naturally acquired immunity can be either active *(triangles)* or passive *(circles)*. (From Herlihy B: *The human body in health and illness*, ed 6, 2018, Saunders.)

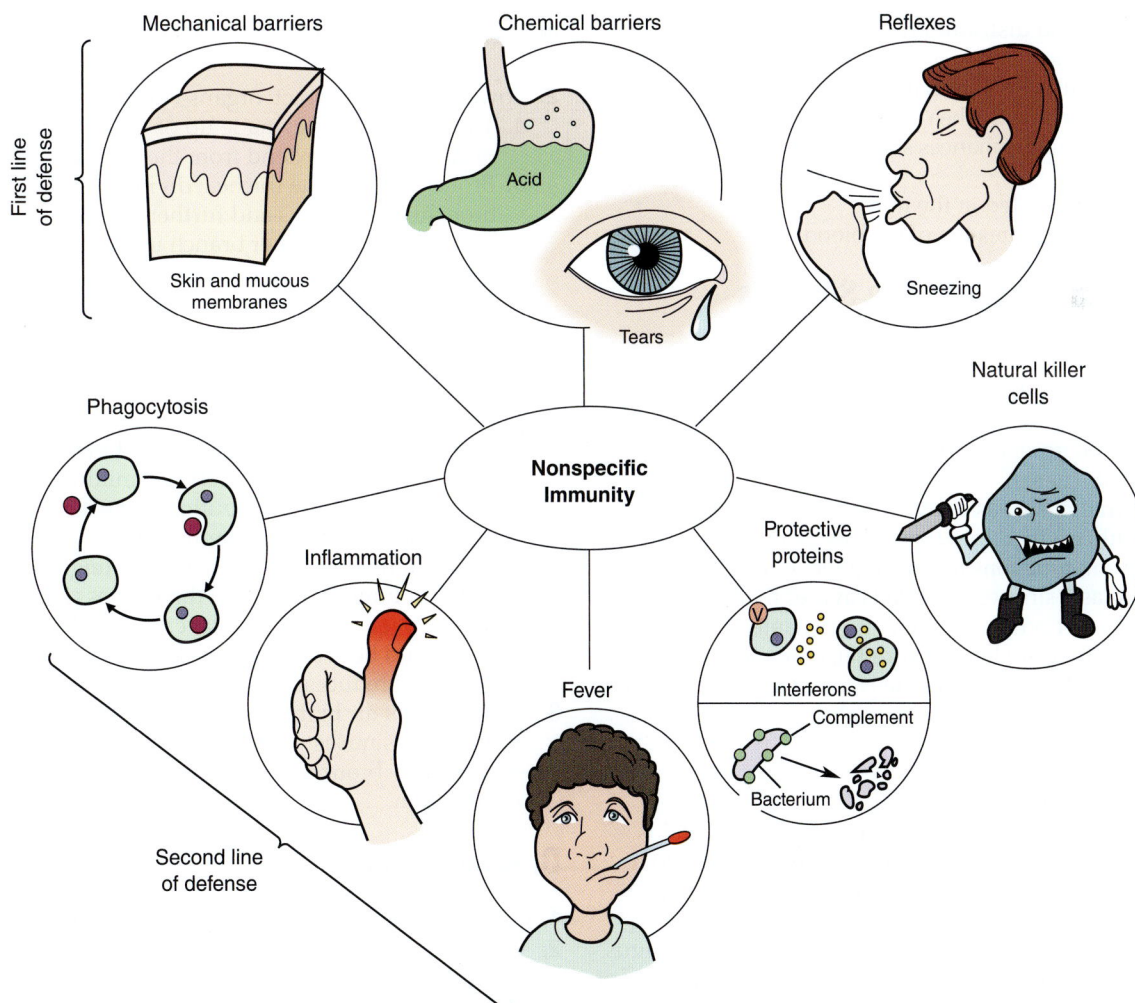

Fig. 2.25 Nonspecific immunity. The first line of defense includes mechanical barriers, chemical barriers, and reflexes. Processes involved in the second line of defense are phagocytosis, inflammation, fever, protective proteins (complement proteins and interferons), and natural killer cells. (From Herlihy B: *The human body in health and illness*, ed 6, 2018, Saunders.)

1) Acquired immunity
   a) Active natural immunity: results when a person has a disease
   b) Active artificial immunity: results when a specific antigen is deliberately introduced into a person (immunization)
   c) Passive natural immunity: results when antibodies are transferred from one person to another (as mother to child)
   d) Passive artificial immunity: results when antibodies that developed in another person or animal are injected into a person
2) Natural immunity: genetic, inborn

XII. Respiratory System

A. General

1. Supplies continuous supply of O_2 to the body
2. Works with the circulatory system to bring O_2 to the entire body and to remove waste products

B. Functions

1. Air exchange and distribution: O_2 carried to tissues and CO_2 carried away
2. Filtration: small hairs in nasal cavity trap substances before air enters the trachea
3. Sound production: enhances sounds produced during speech
4. Sense of smell: located in the nose
5. H regulation: regulates the pH of blood

C. Organs: Divided Into Two Sections (Fig. 2.27)

1. Upper respiratory tract: organs outside of thoracic cavity
   a. Nose
      1) External nose: nasal bones and cartilage; forms nostrils (nares)
      2) Internal nose: nasal cavity; found over roof of mouth; divided into two halves by the nasal septum; functions to warm, filter, and humidify air
      3) Paranasal sinuses: air-filled cavities that surround the nasal cavity and open into it; named for bones in which they are located (frontal, ethmoid, maxillae, sphenoid); produce mucus, reduce the weight of the skull, and influence voice quality
   b. Pharynx
      1) Throat
      2) Has three divisions
         a) Nasopharynx: nearest to nasal cavity; contains adenoids; auditory tubes from ears open into it
         b) Oropharynx: behind the mouth; contains the tonsils
         c) Laryngopharynx: leads to trachea and esophagus
   c. Larynx: voice box; made up of cartilage with ciliated mucous membrane; contains vocal cords; carries air from pharynx to trachea

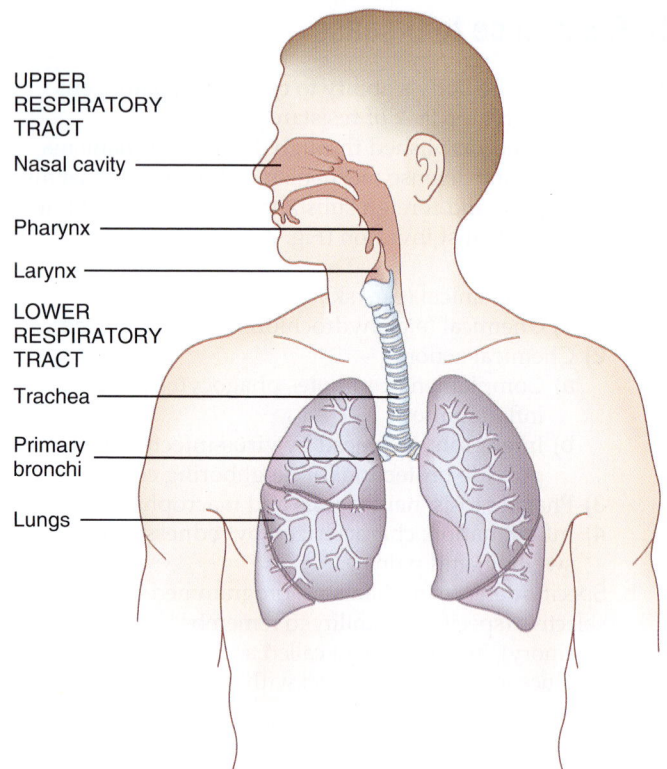

Fig. 2.27 The respiratory tract.

2. Lower respiratory tract: organs within the thorax
   a. Trachea: windpipe; made up of 16–20 C-shaped rings of cartilage that extend from the larynx to the bronchi
   b. Bronchi: end of the trachea; divided into right and left bronchi; enter lungs and further divide into secondary bronchi, which further branch into bronchioles; branches end in alveolar ducts
   c. Alveoli: air sacs; functional units of respiration; resemble clusters of grapes; these form the terminal end of bronchioles; composed of single layers of epithelium surrounded by capillaries; gases exchanged here
   d. Lungs: cone-shaped organs located in thoracic cavity; each contains approximately 300 million alveoli; responsible for air distribution and exchange; bottom portion (base) rests on diaphragm
      1) Left lung divided into two lobes (eight segments)
      2) Right lung divided into three lobes (10 segments)
         a) Covered by double-layered membrane (pleura); fluid between layers (pleural fluid) lubricates and reduces friction during respiration
3. Movement of air in the lungs: air → nose → paranasal cavities and sinuses → pharynx → larynx → trachea → bronchi → bronchioles → alveoli → capillaries → bloodstream

D. Respiration

1. Controlled by respiratory control center of medulla
2. Medulla controls rhythm and depth of inspiration and expiration
3. Monitors O_2, CO_2, and pH of blood, which triggers breathing

4. Involves two processes
   a. Pulmonary ventilation: carries out breathing by means of pressure gradient; has two phases
      1) Inspiration: air drawn into lungs by contraction of diaphragm (makes thoracic cavity larger)
      2) Expiration: air expelled from lungs by relaxation of diaphragm
   b. Cellular respiration: has two phases
      1) External: exchange of gases between alveoli and capillaries
      2) Internal: exchange of gases between capillaries and body cells

XIII. Digestive System

A. General

1. Includes the digestive tract (gastrointestinal [GI] tract, alimentary canal) and accessory organs
2. Digestive tract: long, continuous tube that starts at the mouth and ends at the anus
3. Processes food into molecules small enough to be used by the body

B. Functions

1. Digestion: physical and chemical breakdown of complex foodstuffs into simple nutrients
2. Absorption: passage of simple nutrients through the walls of the small intestine into the blood or lymph
3. Elimination: excretion of indigestible waste from the body in the form of feces

C. Organs (Fig. 2.28)

1. Mouth (oral cavity)
   a. Receives food by ingestion
   b. Breaks down food into small particles by mastication (chewing)
   c. Mixes food with saliva
   d. Lips and cheeks help hold food in place for chewing
   e. Also helps with speech
      1) Palate: separates oral cavity from nasal cavity
         a) Anterior portion (hard palate): supported by bone
         b) Posterior portion (soft palate): made of muscle and connective tissue; ends in fingerlike projection (uvula); uvula and soft palate move upward during swallowing to keep food from entering the nasal cavity
      2) Tongue: moves food around in mouth; helps with speech; covered by papillae; papillae provide friction and contain taste buds
      3) Teeth: used for mastication (chewing)
         a) Two different sets develop
            (1) Deciduous (baby teeth): first 20 teeth, which eventually fall out
            (2) Permanent: set of 32 adult teeth, which replace deciduous teeth

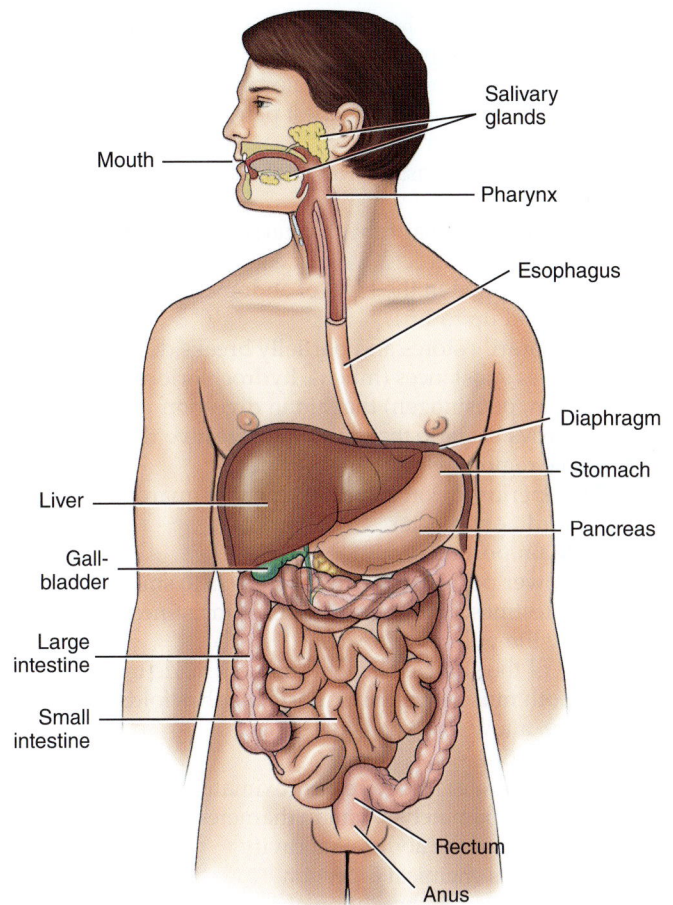

Fig. 2.28 The digestive system. (From Herlihy B: *The human body in health and illness*, ed 6, 2018, Saunders.)

      b) Shape of tooth corresponds to the way it handles food
         (1) Incisors: chisel shaped and sharp edges for biting foods
         (2) Cuspids (canines): conical shaped with points for grasping and tearing foods
         (3) Bicuspids: flat surfaces for crushing and grinding
         (4) Molars: also have flat surfaces for crushing and grinding
      c) Tooth is divided into the following:
         (1) Crown: exposed portion; covered with enamel (hardest surface in the body)
         (2) Neck: narrow portion below crown, protected by gums
         (3) Root: end portion of neck that fits into socket in mandible and maxilla
         (4) Pulp cavity: central core of tooth; contains pulp, which consists of connective tissue, blood vessels, and nerves; surrounded by dentin
      4) Salivary glands
         a) Produce saliva, which contains water, mucus, and enzyme amylase; moistens food; begins chemical digestion
         b) Three pairs of exocrine glands secrete saliva into the mouth

(1) Parotid: largest pair; located in front of the ears (mumps)

(2) Submandibular: located in the floor of the mouth

(3) Sublingual: smallest pair; located under the tongue

2. Pharynx (throat): passageway that transports food to esophagus

3. Esophagus: muscular tube that carries food from pharynx to stomach

4. Stomach: located in the LUQ of abdomen

   a. Can hold up to 1.5 L

   b. Temporarily stores and partially breaks down food

   c. Secretes substances (mucus, hydrochloric acid [HCl], gastrin, pepsinogen) that aid in digestion

   d. Destroys bacteria that enter the digestive tract

   e. Three regions

      1) Superior region (fundus); opening guarded by the cardiac sphincter

      2) Main portion (body)

      3) Lower portion (pylorus); connects to small intestines; opening to the small intestines guarded by the pyloric sphincter

   f. Wall of the stomach has three layers made up of smooth muscle; the innermost layer has folds (rugae), which allow for expansion

5. Small intestine

   a. Coiled tubular structure approximately 6 m in length and approximately 2.5 cm in diameter

   b. Fills most of the abdominal cavity

   c. Completes chemical digestion

   d. Primary site for absorption of nutrients

   e. Has three divisions

      1) Duodenum: upper portion

      2) Jejunum: middle portion

      3) Ileum: end portion

   f. Suspended from the abdominal wall by a fold of peritoneum (mesentery)

   g. Lining contains fingerlike projections (villi); villi contain capillaries and lacteals, which rise off of the surface area and absorb nutrients

6. Large intestine

   a. Folded tube approximately 1.5 m in length and 6 cm in diameter

   b. Absorbs fluid and electrolytes; eliminates waste products

   c. Produces vitamin K (necessary for blood clotting)

   d. Divided into

      1) Cecum: first division connected to ileum of small intestine; contains ileocecal valve; vermiform appendix attached to cecum

      2) Ascending colon: vertical length of colon that runs along the right side of the abdominal cavity

      3) Transverse colon: horizontal length of colon that runs across the abdominal cavity

      4) Descending colon: vertical length of colon that runs along the left side of the abdominal cavity

      5) Sigmoid colon: S-shaped length of colon that connects to the rectum

      6) Rectum: continues to the anal canal; thick muscular wall

      7) Anal canal: continues from the rectum to outside (anus); guarded by two sphincter muscles

7. Peritoneum: serous membrane that covers most of the abdominal organs and holds them in place

   a. Mesentery: holds intestines in coils

   b. Transverse mesocolon: binds transverse colon to posterior abdominal wall

   c. Omentum: sheet of serous membrane that contains fat; protects the abdominal organs

8. Accessory organs

   a. Liver

      1) Accessory organ of digestion

      2) "Can't live without a liver"

      3) Largest gland in the body

      4) Located in the RUQ

      5) Divided into right and left lobes

      6) Filters and destroys wastes and toxic substances

      7) Produces bile, which breaks down (emulsifies) fats

      8) Stores iron; glycogen; and vitamins A, B_{12}, D, E, and K

      9) Produces clotting factors

      10) Recycles iron and hemoglobin from worn-out red blood cells

      11) Controls carbohydrate and lipid metabolism

   b. Gallbladder

      1) Pear-shaped sac attached to inferior surface of liver by cystic duct

      2) Stores, concentrates, and sends bile into the duodenum through the common bile duct (the cystic duct joins the hepatic duct from the liver to form the common bile duct)

   c. Pancreas

      1) Located behind stomach

      2) Endocrine and exocrine functions

         a) Endocrine: beta cells of the islets of Langerhans secrete insulin, which decreases blood glucose levels; alpha cells of the islets of Langerhans secrete glucagon (which increases blood glucose levels)

         b) Exocrine: acinar cells secrete digestive enzymes (amylase, trypsin, peptidase, and lipase)

9. Movement of food: food → mouth → pharynx → esophagus → stomach → duodenum → jejunum → ileum → cecum → ascending colon → transverse colon → descending colon → sigmoid colon → rectum → anus → feces leaves the body

D. Digestion

1. Breakdown of foodstuffs: has two processes

   a. Mechanical digestion: breaks down food, moves it along the canal, and eliminates the waste from the body

      1) Begins with mastication (chewing), which reduces the size of food and mixes the food with saliva to form a bolus

      2) Bolus is swallowed (deglutition)

      3) Wavelike motion of GI tract (peristalsis) moves food along the digestive tract

      4) Food is churned in stomach to mix with gastric juices to form chyme

      5) Chyme is pushed into the duodenum approximately every 20 seconds until empty

6) Chyme mixes with pancreatic liver and intestinal juices
7) Chyme leaves the jejunum approximately 5 hours after entering the small intestine
8) Residue not absorbed enters the large intestine, where excess water is absorbed, and waste (feces) is formed and expelled from the body

b. Chemical digestion: breaks down large complex molecules into smaller molecules for absorption; accomplished by hydrolysis and enzymes
   1) Carbohydrates: initially broken down by amylase; final breakdown by sucrase, lactase, and maltase
   2) Proteins: broken down into amino acids by proteases: pepsin (stomach), trypsin (pancreas), and peptidase (intestines)
   3) Fats: first emulsified by bile in small intestine; finally digested by pancreatic lipase

E. Absorption

1. Process of transporting nutrients from small intestinal mucosa to blood or lymph
2. Most absorption occurs in small intestine
3. Nutrients travel to the liver through the portal system

F. Elimination

1. Solid waste expelled from body by process of defecation
2. Defecation is triggered by stimulation of receptors caused by a full rectum
3. Controlled by the internal sphincter (involuntary) and external sphincter (voluntary)

XIV. Urinary System

A. General

1. Produces and excretes urine from the body
2. Kidneys clean the blood of waste products
3. Plays vital role in electrolyte, water, and acid-base balance

B. Functions

1. Waste elimination: excretes nitrogen-containing liquid waste (urine) from the body
2. Regulation of blood volume: balances water loss and gain
3. Regulation of pH: balances gain and loss of bicarbonate and hydrogen ions
4. Regulation of electrolytes: balances levels through excretion and reabsorption
5. Detoxification: assists liver in neutralizing substances

C. Organs (Fig. 2.29)

1. Kidney: two bean-shaped organs located retroperitoneal between T12 and L3; surrounded by a cushion of fat; two layers
   a. Cortex: outer layer
   b. Medulla: inner layer; contains renal pyramids
      1) Triangle-shaped wedges that contain the nephron
      2) Points of pyramids come together into a cuplike structure (calyx [singular])

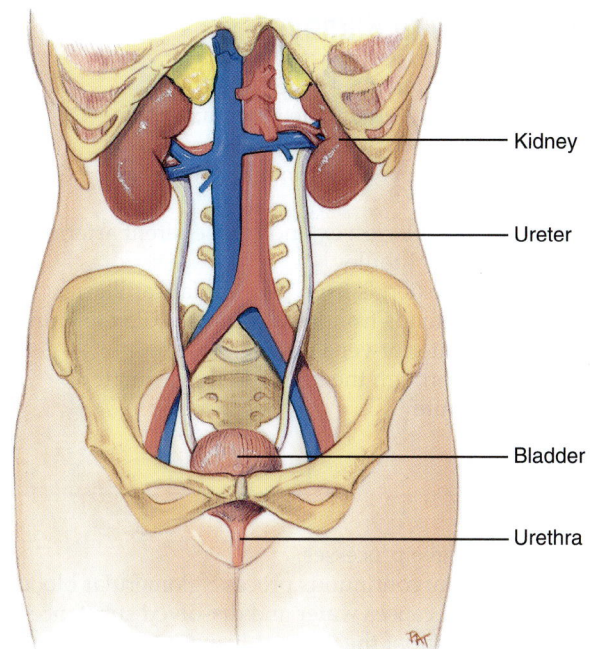

Fig. 2.29 Components of the urinary system. (From Applegate E: *The anatomy and physiology learning system*, ed 4, 2011, Saunders.)

Labels: Kidney, Ureter, Bladder, Urethra

3) Calyces (plural) join together to form renal pelvis, where urine is collected
4) Nephron: microscopic functional unit of kidneys; filters blood and produces urine; composed of the following:
   a) Bowman capsule: cup-shaped structure in renal cortex; holds the glomerulus
   b) Glomerulus: ball-shaped cluster of capillaries that sits in the Bowman capsule; the Bowman capsule and glomerulus make up the renal corpuscle
   c) Proximal convoluted tubule: extension of the Bowman capsule; makes up first part of the renal tubule
   d) Loop of Henle: extends from proximal convoluted tubule
   e) Distal convoluted tubule: extends from loop of Henle
   f) Collecting tubule: tubule formed by union of distal convoluted tubules; convoluted tubules join to form one renal pyramid; pyramids join to form calyx

2. Ureter
   a. Tube that runs from the kidneys into the urinary bladder
   b. Renal pelvis narrows as it leaves the kidney to form the ureter

3. Urinary bladder
   a. Muscular sac located behind the symphysis pubis
   b. Capable of great expansion caused by folds (rugae) in its inner lining
   c. Serves as a temporary storage place for urine

4. Urethra
   a. Tube that carries urine from the bladder to the outside of the body
   b. Opening to outside is urinary meatus

5. Formation of urine: blood (renal artery) → glomerulus → glomerular capsule → renal tubule → renal pelvis → ureter → bladder → urethra → urinary meatus → urine leaves body

D. Blood Flow to Kidneys

1. Renal artery: enters the kidney at hilum
2. Afferent arteriole: enters the Bowman capsule
3. Glomerulus: network of capillaries
4. Efferent arteriole: comes from glomerulus and exits the Bowman capsule
5. Peritubular capillaries: extend from efferent arteriole; surrounds renal tubule
6. Renal venule: extends from peritubular capillaries
7. Renal vein: extends from renal venule; exits the kidney at hilum; joins inferior vena cava
8. Blood flows through the kidneys: approximately 1200 mL/minute

E. Urine

1. Formation
   a. Series of three processes
      1) Filtration: continuous process; glomerular blood pressure causes water and dissolved substances to filter out of the glomeruli and into the Bowman capsule
      2) Reabsorption: movement of substances out of renal tubules into blood in peritubular capillaries; water, nutrients, and electrolytes reabsorbed
      3) Secretion: movement of substances not reabsorbed into urine into collecting tubules
2. Composition
   a. Water: 95% of urine
   b. Nitrogenous waste products: urea, ammonia, uric acid, and creatinine (end products of protein metabolism)
   c. Electrolytes: sodium, potassium, phosphate, sulfates, ammonium, bicarbonate, and chloride
   d. Toxins
   e. Pigment: urochrome

F. Body Fluids

1. Constitute about 60% of body weight in nonobese men (less in women)
2. Not evenly distributed; separated into compartments
3. Fluid can move back and forth between compartments
4. Fluid intake should equal fluid output
5. Kidneys are the main regulators of fluid loss under the control of antidiuretic hormone (ADH)

XV. Endocrine System

A. General

1. Body's slower-acting control system
2. Made up of glands that secrete substances (hormones)
3. Hormones travel through the bloodstream to target organs and cells

B. Functions

1. Control: regulates internal body functions and processes
2. Communication: complements the nervous system; directs communication among the body systems for optimal functioning

C. Hormones

1. Chemical substances secreted from the endocrine glands
2. Each is unique in composition and action
3. Classified as either steroid or protein
4. Tropic hormones: stimulate other endocrine glands to secrete their hormones
5. Sex hormones: stimulate reproductive tissue
6. Anabolic hormones: stimulate cells to grow and repair
7. Prostaglandins: tissue hormones that regulate cellular activity

D. Glands (Fig. 2.30)

1. Pituitary gland: master gland; hypophysis
   a. Located on the inferior surface of the brain
   b. Connected to the hypothalamus by stalk (infundibulum)
   c. Divided into two sections
      1) Anterior hypophysis (adenohypophysis) (Fig. 2.31): secretes
         a) Growth hormone: promotes tissue growth; stimulates fat metabolism; helps maintain blood glucose levels
         b) Prolactin: promotes development of the breast and milk secretion; works with luteinizing hormone during menstrual cycle
         c) Thyroid-stimulating hormone: stimulates development and hormone production of thyroid gland

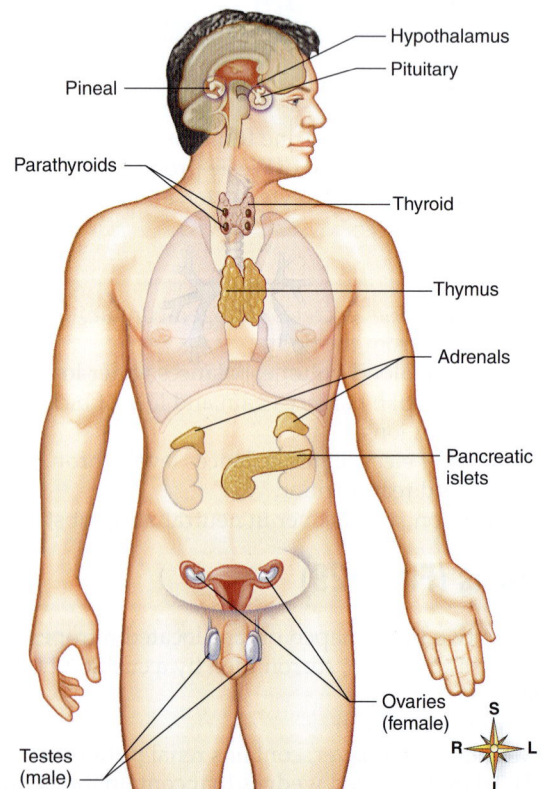

Fig. 2.30 Major endocrine glands of the body. (From Patton KT, Thibodeau GA: *The human body in health and disease*, ed 7, 2020, Mosby.)

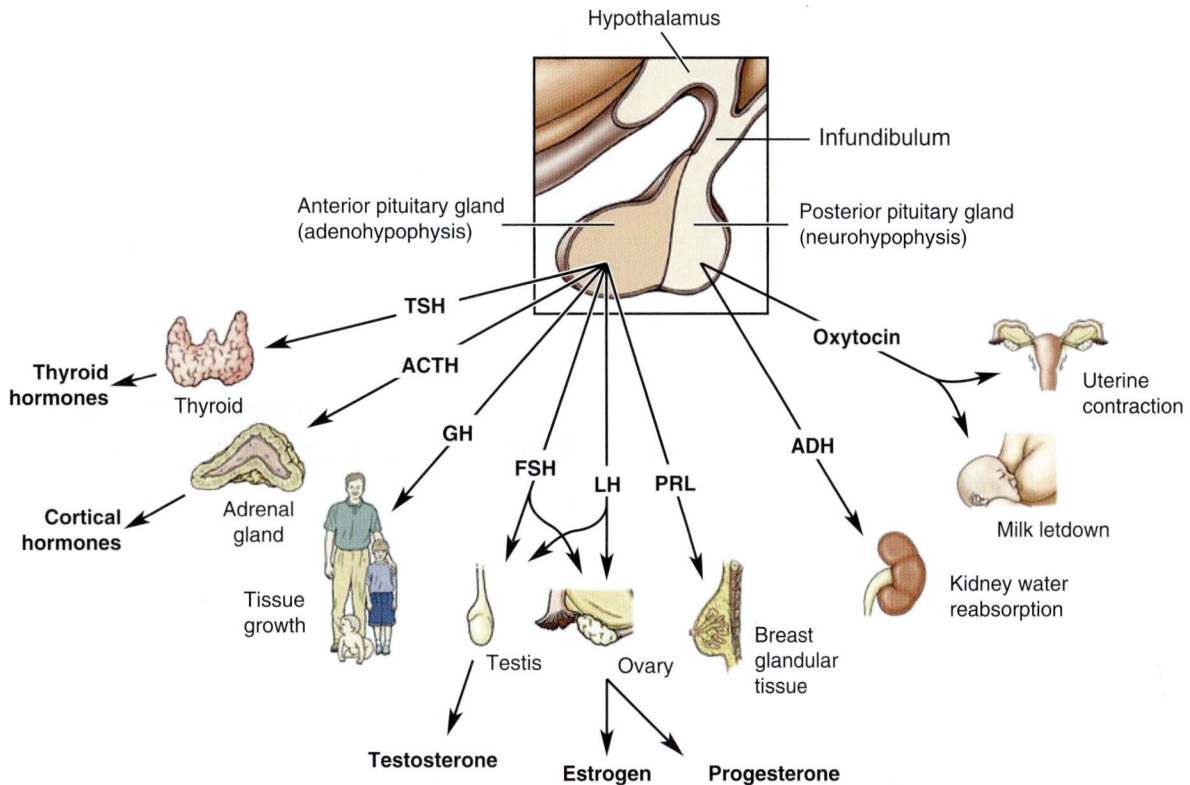

Fig. 2.31 Pituitary gland. Hormones secreted by the anterior and posterior pituitary glands. Target organs are also shown. *ACTH*, Adrenocorticotropic hormone; *ADH*, antidiuretic hormone; *FSH*, follicle-stimulating hormone; *GH*, growth hormone; *LH*, luteinizing hormone; *MSH*, melanocyte-stimulating hormone; *PRL*, prolactin; *TSH*; thyroid-stimulating hormone. (From Herlihy B: *The human body in health and illness*, ed 6, 2018, Saunders.)

d) Adrenocorticotropic hormone (ACTH): stimulates development and hormone production of adrenal cortex
e) Follicle-stimulating hormone
 (1) In females: stimulates follicle development and secretion of estrogen
 (2) In males: stimulates sperm production
f) Luteinizing hormone
 (1) In females: stimulates secretion of estrogen and progesterone
 (2) In males: stimulates secretion of testosterone
g) Melanocyte-stimulating hormone: regulates normal color of the skin; helps regulate response of the adrenal gland to ACTH
2) Posterior pituitary (neurohypophysis)
 a) Does not manufacture hormones
 b) Stores and releases hormones made in the hypothalamus
  (1) ADH: prevents excessive formation of urine
  (2) Oxytocin: stimulates the uterus to contract during childbirth; causes letdown of milk
2. Pineal gland
 a. Pinecone-shaped gland located behind the hypothalamus
 b. Produces melatonin that regulates the body's "biological clock"
3. Thyroid gland
 a. Butterfly-shaped gland located in the neck, lateral and anterior to the trachea
 b. Secretes two hormones

1) Thyroxine (tetraiodothyronine [T_4]) and triiodothyronine (T_3): regulate metabolism of the body; iodine is needed for synthesis
2) Calcitonin: stimulates movement of calcium from the blood to the bone
4. Parathyroid gland
 a. Four pea-shaped glands embedded in the thyroid gland
 b. Secretes parathormone (PTH), which causes calcium to leave bone and enter the bloodstream
5. Adrenal glands
 a. Located on top of each kidney
 b. Composed of two regions
  1) Adrenal cortex: outer region; secretes corticosteroids
   a) Aldosterone: regulates mineral salts
   b) Cortisol: regulates blood pressure
   c) Androgen and estrogen: minor sex hormones
  2) Adrenal medulla: inner region; secretes hormones that are important in the sympathetic and parasympathetic nervous systems
   a) Epinephrine
   b) Norepinephrine
6. Pancreas
 a. Elongated gland that extends posterior to the stomach
 b. Produces glucagon; from alpha cells; stimulates conversion of glycogen to glucose in the liver
 c. Produces insulin; from beta cells; decreases glucose levels in blood
 d. Produces somatostatin; from delta cells; regulates other pancreatic cells

7. Gonads
   a. Testes in males: secrete testosterone, which stimulates the development of male sex characteristics
   b. Ovaries in females
      1) Secrete estrogen: from follicles; stimulates development of female sex characteristics
      2) Secrete progesterone: from corpus luteum; maintains pregnancy
8. Thymus
   a. Located in mediastinum below the sternum
   b. Largest in the children; atrophies during adolescence
   c. Produces thymosin; stimulates T lymphocytes for immunity
9. Placenta: produces human chorionic gonadotropin (HCG) during pregnancy
10. Prostaglandins
   a. Potent chemical regulators
   b. Produced in minute amounts and found throughout the body
   c. Cannot be stored
   d. Many actions
      1) Affect smooth muscle contraction
      2) Moderate hormone actions
      3) Involved in blood-clotting mechanisms
      4) Promote many aspects of inflammatory response
      5) Inhibit gastric secretion of HCl
      6) Elevated levels associated with premenstrual syndrome (PMS) and premature labor

XVI. Reproductive System

A. General

1. Produces offspring for the survival of the species

B. Functions

1. Production of egg and sperm cells
2. Nurturing of developing offspring
3. Production of hormones

C. Organs and Structures of the Male Reproductive System (Fig. 2.32)

1. Testes
   a. Essential organs (gonads)
   b. Produces sperm (male gamete)
   c. Glandular structures located outside of the body in the scrotum
   d. Made up of seminiferous tubules (sperm development) and interstitial cells (produces testosterone)
2. Epididymis
   a. Continuation of seminiferous tubules
   b. Lies on the superior surface of the testes
   c. Secretes part of seminal fluid

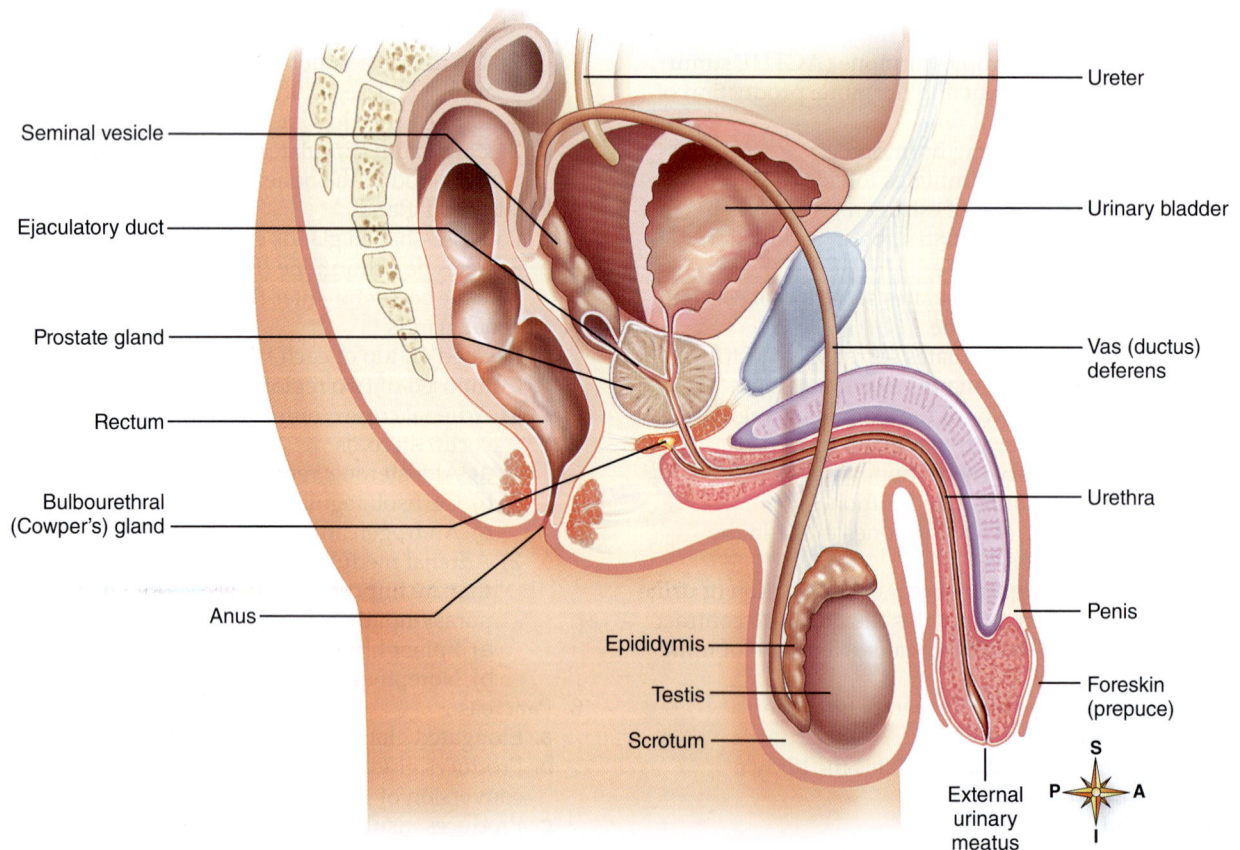

Fig. 2.32 Male reproductive organs. (From Patton KT, Thibodeau GA: *The human body in health and disease*, ed 7, 2020, Mosby.)

3. Vas deferens
   a. Extension of the epididymis
   b. Passes through the inguinal canal into the abdominal cavity; arches over the bladder and joins the seminal vesicles
   c. Site of male sterilization (vasectomy)
4. Seminal vesicles
   a. Bilateral pouches behind the urinary bladder
   b. Secrete a nutrient-rich fluid that nourishes sperm
5. Ejaculatory duct
   a. Formed by the union of the vas deferens and seminal vesicles
   b. Passes through the prostate gland and enters the urethra
   c. Propels sperm and seminal fluid into the urethra during orgasm
6. Prostate gland
   a. Doughnut-shaped gland that encircles the base of the urethra on the posterior surface of the bladder
   b. Secretes alkaline fluid that protects sperm from the acidity of the vagina
7. Bulbourethral gland (Cowper gland)
   a. Pea-shaped glands located on both sides of the urethra
   b. Secretes lubrication during intercourse
8. Scrotum
   a. Pouch of skin suspended from the perineal area
   b. Holds the testes and epididymis
   c. Keeps the testes away from the body; body temperature is too high for sperm production
9. Penis
   a. External male genitalia
   b. Composed of three cylinders of erectile tissue
   c. During sexual arousal, erectile tissue fills with blood and becomes erect
   d. Contains the urethra
   e. Distal end covered by the prepuce (foreskin), which is removed by circumcision

D. Organs and Structures of the Female Reproductive System (Fig. 2.33)

1. Ovaries
   a. Essential organs (gonads)
   b. Produce ova (female gamete)
   c. Almond-shaped glands located in the pelvic cavity
   d. Contain ovarian (graafian) follicles where ova develop
   e. Produce estrogen and progesterone
2. Uterus
   a. Pear-shaped muscular organ located in the pelvic cavity between the bladder and rectum
   b. Three divisions
      1) Fundus: upper region
      2) Body: large central region
      3) Cervix: lower neck region; opens to the vagina
   c. Three layers
      1) Endometrium: inner layer; the fertilized ovum implants and grows here; sheds monthly (menstruation; menses)
      2) Myometrium: middle muscular layer
      3) Perimetrium (epimetrium): outer layer
   d. Contracts to deliver the fetus
3. Fallopian tubes (oviducts)
   a. Attached to the upper, outer sides of the uterus
   b. Serve as the site of fertilization; the fertilized ovum travels through the tube into the uterus for implantation
   c. Distal ends contain fingerlike structures (fimbriae); gentle movement of fimbriae draws the ovum into the tube after release from the ovary
   d. Site of female sterilization (tubal ligation)
4. Vagina
   a. Tubular structure that extends from the cervix to the outside
   b. Located between the rectum and urethra
   c. Capable of great expansion
   d. Serves as the birth canal and means of shedding menstrual tissues

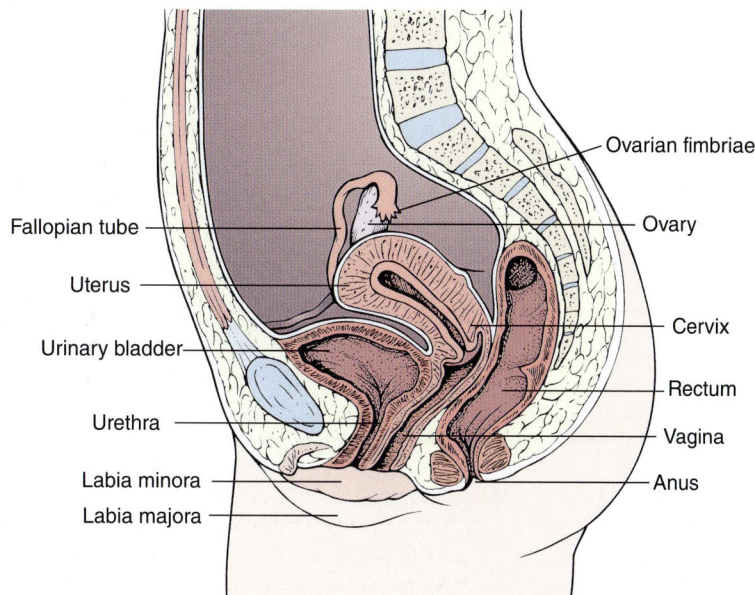

Fig. 2.33 Normal female reproductive system. (From Frazier MS, Drzymkowski JW: *Essentials of human diseases and conditions*, ed 6, 2016, Elsevier.)

5. Vulva
   a. External genitalia
   b. Includes
      1) Mons pubis: fat pad that covers the symphysis pubis
      2) Labia majora: two large folds of skin extending from the mons pubis to the anus
      3) Labia minora: two small folds of skin medial to the labia majora
      4) Clitoris: small nodule of erectile tissue superior to the labia majora; plays a role in sexual arousal
      5) Bartholin glands: located at the entrance to the vagina; secrete lubricating fluid during intercourse
6. Perineum: region between the vaginal opening and the rectum; may be cut (episiotomy) or torn during childbirth
7. Breasts
   a. Mammary glands
   b. Fatty tissue and milk glands that overlie the pectoral muscles
   c. Produce milk (lactation) for offspring
   d. Nipple is a protrusion for delivery of milk
   e. Areola is the dark area that surrounds nipple

E. Reproductive Cycle

1. Ovarian cycle: ovum develops and matures in the ovary
2. Menstrual cycle
   a. Menses: days 1–5; if the ovum is not fertilized, the endometrium is shed
   b. Postmenstrual: days 6–13; the endometrium thickens as the ovum matures in the ovary; estrogen levels increase
   c. Ovulation: day 14; the mature ovum is released from the ovary
   d. Premenstrual: days 15–28; the corpus luteum develops on the ovary where the ovum was released and secretes progesterone; endometrium thickens in preparation for a fertilized ovum

F. Pregnancy

1. Ovulation: release of ovum
2. Insemination: sperm are released into the vagina and travel through the cervix and uterus into the fallopian tube
3. Conception: fertilization; union of sperm and egg; occurs in the fallopian tube; results in a zygote with 46 chromosomes (23 from ovum, 23 from sperm)
4. Zygote divides and implants in the uterine wall; becomes an embryo at the 3rd week of development until the end of the 8th week; becomes a fetus at the 9th week until birth
5. Placenta: highly vascular disk-shaped organ; develops from embryonic and maternal tissues; attaches the developing fetus to the uterus; performs nutrition, excretory, and respiratory functions; excretes HCG for continued pregnancy
6. Gestation: lasts approximately 40 weeks; three 3-month trimesters
7. Parturition: childbirth; occurs in three stages
   a. Onset of contractions to cervical dilation (10 cm)
   b. Dilation to birth of the fetus
   c. Expulsion of the placenta

Diseases and Disorders

I. Introduction to Disease

A. Disease Terminology

1. Acute: when signs and symptoms appear suddenly, persist for a short time, and then disappear
2. Anomaly: a deviation from normal
3. Asymptomatic: showing no symptoms
4. Chronic: diseases that develop slowly, last for a long time
5. Communicable: can be transmitted from one person to another
6. Congenital disorder: abnormal condition that exists at birth
7. Disease: abnormality in body function that threatens health
8. Endemic: disease that is native to a local region
9. Epidemic: disease that spreads to many individuals at the same time
10. Etiology: study of the cause of disease
11. Functional: disease with no detectable physical changes to explain the symptoms being experienced by the patient
12. Health: physical, mental, and social well-being; no disturbance in homeostasis
13. Hereditary disorder: condition caused by a defective gene
14. Idiopathic: diseases without a known or recognizable cause
15. Nosocomial: hospital-acquired infection that was not present on admission
16. Organic: disorder in which there are physical changes that explain symptoms being experienced by the patient
17. Pandemic: epidemic that affects a large geographic region
18. Pathogen: microorganism that causes disease
19. Pathology: study of disease
20. Sign: objective abnormalities seen by someone besides the patient
21. Somatoform: presence of physical symptoms that suggest a general medical condition but are not explained by the patient's actual condition
22. Symptom: subjective abnormality felt by the patient
23. Syndrome: collection of different signs and symptoms

B. Causes of Diseases

1. Disturbances of homeostasis and how the body responds
2. Genetic mechanism
3. Pathogenic organisms
4. Tumors and cancer
5. Physical and chemical agents
6. Malnutrition
7. Autoimmunity
8. Inflammation
9. Degeneration
10. Trauma

C. Risk Factors (Predisposing Conditions)

1. Genetic factors
2. Age
3. Lifestyle
4. Stress
5. Environmental factors
6. Preexisting conditions

II. Diseases, Disorders, and Conditions of Body Systems

A. Diseases and Disorders of the Integumentary System

1. Abrasion: scrape
2. Abscess: localized collection of pus within a circumscribed area; associated with tissue destruction
3. Acne vulgaris: inflammation of a sebaceous gland; characterized by papules, pustules, and comedos

4. Actinic keratosis: premalignant lesion of the skin caused by excess exposure to sunlight
5. Albinism: whiteness of skin caused by lack of melanin
6. Alopecia: baldness
   a. Alopecia areata: characterized by well-defined bald areas usually on the scalp and face
   b. Alopecia capitis totalis: characterized by the loss of all the hair on the scalp
   c. Alopecia universalis: total loss of hair on all parts of the body
7. Avulsion: torn-away tissue
8. Bulla: large vesicle
9. Burn: tissue injury resulting from thermal, chemical, electrical, or radioactive agents
   a. First degree: superficial involvement of epidermis; characterized by erythema, tenderness, and pain
   b. Second degree: partial thickness involves epidermis and dermis; characterized by vesicles
   c. Third degree: full-thickness burn that involves epidermis, dermis, and injury to underlying tissues; characterized by charring, tissue damage, and loss of fluid
   d. Rule of nines for adults: method of determining percentage of body surface area affected:
      1) Head and neck = 9%
      2) Torso = 36%
      3) Arms = 18%
      4) Legs = 36%
      5) Genitals = 1%
10. Callus: thickened area of the epidermis caused by pressure or friction
11. Carcinoma: skin cancer; caused by exposure to UV rays and radiation
    a. Basal cell: malignant tumor of the basal cell layer of the epidermis
    b. Squamous cell: malignant tumor of the squamous epithelial cells of the epidermis
    c. Malignant melanoma: cancerous growth of melanocytes
12. Cellulitis: infection of connective tissue with severe inflammation within the skin layers
13. Chloasma: pigmentation disorder characterized by brownish spots on the face; mask of pregnancy
14. Comedo (pl. *comedos*): papule having a small, dark central region (blackhead) or pale region (whitehead)
15. Contusion: injury that does not break the skin; characterized by swelling, pain, and discoloration
16. Cyanosis: blue coloration of the skin caused by lack of oxygen
17. Cyst: raised or flat fluid-filled or solid-filled sac
18. Decubitus ulcer: bedsore; open lesion caused by poor or no circulation to the area resulting from pressure against the tissue
19. Dermatitis: inflammation of the skin; characterized by pruritus, various lesions, and erythema
    a. Seborrheic dermatitis: chronic dermatitis; caused by an increase in sebaceous secretions; characterized by greasy scales, pruritus, and dandruff
    b. Atopic dermatitis: inflammation with rash
    c. Contact dermatitis: inflammation caused by irritant
20. Eczema: dry, leathery vesicles in adults; characteristic pattern on the face, neck, elbows, and knees

21. Dermatophytosis: superficial fungal infection; lesions are round, scaly, or ring shaped
    a. Tinea corporis: ringworm; involves exposed skin
    b. Tinea unguium: involves toenail
    c. Tinea pedis: athlete's foot
    d. Tinea cruris: jock itch
22. Diaphoresis: excessive sweating
23. Ecchymosis: purplish area caused by bleeding within the skin; a bruise
24. Eczema: an acute or chronic skin inflammation characterized by redness, scales, crusts, and itching
25. Erythema: redness caused by local inflammation or irritation
26. Excoriation: scratch
27. Fissure: crack, groove, or crevice
28. Furuncle: boil; pus-containing abscess that involves the entire hair follicle and adjacent subcutaneous tissue
29. Hematoma: bruise; caused by collection of blood under the tissue from a blood vessel injury
30. Hemangioma: benign tumor made up of blood vessels
31. Herpes simplex: cold sore or fever blister; small, painful vesicles that erupt around the mouth, lips, nose, or mucus membranes; caused by herpes simplex virus type 1
32. Herpes zoster: shingles; acute inflammatory eruption of painful vesicles along the course of a peripheral nerve; caused by herpes zoster virus
33. Hirsutism: excessive hairiness
34. Impetigo: infectious bacterial infection caused by staphylococci or streptococci; vesicles dry to form crusts especially around the mouth and nose
35. Infestation: parasite found on an external surface
36. Jaundice: yellowing of the skin; can be caused by liver, blood, or gallbladder disorders
37. Keloid: abnormal scar formation
38. Lesion: any injury, wound, or area of disease
39. Lipoma: benign fatty deposit under the skin
40. Macule: flat lesion (freckle)
41. Nevus (pl. *nevi*): mole
42. Nodule: raised lesion made of a solid tissue mass
43. Onychocryptosis: ingrown toenail
44. Onychomycosis: fungal infection of the nail
45. Papule: firm, raised lesion (pimple)
46. Pediculosis: infestation by lice (genus: *Pediculus*)
    a. Pediculosis capitis: head lice
    b. Pediculosis corporis: body lice
    c. Pediculosis palpebrarum: infestation of eyebrows and lashes
    d. Pediculosis pubis: "crabs," genital lice
47. Petechiae: small pinpoint hemorrhages; smaller versions of bruises
48. Polyp: cyst on a stalk
49. Port-wine stain: large, reddish purple discoloration of the face or neck; present at birth and does not resolve without treatment
50. Pruritus: itching
51. Psoriasis: chronic disease characterized by red lesions and silvery scales; may be autoimmune
52. Pustule: pus-filled vesicle
53. Rosacea: chronic condition of unknown cause that produces redness, tiny pimples, and broken blood vessels

54. Scabies: skin infection caused by infestation with the itch mite
55. Scleroderma: thick, dense, fibrous skin
56. Sebaceous cyst: cyst of a sebaceous gland containing yellow, fatty material
57. Skin tags: small, flesh-colored, or light brown growths that hang from the body by fine stalks; acrochordon
58. Ulcer: open sore
59. Urticaria: hives; usually caused by allergic reaction
60. Verruca (pl. *verrucae*): warts; caused by papillomavirus
61. Vesicle: fluid-filled lesion (blister)
62. Vitiligo: white patches on skin caused by lack of melanin production
63. Wheal: circular, raised lesion having central pallor and circumscribed redness
64. Xeroderma: excessively dry skin

B. Diseases and Disorders of the Skeletal System

1. Abnormal spinal curvatures
   a. Scoliosis: abnormal lateral curvature of the spine
   b. Kyphosis: humpback; abnormal outward curvature of the spine
   c. Lordosis: swayback; abnormal inward curvature of the spine
2. Arthralgia: pain in a joint or joints
3. Arthritis: inflammation of the joints
   a. Osteoarthritis: chronic inflammation of joint; results in degeneration of cartilage, which causes hypertrophy of bone
   b. Rheumatoid arthritis: chronic, systemic inflammatory disease of joint; causes erosion of cartilage
   c. Juvenile rheumatoid arthritis: affects children; characterized by pain and swelling in joints, skin rash, fever, slowed growth, and fatigue
   d. Gouty arthritis: associated with the formation of uric acid crystals in the joint; gout
4. Ankylosing spondylitis: rheumatoid arthritis of the spine
5. Bursitis: inflammation of the bursa (thin sac that helps tendons and muscles move over bones)
6. Crepitation: crackling sensation that is felt and heard when the ends of a broken bone move together; crepitus
7. Ewing sarcoma: cancer usually occurring in the diaphyses of the long bones in the arms and legs of children and adolescents
8. Fracture: crack or break in a bone
   a. Simple (closed): fracture with no external wound
   b. Compound (open): fracture with external break in the skin
   c. Greenstick: incomplete break
   d. Comminuted: shattering of the bone (bone fragments)
   e. Impacted: one broken end forced into the other
   f. Spiral: resembles a spiral
9. Lumbago: pain in the lumbar region; low back pain
10. Neoplasms
    a. Osteosarcoma: malignant tumor of connective tissue arising from the bone
    b. Osteochondroma: tumor of bone and cartilage
    c. Chondrosarcoma: tumor of cartilage

11. Osteomalacia: condition of softening of bones; known as rickets in children; caused by low level of vitamin D
12. Osteomyelitis: inflammation of bone, usually following compound fracture or symptoms
13. Osteoporosis: condition of porous, brittle bones, especially in menopausal and postmenopausal females; caused by low levels of calcium and potassium
14. Paget disease: osteitis deformans; chronic metabolic disease causing bones to thicken and soften
15. Spina bifida: congenital abnormality characterized by failure of vertebrae to close around the spinal cord
16. Subluxation: partial displacement of a bone from its joint
17. Talipes: clubfoot

C. Diseases and Disorders of the Muscular System

1. Carpal tunnel syndrome: inflammation of the tendons passing through the carpal tunnel of the wrist
2. Contracture: abnormal shortening of muscle tissues making the muscle resistant to stretching
3. Fibromyalgia: chronic pain condition associated with tenderness and stiffness that affects muscles, joints, and tendons throughout the body
4. Fasciitis: inflammation of a fascia
5. Intermittent claudication: complex of symptoms including cramplike pain of the leg muscles caused by poor circulation
6. Muscular dystrophy: congenital disorder; characterized by progressive wasting of muscle tissue
   a. Becker muscular dystrophy: less severe form that does not appear until early adolescence or adulthood
   b. Duchenne muscular dystrophy: severe form that appears between 2 and 6 years of age
7. Myalgia: muscle pain or tenderness
8. Myasthenia gravis: chronic, progressive neuromuscular disease; may be autoimmune; characterized by muscle weakness, dysphagia, and blepharoptosis
9. Rotator cuff tendinitis: inflammation of the tendons of the rotator cuff
10. Shin splint: pain caused by the muscle tearing away from the tibia
11. Spasm: sudden, violent involuntary contraction of a muscle or a group of muscles; cramp
12. Sprain: acute partial tear of a muscle, tendon, or ligament
13. Strain: result of overuse, overstretching, or excessive forcible stretching of a muscle
14. Tendinitis (sometimes spelled *tendonitis*): inflammation of tendon

D. Diseases and Disorders of the Brain and Nervous System and Psychiatric Disorders

1. Addiction: compulsive, uncontrollable dependence on a substance, habit, or action to the degree that stopping causes severe emotional, mental, or physiologic reactions
2. Alcoholism: chronic dependence or abuse of alcohol with specific signs and symptoms of withdrawal
3. Alzheimer disease: senile dementia; chronic organic brain syndrome; characterized by degeneration of nervous tissue resulting in lowered intellectual functioning and untimely death

4. Amnesia: disturbance in memory marked by total or partial inability to recall past experiences
5. Amyotrophic lateral sclerosis (ALS): also known as Lou Gehrig disease; affects motor neurons; characterized by muscle atrophy and weakness
6. Anxiety state: feeling of apprehension, tension, or uneasiness that stems from the anticipation of danger, largely unknown or unrecognized
7. Aphasia: inability to speak, write, or comprehend speech or the spoken word; often follows a stroke
8. Ataxia: inability to coordinate muscles for voluntary movement
9. Attention-deficit disorder: characterized by a child having a short attention span and impulsiveness that are inappropriate for the child's developmental age
10. Attention-deficit/hyperactivity disorder (ADHD): characterized by a pattern of inattention and hyperactivity that are inappropriate for the child's developmental age
11. Autism: characterized by a young child's inability to develop normal social relationships; child behaves in compulsive and ritualistic ways and frequently has poor communication skills; autism spectrum disorder
12. Bipolar disorder: major affective disorder characterized by intense mood swings from a hyperactive (manic) state to a depressive state
13. Cephalalgia: pain in the head; headache
14. Cerebral palsy: caused by congenital brain defects or injury at birth; characterized by loss of sensation or control of muscle movements
15. Concussion: violent shaking or jarring of the brain
16. Conscious: state of being awake, aware, and responding appropriately
17. Convulsion: sudden, violent, involuntary contraction of muscles caused by a disturbance in brain function; seizure
    a. Clonic: state marked by alternate contraction and relaxation of muscles resulting in jerking movements of the face, trunk, and extremities
    b. Tonic: state of continuous muscular contraction that results in rigidity and violent spasms
18. Dementia: slowly progressive decline in mental abilities including impaired memory, thinking, and judgment
19. Dyslexia: learning disability characterized by difficulty using and interpreting written forms of communication
20. Encephalitis: inflammation of the brain
21. Epilepsy: abnormal electrical activity of the brain; characterized by random, intense electrical discharges that result in seizure activity
    a. Grand mal: more severe form; characterized by generalized tonic-clonic seizures
    b. Petit mal: milder form; characterized by a sudden, temporary loss of consciousness lasting only seconds
22. Guillain-Barré syndrome: acute, rapidly progressive disease of the spinal nerves
23. Hallucination: sense perception that has no basis in external stimulation
24. Huntington chorea: Huntington disease; hereditary degenerative disease of the cerebral cortex; progressive atrophy of the brain occurs
25. Hydrocephalus: excessive amount of cerebrospinal fluid (CSF) causing macroencephaly
26. Insomnia: abnormal inability to sleep

27. Lethargy: lowered level of consciousness characterized by listlessness, drowsiness, and apathy
28. Major depressive disorder: prolonged period during which there is either a depressed mood or the loss of interest or pleasure in activities
29. Manic episode: distinct period during which there is an abnormally and persistently elevated, expansive, and irritable mood
30. Meningitis: inflammation of meninges; can be caused by virus or bacteria
31. Mental retardation: significantly below-average general intellectual functioning accompanied by significant limitation in adaptive functioning
32. Migraine: periodic severe headaches; accompanied by nausea and vomiting, auras, and throbbing pain
33. Multiple sclerosis (MS): chronic inflammation of central nervous system; attacks myelin sheath, causing sensory and motor abnormalities
34. Munchausen syndrome: characterized by the "patient" repeatedly making up clinically convincing simulations of disease for the purpose of gaining attention
    a. Munchausen syndrome by proxy: occurs when parent falsifies an illness in a child by making up or creating symptoms and then seeking medical care; form of child abuse
35. Narcolepsy: syndrome characterized by recurrent uncontrollable drowsiness and sleep
36. Neuralgia: pain in a nerve or nerves
37. Neuritis: inflammation of peripheral nerves
38. Obsessive-compulsive disorder (OCD): pattern of specific behaviors that are caused by obsessions and compulsions
39. Panic attack: mental state that includes intense feelings of apprehension, fearfulness, terror, and impending doom and physical symptoms that include shortness of breath and heart palpitations
40. Paralysis: loss of voluntary muscular control and sensation to a body part or organ
    a. Hemiplegia: paralysis of one side of body, often caused by stroke (cerebrovascular accident [CVA])
    b. Paraplegia: paralysis of trunk and lower extremities, caused by spinal cord injury; the area below the injury is paralyzed
    c. Quadriplegia: paralysis of all four extremities
    d. Bell palsy: paralysis of muscles on one side of face
41. Parkinson disease: chronic disease; characterized by tremors and muscle rigidity
42. Poliomyelitis: viral infection of the gray matter of the spinal cord that may result in paralysis
43. Postpolio syndrome (PPS): recurrence later in life of some polio symptoms in individuals who have had polio and recovered from it
44. Posttraumatic stress disorder (PTSD): development of symptoms such as sleep disorders and anxiety after a psychologically traumatic event
45. Schizophrenia: psychotic disorder characterized by delusions, hallucinations, incoherent disorganized speech, and disruptive or catatonic behavior
46. Sciatica: inflammation of the sciatic nerve; results in pain along the course of the nerve through the thigh and leg
47. Sleep apnea: intermittent short periods of breathing cessation during sleep; can be life-threatening

48. Stroke: CVA; "brain attack"; caused by occlusion or hemorrhage of blood vessels supplying the brain; results in impairment and paralysis of the affected side
    a. Hemorrhagic stroke: damage to brain tissue caused by the rupture of a blood vessel within the brain; brain bleed
    b. Ischemic stroke: damage to the brain caused by narrowing or blockage of the carotid artery; CVA
49. Syncope: fainting
50. Tic douloureux: inflammation of the trigeminal nerve characterized by sudden, intense, sharp pain on one side of the face; trigeminal neuralgia
51. Transient ischemic attack (TIA): "mini" stroke; temporary, recurrent episodes of impaired neurologic activity; caused by lack of blood flow to the brain

E. Diseases and Disorders of the Eye

1. Amblyopia: dimness of vision or partial loss of sight without detectable disease of the eye
2. Astigmatism: irregular focusing of light rays caused by a nonspheroid cornea
3. Blepharitis: inflammation of the eyelids
4. Blepharoptosis: drooping of the eyelid
5. Blindness: inability to see
6. Cataract: opaqueness, cloudiness of the lens of the eye
7. Chalazion: a localized swelling of the eyelid resulting from obstruction of one of the oil-producing glands of the eyelid
8. Conjunctivitis: pinkeye; inflammation of the conjunctiva
9. Corneal abrasion: an injury, such as a scratch or irritation, to the outer layers of the cornea
10. Detached retina: retina is pulled away from its normal position of being attached to the choroid in the back of the eye
11. Diplopia: double vision
12. Exophthalmos: abnormal protrusion of the eye
13. Glaucoma: accumulation of fluid in the eye; increases pressure, which can cause damage to the retina and the optic nerve
14. Hordeolum: stye; infection of the sebaceous gland of the eye
15. Hyperopia: farsightedness; ability to see far objects clearly but not near objects
16. Keratitis: inflammation of the eyelids
17. Macular degeneration: degenerative disease in the center of the field of vision (macula lutea); affects central vision, not peripheral
18. Myopia: nearsightedness; ability to see near objects clearly but not far objects
19. Nyctalopia: difficulty seeing at night
20. Nystagmus: repetitive involuntary movement of the eye
21. Presbyopia: inability to focus quickly; caused by age-related loss of lens elasticity
22. Refractive disorder: the lens of the eye and cornea do not bend light, so they do not focus properly on the retina
23. Retinal detachment: partial or complete separation of the retina from the choroid; results in blindness
24. Retinopathy: any condition of the retina
25. Strabismus: "lazy eye"; inability of both eyes to focus on the same thing
26. Xerophthalmia: drying of the eye surfaces; can result in the loss of the conjunctiva and cornea

F. Diseases and Disorders of the Ear

1. Deafness: inability to hear
    a. Conductive: outer or middle ear does not conduct sound vibrations to the inner ear
    b. Noise induced: damage to the sensitive hairlike cells of the inner ear caused by repeated exposure to intense noise
    c. Sensorineural: caused by problems affecting the inner ear; nerve deafness
2. Impacted cerumen: solidified earwax compacted within ear canal
3. Ménière disease: chronic disease of the inner ear; characterized by vertigo, tinnitus, progressive hearing loss, and sensation of fullness or pressure in the ear
4. Myringitis: inflammation of the tympanic membrane
5. Otalgia: pain in the ear; earache
6. Otitis: inflammation of the ear
    a. Otitis externa: inflammation of the outer ear
    b. Otitis media: inflammation of the middle ear
7. Otosclerosis: bone formation around the oval window and stapes; causes partial to complete deafness
8. Presbycusis: progressive age-related hearing loss
9. Ruptured tympanic membrane: an opening in the eardrum caused by middle ear inflammation resulting from sharp objects in the canal or a blow to the ear; major risk is infection developing in the middle ear
10. Tinnitus: ringing in ears
11. Vertigo: dizziness

G. Diseases and Disorders of the Blood

1. Anemia: abnormal decrease in hemoglobin, red blood cell (RBC) count, or hematocrit
    a. Aplastic anemia: marked absence of all formed elements
    b. Cooley anemia: group of genetic disorders characterized by short-lived RBCs that lack the normal ability to produce hemoglobin; thalassemia
    c. Hemolytic anemia: RBCs are destroyed faster than they can be replaced
    d. Megaloblastic anemia: bone marrow produces large, abnormal RBCs with reduced capacity to carry oxygen
    e. Pernicious anemia: characterized by lack of intrinsic factor, which is needed for absorption of vitamin B_{12}
    f. Sickle cell anemia: genetic disorder that causes abnormal hemoglobin that results in RBCs assuming an abnormal sickle shape
2. Dyscrasia: any abnormal or pathologic condition of blood
3. Erythrocytosis: an abnormal increase in the number of circulating RBCs
4. Hemophilia: hereditary bleeding disorder in which one of the factors to clot the blood is missing
5. Hemorrhage: loss of a large amount of blood in a short time
6. Leukemia: malignant neoplasm of blood-forming organs; usually involves one specific type of blood cell
    a. Acute lymphocytic leukemia (ALL): characterized by an overproduction of immature lymphatic cells
    b. Chronic lymphocytic leukemia (CLL): slowly progressive disease of the lymphocytes

c. Acute myelogenous leukemia (AML): rapidly progressive neoplasm of granulocytic cells

d. Chronic myelogenous leukemia (CML): slowly progressing neoplasm that arises from a hematopoietic stem cell

7. Leukopenia: abnormal decrease in the number of white blood cells (WBCs)
8. Polycythemia: abnormal increase in hemoglobin, RBC count, or hematocrit
9. Septicemia: presence of pathogenic microorganisms or their toxins in the blood; blood poisoning
10. Thrombocytopenia: decrease in thrombocytes; results in decrease in clotting capabilities

H. Diseases and Disorders of the Lymphatic System and Immunity

1. Acquired immunodeficiency syndrome (AIDS): suppression or deficiency of immune system caused by the human immunodeficiency virus (HIV)
2. Anaphylaxis: severe response to a foreign substance
3. Autoimmune disorder: disorder of the immune system in which the body attacks itself
4. Hodgkin lymphoma: malignant condition of lymphatic tissue in spleen and nodes
5. Inflammation: localized response to tissue injury or destruction
6. Lymphadenitis: inflammation of the lymph nodes; swollen glands
7. Lymphedema: abnormal accumulation of lymph caused by obstruction of vessels; occurs in the extremities
8. Lymphoma: malignancy that develops in the lymphatic system
9. Mononucleosis: acute infectious disease caused by Epstein-Barr virus by direct oral contact
10. Multiple myeloma: cancer of plasma cells (type B lymphocytes) that produce antibodies
11. Non-Hodgkin lymphoma: all lymphomas other than Hodgkin lymphoma
12. Systemic lupus erythematosus (SLE): autoimmune disease that can affect the skin, joints, kidneys, blood cells, brain, heart, and lungs

I. Diseases and Disorders of the Cardiovascular System

1. Angina pectoris: chest pain; usually caused by a lack of blood supply to the heart
2. Arrhythmia: dysrhythmia; irregularity or loss of normal rhythm of the heartbeat
3. Aneurysm: abnormal ballooning of a vessel wall
4. Atherosclerosis: formation of fatty plaques along the vessel walls, causing them to narrow; can be the cause of arteriosclerosis
5. Arteriosclerosis: hardening of the arteries; walls of vessels become thick and lose elasticity
6. Bradycardia: abnormally slow heart rate (<60 beats per minute)
7. Cardiac arrest: unexpected stoppage of the heart function; may follow myocardial infarction (MI)
8. Cardiomyopathy: noninflammatory disease of the heart muscle

9. Carditis: inflammation of the heart
10. Congestive heart failure (CHF): characterized by the inability of the heart to keep blood circulating; results in generalized edema
11. Coronary artery disease: atherosclerosis of the coronary arteries that may cause angina, myocardial infarction, and sudden death
12. Coronary thrombosis: thrombus blocking a coronary artery
13. Embolism: blood clot, air, fat globule, or piece of tissue that has broken loose and entered the circulation; pl. *emboli*
14. Endocarditis: inflammation of endocardium, including valves
15. Fibrillation: rapid, random, and ineffective contractions of the heart
    a. Atrial fibrillation: atria beat faster than the ventricles
    b. Ventricular fibrillation: irregular contractions of the ventricles; can be fatal if not reversed by electrical defibrillation
16. Flutter: cardiac arrhythmia in which the atrial contractions are rapid but regular
17. Infarct: localized area of tissue death caused by an interruption of the blood supply
18. Hypertension (HTN): high blood pressure (> 130/80 mm Hg)
19. Mitral stenosis: narrowing of mitral valve that prevents normal flow of blood from the atrium to the ventricle
20. Mitral valve prolapse: protrusion of one or both cusps of the mitral valve back into the left atrium
21. MI: heart attack; caused by occlusion of coronary vessels that decreases the blood supply to the heart; tissue without blood supply necroses
22. Myocarditis: inflammation of the myocardium
23. Palpitation: pounding or racing heart
24. Patent ductus arteriosus: abnormal opening between the aorta and the pulmonary artery
25. Pericarditis: inflammation of the pericardium
26. Phlebitis: inflammation of a vein
27. Rheumatic heart disease: can be caused by streptococci; causes inflammation of the heart and scarring of the valves; can be the result of rheumatic fever or MI
28. Tachycardia: abnormally rapid heart rate (>100 beats per minute)
29. Tetralogy of Fallot: congenital heart abnormality; characterized by four abnormalities—ventricular septal defect, pulmonary stenosis, displacement of the aorta to the right, ventricular enlargement
30. Thrombophlebitis: inflammation of a vein accompanied by clot formation
31. Thrombus: blood clot
32. Varicosity (varicose veins): large, twisted, superficial vein; can occur in the lower legs, rectum, or esophagus

J. Diseases and Disorders of the Respiratory System

1. Acute respiratory distress syndrome (ARDS): type of lung failure resulting from many different disorders that cause pulmonary edema
2. Allergic rhinitis: allergic reaction to airborne allergens that causes an increased flow of mucus

3. Allergy: overreaction by the body to a particular antigen
4. Anoxia: lack of oxygen
5. Apnea: lack of breathing
6. Asphyxia: decrease in oxygen intake
7. Asthma: spasms of bronchus; results in dyspnea and wheezing
8. Atelectasis: partial or complete collapse of alveoli
9. Bradypnea: abnormally slow rate of respiration (< 10 breaths per minute)
10. Bronchiectasis: chronic dilation of bronchi or bronchioles
11. Bronchitis: inflammation of bronchi; may be chronic or acute
12. Bruit: abnormal sound or murmur heard on auscultation
13. Carcinoma: malignant tumor of the lung or respiratory system
14. Cheyne-Stokes respiration: alternating episodes of tachypnea and apnea; usually precedes death
15. Chronic obstructive pulmonary disease (COPD) and chronic obstructive lung disease (COLD): a group of disorders characterized by progressive, irreversible obstruction of airflow; major disorders observed include chronic bronchitis, emphysema, and asthma
16. Croup: acute viral infection characterized by a barklike cough
17. Cystic fibrosis: genetic disorder in which the lungs are clogged with large quantities of abnormally thick mucus
18. Dyspnea: painful or difficulty breathing
19. Emphysema: loss of elasticity and enlargement of alveoli
20. Epistaxis: nosebleed
21. Eupnea: easy, normal breathing
22. Hemoptysis: spitting of blood or blood-stained sputum
23. Hyperpnea: increase in the volume of breathing
24. Hypoxia: decrease in oxygen
25. Infectious mononucleosis: "mono"; acute viral infection caused by Epstein-Barr virus; may include upper respiratory symptoms
26. Influenza: acute, highly contagious viral respiratory infection; spread by respiratory droplets
27. Laryngitis: inflammation of larynx; causes loss of voice
28. Legionnaires' disease: Legionellosis; type of pneumonia caused by the bacterium *Legionella pneumophila*
29. Mycoplasma pneumonia: milder but longer-lasting form of pneumonia caused by the fungus *Mycoplasma pneumoniae*; "walking pneumonia"
30. Orthopnea: breathing facilitated by an upright position
31. Pertussis: whooping cough; lung disease caused by *Bordetella pertussis* bacterium; characterized by "whoop"-sounding cough
32. Pharyngitis: inflammation of the throat
33. Pleurisy: inflammation of the pleural membranes
34. Pneumonia: inflammation of the bronchioles and alveoli; can be viral or bacterial; air sacs fill with pus and other liquid
35. Pneumonitis: inflammation of the lungs
36. Pneumothorax: collection of air in the pleural cavity; may cause the lung to collapse
37. Pulmonary edema: accumulation of fluid in lung tissue
38. Pulmonary embolism: clot located in the pulmonary artery or one of its branches; restricts blood flow to the lungs
39. Rales: crackling sounds on inspiration

40. Respiratory acidosis: decreased pH level of body caused by inadequate removal of carbon dioxide by the lungs; can progress to tissues outside of the lungs
41. Respiratory alkalosis: increased pH levels caused by excessive removal of carbon dioxide by the lungs
42. Rhinitis: inflammation of the nose
43. Rhinorrhea: excessive flow of mucus from the nose; runny nose
44. Rhonchus: added lung sound with a musical pitch occurring on inspiration; wheezing
45. Respiratory syncytial virus pneumonia (RSV): inflammatory and infectious condition of the lungs; most common in infants and young children
46. Sinusitis: inflammation of paranasal sinuses
47. Smoker's respiratory syndrome: group of symptoms seen in smokers including cough, wheezing, vocal hoarseness, pharyngitis, difficulty breathing, and susceptibility to respiratory infections
48. Stridor: high-pitched sounds on inspiration caused by obstruction
49. Suffocation: prevention of breathing by external causes
50. Tachypnea: abnormal, rapid breathing
51. Tonsillitis: inflammation of the tonsils
52. Tuberculosis (TB): communicable lung disease caused by *Mycobacterium tuberculosis*; characterized by tubercles in the tissue
53. Upper respiratory infection (URI): acute inflammatory process affecting mucus membranes that line the upper respiratory tract

K. Diseases and Disorders of the Digestive System

1. Amebic (or amoebic) dysentery: intestinal infection caused by the ameba *Entamoeba histolytica*
2. Anorexia: lack of appetite
3. Anorexia nervosa: eating disorder characterized by a refusal to maintain a minimally normal body weight and an intense fear of gaining weight
4. Appendicitis: inflammation of the appendix
5. Bruxism: involuntary grinding or clenching of the teeth; usually occurs during sleep; is associated with stress and tension
6. Bulimia: eating disorder characterized by episodes of binge eating followed by self-induced vomiting
7. Celiac sprue: malabsorption syndrome; characterized by intolerance to gluten and damage to intestinal mucosa
8. Cholecystitis: inflammation of the gallbladder
9. Cholelithiasis (gallstones): caused by collection of solid cholesterol or calcium in the gallbladder or bile ducts
10. Cirrhosis: degenerative disease of the liver
11. Colitis: inflammation of the colon
12. Constipation: hard stools resulting in difficulty in defecating
13. Crohn disease: common chronic inflammatory disease of the gastrointestinal tract; walls of the bowel become edematous and inflamed
14. Dehydration: condition in which fluid loss exceeds fluid intake; disrupts normal electrolyte balance of the body
15. Dental calculus: hardened dental plaque on the teeth that irritates the surrounding tissues

16. Dental caries: disease process that destroys the enamel and dentin of the tooth; tooth decay; cavities
17. Dental plaque: soft deposit consisting of bacteria and bacterial by-products that build up on the teeth; major cause of dental caries and periodontal disease
18. Diarrhea: loose, watery stools
19. Diverticulitis: inflammation of pouches (diverticula) in the colon
20. Diverticulosis: progressive condition characterized by defects in the muscular wall of the large intestine
21. Dyspepsia: indigestion
22. Dysphagia: difficulty in swallowing
23. *E. coli*: intestinal infection caused by *Escherichia coli*; characterized by fever, diarrhea, vomiting, and dehydration
24. Emaciated: abnormally thin
25. Emesis: vomiting
26. Eructation: belching
27. Esophageal reflux: upward flow of stomach acid into the esophagus; gastroesophageal reflux disease (GERD)
28. Esophageal varices: enlarged and swollen veins at the lower end of the esophagus
29. Gallstone: hard deposit that forms in the gallbladder and bile ducts
30. Gastritis: inflammation of the stomach
31. Gastroenteritis: inflammation of stomach and intestines
32. Gingivitis: inflammation of the gums
33. Halitosis: unpleasant breath odor; bad breath
34. Hematemesis: vomiting blood
35. Hemorrhoids: inflammation and dilation of surface veins in the rectum and anus
36. Hepatitis: inflammation of the liver; can be acute or chronic
    a. Hepatitis A: highly contagious acute infection of the liver; caused by hepatitis A virus (HAV); transmitted through fecal-oral route
    b. Hepatitis B: caused by hepatitis B virus (HBV); transmitted through contact with blood, semen, saliva, and vaginal secretions
    c. Hepatitis C: caused by hepatitis C virus (HCV); transmitted through blood and body fluids
37. Hernia: a protrusion of a part of the intestine into an adjacent area or cavity
    a. Hiatal hernia: protrusion of part of the stomach through the esophageal sphincter in the diaphragm
    b. Inguinal hernia: protrusion of a small loop of bowel through a weak place in the lower abdominal wall or groin
38. Intussusception: telescoping of one part of the intestine onto another part just below it
39. Irritable bowel syndrome (IBS): collection of symptoms with no organic cause; characterized by abdominal pain, constipation, and diarrhea
40. Jaundice: yellow discoloration of the skin and tissues caused by greater than normal amounts of bilirubin in the blood
41. Malabsorption syndrome: disease process that inhibits absorption of nutrients
42. Malnutrition: lack of proper food or nutrients; can be due to shortage of food, improper absorption, or distribution of nutrients
43. Melena: black stools containing digested blood
44. Mumps: inflammation of parotid salivary glands
45. Nausea: sensation that leads to the urge to vomit
46. Obesity: an excessive accumulation of fat in the body
47. Pancreatitis: inflammation of the pancreas
48. Periodontal disease: inflammation of the tissues that surround and support teeth
49. Phenylketonuria: genetic disorder in which an essential digestive enzyme is missing
50. Pica: eating disorder characterized by persistent eating of nonnutritional substances
51. Regurgitation: return of swallowed food into the mouth
52. Stomatitis: inflammation of mouth
53. Thrush: yeast infection of the mouth; caused by *Candida albicans*
54. Ulcer: lesion in the mucosa of the stomach or intestine
    a. Duodenal ulcer: peptic ulcer occurring in the upper part of the small intestine
    b. Peptic ulcer: lesion of the mucus membranes of the digestive system caused by the bacterium *Helicobacter pylori*
55. Vincent angina: trench mouth; ulcerations of the mucosa of the mouth
56. Volvulus: twisting of the intestine on itself that causes an obstruction

L. Diseases and Disorders of the Urinary System

1. Albuminuria: protein in the urine
2. Anuria: no urine produced
3. Bacteriuria: bacteria in the urine
4. Cystitis: inflammation of the bladder
5. Calculi: kidney stones
6. Diuresis: increased excretion of urine
7. Dysuria: difficult or painful urination
8. Enuresis: involuntary discharge of urine
9. Glycosuria: glucose in the urine
10. Hematuria: blood in the urine
11. Incontinence: voiding urine involuntarily
12. Ketonuria: ketones in the urine
13. Nephrolithiasis (renal calculi): kidney stones
14. Nocturia: excessive urination at night
15. Oliguria: scanty urine output
16. Polycystic kidney disease: collecting tubular disease characterized by swollen, fluid-filled sacs; tubules are unable to empty into the renal pelvis
17. Polyuria: excessive urination
18. Proteinuria: protein in the urine
19. Pyuria: pus in the urine
20. Renal failure: kidneys fail to function; may be chronic or acute
21. Urethritis: inflammation of the urethra
22. Urinary tract infection (UTI): mostly caused by gram-negative bacteria; can occur in any organ in the urinary tract

M. Diseases and Disorders of the Endocrine System

1. Acromegaly: hypersecretion of growth hormone (GH) after puberty

2. Addison disease: hyposecretion of cortisol; characterized by hypotension and increased skin pigmentation
3. Adenitis: inflammation of a gland
4. Adenoma: benign tumor of a gland
5. Cretinism: hypothyroidism caused by hyposecretion of thyroxine during infancy; characterized by slow growth, impaired intelligence, and delayed development of secondary sex characteristics
6. Cushing syndrome: hypersecretion of cortisol; characterized by "moon face," acne, and fatty deposits on the upper back
7. Diabetes insipidus: hyposecretion of antidiuretic hormone; characterized by polyuria and polydipsia
8. Diabetes mellitus: hyperglycemia; hyposecretion of insulin; characterized by polyuria, polyphagia, and polydipsia
   a. Gestational: occurs during pregnancy and usually disappears after delivery
   b. Type 1: insulin deficiency disorder; pancreas produces little or no insulin; insulin-dependent diabetes mellitus
   c. Type 2: insulin resistance disorder; insulin is produced, but the body does not respond to it; non–insulin-dependent diabetes mellitus
9. Dwarfism: hyposecretion of GH; characterized by abnormally small size
10. Giantism: hypersecretion of GH; characterized by abnormally large size
11. Goiter: enlargement of thyroid gland; caused by iodine deficiency
12. Graves disease: hyperthyroidism caused by hypersecretion of thyroxine; characterized by weight loss, exophthalmia, nervousness, diaphoresis, and heat intolerance
13. Hypoglycemia: abnormally low blood glucose level in the blood
14. Myxedema: hyposecretion of thyroxine later in life; characterized by fatigue, weight gain, and cold intolerance
15. Polydipsia: excessive thirst

N. Diseases and Disorders of the Female Reproductive System

1. Amenorrhea: absence of menstruation
2. Anteversion: abnormal tipping, tilting, or turning forward of the entire uterus
3. Bacterial vaginosis: bacterial infection of the vagina
4. Breast augmentation: mammoplasty to increase breast size
5. Cervical dysplasia: abnormal growth of cells of the cervix; can be precancerous
6. Cervicitis: inflammation of the cervix
7. Ductal carcinoma in situ: breast cancer at the earliest stage before the cancer has broken through the walls of the duct
8. Dysmenorrhea: painful menstruation
9. Dyspareunia: painful intercourse
10. Endometriosis: growth of endometrial tissue outside of the uterus, usually within the pelvic cavity
11. Fibrocystic breast: presence of single or multiple cysts in the breast

12. Fibroid: benign tumor that is found in the muscle of the uterus
13. Infertility: inability of a couple to achieve pregnancy after 1 year of regular, unprotected intercourse
14. Invasive ductal carcinoma: form of cancer that starts in the milk duct, breaks through the duct wall, and invades the fatty tissue of the breast
15. Invasive lobular carcinoma: form of cancer that starts in the milk glands, breaks through the wall of the gland, and invades the fatty tissue of the breast
16. Leukorrhea: profuse white discharge from the uterus and vagina
17. Mastitis: inflammation of the breast
18. Menorrhagia: excessive amount of menstrual flow over a longer duration than a normal period
19. Mittelschmerz: pain experienced at the time of ovulation
20. Oligomenorrhea: markedly reduced menstrual flow and abnormally infrequent menstruation
21. Oophoritis: inflammation of the ovary
22. Ovarian cyst: solid or fluid-filled cyst found on the ovary
23. Pelvic inflammatory disease (PID): acute or chronic infection of the female reproductive tract
24. Premenstrual syndrome (PMS): various symptoms that occur before the menstrual period; can include fatigue, irritability, depression, swollen and tender breasts, edema, or cramping
25. Polycystic ovary syndrome: enlargement of the ovaries caused by the presence of many cysts
26. Retroflexion: abnormal tipping of the uterus with the body bent, forming an angle with the cervix
27. Sexually transmitted disease (STD): sexually transmitted infection (STI)
   a. Trichomonas: parasitic infection caused by *Trichomonas vaginalis*
   b. Gonorrhea: highly contagious bacterial infection caused by *Neisseria gonorrhoeae*
   c. Syphilis: highly contagious infection caused by the spirochete *Treponema pallidum*
   d. Genital herpes: highly contagious viral infection caused by herpes simplex virus type 2
   e. Genital warts: highly contagious growths caused by human papillomavirus
   f. Chlamydia: highly contagious bacterial infection caused by *Chlamydia trachomatis*
28. Uterine prolapse: falling or sinking of the uterus until it protrudes through the vaginal opening
29. Vaginal candidiasis: vaginal yeast infection caused by *C. albicans*
30. Vaginitis: inflammation of the vagina

O. Diseases and Disorders of Pregnancy and Childbirth

1. Abortion: termination of a pregnancy; can be spontaneous (miscarriage) or therapeutic
2. Abruptio placentae: placenta prematurely separates from uterine wall
3. Breech presentation: abnormal birth position in which the buttocks or feet are presented first
4. Eclampsia (toxemia): serious condition of pregnancy characterized by maternal HTN, edema, and proteinuria; if untreated, may result in seizures and coma

5. Ectopic pregnancy: implantation of fertilized ovum outside of the uterus; usually in the fallopian tube
6. Hyperemesis gravidarum: excessive vomiting during pregnancy
7. Lochia: vaginal discharge during the first 1 to 2 weeks after childbirth
8. Nulligravida: a female who has never been pregnant
9. Placenta previa: placenta implants over the cervix
10. Stillbirth: fetus that dies before delivery
11. Twins: two fetuses developing within the uterus at the same time
    a. Fraternal: two embryos resulting from the fertilization of separate ova by separate sperm
    b. Identical: two embryos resulting from the fertilization of a single ovum by a single sperm that has been separated into two separate parts

P. Diseases and Disorders of the Male Reproductive System

1. Anorchism: congenital absence of one or both testicles
2. Azoospermia: absence of sperm in the semen
3. Balanitis: inflammation of the glans penis
4. Benign prostatic hypertrophy (BPH): abnormal growth of prostatic cells causing enlargement of gland
5. Cryptorchidism: undescended testes; testes remain in abdomen
6. Epispadias: congenital abnormality in which the opening of the urethra is on the upper surface of the penis
7. Gynecomastia: excessive mammary development in a male
8. Hydrocele: accumulation of fluid in the scrotum
9. Hypospadias: abnormal congenital opening of the urethra on the underside of the penis
10. Impotence: inability to develop or sustain an erection
11. Oligospermia: abnormally low number of sperm in the ejaculate; low sperm count
12. Orchitis: inflammation of the testes
13. Phimosis: narrowing at the opening of the foreskin so that it cannot be retracted to expose the glans
14. Prostatitis: inflammation of the prostate
15. Varicocele: varicose vein of the testicles; may cause infertility

Q. Tumors and Cancer

1. Benign: tumors that remain localized within the tissues from which they arose
   a. Papilloma: type of tumor that forms fingerlike projections (wart)
   b. Adenoma: tumors of glandular epithelium
   c. Nevus: small, pigmented tumors of the skin (mole)
   d. Lipoma: tumors from adipose tissue
   e. Osteoma: tumor from bone tissue
   f. Chondroma: tumor from cartilage
2. Carcinoma: malignant tumors that originate from epithelial tissues
3. Malignant: tumors that spread to other regions of the body; cancer
   a. Melanoma: cancer that involves melanocytes
   b. Adenocarcinoma: malignant tumors of glandular tissue
   c. Lymphoma: cancer of the lymphatic tissue
   d. Osteosarcoma: cancer of bone tissue
4. Metastasis: spreading of malignant cells
5. Neoplasm: "new growth"; abnormal growth of cells
6. Sarcoma: malignant tumor that arises from connective tissue

R. Diseases and Disorders Caused by Pathogens

1. TB
   a. Cause: *Mycobacterium tuberculosis*
   b. Transmission: inhalation
   c. Symptoms/signs: cough, hemoptysis, sweats, weight loss
   d. Tests/specimens: sputum culture, radiographs, skin tests
   e. Prevention/immunization: Bacillus Calmette–Guérin (BCG) vaccine
2. UTI
   a. Cause: *E. coli, Proteus, Pseudomonas aeruginosa*
   b. Transmission: ascends the urethra from contaminated area
   c. Symptoms/signs: frequency, burning, blood in urine, flank pain, fever
   d. Tests/specimens: clean-catch urine for culture
   e. Prevention/immunization: good personal hygiene
3. Legionnaires' disease
   a. Cause: *L. pneumophila*
   b. Transmission: grows in water (air-conditioning systems)
   c. Symptoms/signs: pneumonia-like symptoms
   d. Tests/specimens: sputum, blood
   e. Prevention/immunization: isolation
4. Tetanus (lockjaw)
   a. Cause: *Clostridium tetani*
   b. Transmission: open wounds, fractures, punctures
   c. Symptoms/signs: toxin affects motor nerves; muscle spasms, convulsions, rigidity
   d. Tests/specimens: blood
   e. Prevention/immunization: diphtheria, tetanus, and acellular pertussis (DTaP) vaccine in childhood; tetanus and diphtheria (Td) every 10 years
5. Gangrene
   a. Cause: *Clostridium botulinum*
   b. Transmission: wounds
   c. Symptoms/signs: gas and watery exudates from wound; blackened tissue
   d. Tests/specimens: swab; aspirate of wound for culture
   e. Prevention/immunization: proper wound care
6. Botulism
   a. Cause: *C. botulinum*
   b. Transmission: improperly cooked canned foods
   c. Symptoms/signs: neurotoxin affects speech, swallowing, vision; paralysis of respiratory muscles; death
   d. Tests/specimens: contaminated food, blood
   e. Prevention/immunization: botulinum antitoxin; boiling canned goods before eating

7. Diphtheria
   a. Cause: *Corynebacterium diphtheriae*
   b. Transmission: respiratory secretions
   c. Symptoms/signs: sore throat, fever, headache, gray membrane in back of throat
   d. Tests/specimens: swabs; gram stain; culture; Schick test
   e. Prevention/immunization: DTaP in childhood; Td, TdaP for adults

8. Whooping cough (pertussis)
   a. Cause: *Bordetella pertussis*
   b. Transmission: respiratory secretions
   c. Symptoms/signs: upper respiratory tract symptoms; high-pitched crowing "whoop"
   d. Tests/specimens: swabs for culture
   e. Prevention/immunization: DTaP in childhood, TdaP for adults

9. Pneumonia
   a. Cause: *Streptococcus pneumoniae*
   b. Transmission: direct contact, droplets
   c. Symptoms/signs: productive cough, fever, chest pain
   d. Tests/specimens: culture; gram stain
   e. Prevention/immunization: vaccine

10. Strep throat
    a. Cause: *Streptococcus pyogenes* (group A strep)
    b. Transmission: direct contact, droplets, fomites
    c. Symptoms/signs: severe sore throat, fever, malaise
    d. Tests/specimens: direct swab; rapid strep tests
    e. Prevention/immunization: none

11. Wound infection, abscesses, boils
    a. Cause: *Staphylococcus aureus*
    b. Transmission: direct contact with carriers, fomites, poor handwashing
    c. Symptoms/signs: area red, warm, swollen; pus; pain; ulceration
    d. Tests/specimens: deep swab; aspirate of drainage
    e. Prevention/immunization: none

12. Food poisoning
    a. Cause: *S. aureus*
    b. Transmission: poor hygiene, improper refrigeration of foods
    c. Symptoms/signs: vomiting, abdominal cramps, diarrhea
    d. Tests/prevention: suspected foods, stool
    e. Prevention/immunization: refrigerate food to prevent toxin production

13. Toxic shock
    a. Cause: *S. aureus*
    b. Transmission: use of absorbent pack material (tampons, nasal packs)
    c. Symptoms/signs: fever, headache, vomiting, delirium, low blood pressure
    d. Tests/prevention: swab, blood
    e. Prevention/immunization: change tampons and packing materials often

14. Gonorrhea
    a. Cause: *N. gonorrhoeae*
    b. Transmission: sexually transmitted
    c. Symptoms/signs: females, pelvic pain, discharge; males, may be asymptomatic, urethral discharge, pain on urination
    d. Tests/specimens: swab of cervix, urethra; rectal and pharyngeal swabs
    e. Prevention/immunization: avoid unprotected sex; abstinence

15. Meningococcal meningitis
    a. Cause: *Neisseria meningitidis*
    b. Transmission: respiratory secretions
    c. Symptoms/signs: high fever, headache, projectile vomiting, delirium, neck and back rigidity
    d. Tests/specimens: nasopharyngeal swabs, CSF culture, blood
    e. Prevention/immunization: vaccine; prophylactic antibiotics

16. Syphilis
    a. Cause: *T. pallidum* (spirochete)
    b. Transmission: sexually transmitted
    c. Symptoms/signs: painless sore (chancre), generalized rash
    d. Tests/specimens: blood for VDRL (Venereal Disease Research Laboratory), RPR (Rapid Plasma Reagin), FTA-ABS (Fluorescent Treponemal Antibody – absorption test)
    e. Prevention/immunization: avoid unprotected sex; abstinence

17. Lyme disease
    a. Cause: *Borrelia burgdorferi* (spirochete)
    b. Transmission: tick bite
    c. Symptoms/signs: fever, joint pain, red bull's-eye rash
    d. Tests/specimens: swab for culture
    e. Prevention/immunization: avoid tick-infested areas

18. Pyloric ulcers
    a. Cause: *H. pylori*
    b. Transmission: unknown
    c. Symptoms/signs: burning pain in stomach especially between meals
    d. Tests/specimens: blood, stool
    e. Prevention/immunization: unknown

19. Rocky Mountain spotted fever
    a. Cause: *Rickettsia rickettsii*
    b. Transmission: tick bite
    c. Symptoms/signs: headache, fever, chills, characteristic rash on trunk and extremities
    d. Tests/specimens: blood, skin biopsy

20. Atypical pneumonia ("walking pneumonia")
    a. Cause: *M. pneumoniae*
    b. Transmission: respiratory secretions
    c. Symptoms/signs: fever, cough, chest pain
    d. Tests/specimens: blood, sputum culture

21. Nongonococcal urethritis and vaginitis
    a. Cause: *C. trachomatis*
    b. Transmission: sexual
    c. Symptoms/signs: may be asymptomatic
    d. Tests/specimens: swabs for DNA probe, serologic testing

22. Inclusion conjunctivitis, pneumonia
    a. Cause: *C. trachomatis*
    b. Transmission: infected mother during birth
    c. Symptoms/signs: severe conjunctivitis in newborns; afebrile pneumonia in newborns
    d. Tests/specimens: swabs for DNA probe, serologic testing

23. Thrush (oral yeast), vulvovaginal candidiasis, or monilia (vaginal yeast)
    a. Cause: *Candida* species (yeast)
    b. Transmission: oral—during birth; other—following antibiotic therapy, oral birth control, diabetes
    c. Symptoms/signs: white, cheesy growth
    d. Tests/specimens: swab for KOH (potassium hydroxide) preparation; cultures
24. Pinworm
    a. *Enterobius vermicularis* (roundworm)
    b. Transmission: fecal-oral
    c. Symptoms/signs: severe rectal itching
    d. Tests/specimens: clear tape applied to perianal area
25. Scabies
    a. Cause: *Sarcoptes scabiei* (itch mite)
    b. Transmission: direct contact, clothing, bedding
    c. Symptoms/signs: nocturnal itching; skin lesions
    d. Tests/specimens: skin scrapings for parasite
26. Lice
    a. Cause: *Pediculus* species
    b. Transmission: direct contact, clothing, bedding
    c. Symptoms/signs: intense itching; skin lesions
    d. Tests/specimens: finding adult lice or eggs (nits) on body or hair
27. Smallpox
    a. Cause: Variola major virus
    b. Transmission: direct contact, fomites
    c. Symptoms/signs: vesicles on entire body including soles and palms
    d. Tests/specimens: none
    e. Prevention/immunization: eradicated; vaccine still available
28. Infectious mononucleosis
    a. Cause: Epstein-Barr virus
    b. Transmission: direct, airborne
    c. Symptoms/signs: sore throat, malaise, lymph gland involvement
    d. Tests/specimens: serology for heterophile antibodies; complete blood count (CBC)
    e. Prevention/immunization: avoid direct contact
29. Influenza
    a. Cause: myxovirus influenza A and B
    b. Transmission: droplets, fomites
    c. Symptoms/signs: fever, body aches, cough
    d. Tests/specimens: nasopharyngeal swab, nasal wash
    e. Prevention/immunization: immunization for old, young, and debilitated individuals
30. Warts (verrucae)
    a. Cause: human papillomavirus
    b. Transmission: direct and indirect contact
    c. Symptoms/signs: circumscribed outgrowths on skin
    d. Tests/specimens: scrapings
    e. Prevention/immunization: none

31. Rabies
    a. Cause: rhabdovirus
    b. Transmission: contact with saliva on infected animal
    c. Symptoms/signs: fever, uncontrollable excitement, spasms of the throat, profuse salivation
    d. Tests/specimens: direct fluorescent antibody from brain or hair follicle
    e. Prevention/immunization: vaccine available; vaccinate pets
32. Mumps
    a. Cause: paramyxovirus
    b. Transmission: direct contact
    c. Symptoms/signs: pain and swelling of salivary glands, fever
    d. Tests/specimens: serum titers
    e. Prevention/immunization: measles, mumps, rubella (MMR) vaccine
33. Measles (variola)
    a. Cause: paramyxovirus
    b. Transmission: direct contact, droplets
    c. Symptoms/signs: fever, nasal discharge, red eyes, Koplik's spots, rash
    d. Tests/specimens: serum titers
    e. Prevention/immunization: MMR vaccine
34. German measles (rubella)
    a. Cause: rubella virus
    b. Transmission: direct contact, droplets
    c. Symptoms/signs: rash, swollen lymph glands; can cause severe birth defects
    d. Tests/specimens: serum titer
    e. Prevention/immunization: MMR vaccine
35. Chickenpox (varicella)
    a. Cause: herpesvirus varicella zoster
    b. Transmission: direct contact
    c. Symptoms/signs: slight fever, malaise, clear vesicles
    d. Tests/specimens: clinical signs
    e. Prevention/immunization: varicella vaccine
36. Common cold
    a. Cause: rhinovirus
    b. Transmission: direct, droplets
    c. Symptoms/signs: headache, fever, runny nose, congestion
    d. Tests/specimens: none
    e. Prevention/immunization: good hygiene
37. Polio
    a. Cause: poliovirus
    b. Transmission: direct contact
    c. Symptoms/signs: fever, headache, stiff neck and back, paralysis of muscles
    d. Tests/specimens: none
    e. Prevention/immunization: inactivated poliovirus (IPV) vaccine

4

Growth and Development

I. Major Theorists

A. Sigmund Freud

1. Provided the foundation from which many other psychological theories developed
2. Believed that infancy and childhood are the critical periods for psychological development
3. Psychoanalytical theory: theory of personality development that includes
   a. Levels of awareness
      1) Conscious: experiences within one's immediate awareness; reality based
      2) Subconscious: stores memories, thoughts, and feelings
      3) Unconscious: closed to one's awareness
   b. Components of the personality
      1) Id: body's basic primitive urges
      2) Ego: closely related to reality
      3) Superego: further development of ego; makes judgments; controls and punishes
   c. Psychosexual stages of development
      1) Oral stage: birth to end of first year of life; mouth is the source of all comfort and pleasure
      2) Anal stage: end of first year of life to third year; elimination gives pleasure and satisfaction
      3) Phallic stage: ages 3–6 years; associates pleasure and conflict with genital organs; Oedipus complex (boy's unconscious sexual attraction to his mother) and Electra complex (girl's unconscious sexual attraction to her father) develop
      4) Latency stage: ages 6–12 years; sexual urges are dormant; peer relationships develop with the same sex
      5) Genital stage: begins at puberty; body is preparing for reproduction; sexual attraction and heterosexual relationships begin

B. Erik Erikson

1. Broadened Freud's theory of personality development
2. Psychosocial theory: eight stages with goals
   a. Trust versus mistrust: birth to 18 months; to develop a basic trust in the mothering figure and to be able to generalize it to others
   b. Autonomy versus shame and doubt: age 18 months to 3 years; to gain self-control and independence within the environment
   c. Initiative versus guilt: age 3–6 years; to develop a sense of purpose and the ability to initiate and direct one's own activities
   d. Industry versus inferiority: age 6–11 years; to achieve a sense of self-confidence by learning, competing, performing successfully, and receiving recognition from others
   e. Identity versus role confusion: age 12–20 years; to integrate the tasks mastered in the previous stages into a secure sense of self
   f. Intimacy versus isolation: age 20–30 years; to form an intense, lasting relationship or a commitment to another person, cause, institution, or creative effort
   g. Generativity versus stagnation: age 30–65 years; to achieve the life goals established for oneself while considering the welfare of future generations
   h. Ego integrity versus despair: age 65 to death; to review one's life and derive meaning from both positive and negative events while achieving a positive sense of self-worth

C. Jean Piaget

1. Cognitive development
2. Concerned with acquisition of intellect and development of thought processes
3. Believed that the child's cognitive abilities progress through four stages

a. Sensorimotor stage: birth to 2 years; acquires knowledge through exploration of the environment; attaches meaning and recognition of things
b. Preoperational stage: age 2–6 years; develops language; child sees self as the center of the universe
c. Concrete operational stage: age 6–12 years; begins to solve problems and to think logically; becomes less egocentric and more social
d. Formal operational stage: age 12–15 years; ability to think logically in hypothetical and abstract terms; cognitive maturity achieved

D. Abraham Maslow

1. Described human behavior as being motivated by needs that are ordered in a hierarchy
2. Believed people must meet their most basic needs before they can move up the hierarchy to any higher level
3. Hierarchy begins at the bottom with basic survival needs and moves to the top with more complex needs
   a. Physiologic needs: basic fundamental needs; includes food, water, elimination, air, sleep, exercise, shelter, and sexual expression
   b. Safety and security: needs for avoiding harm and maintaining comfort, order, structure, physical safety, protection, and freedom from fear
   c. Love and belonging: needs for giving and receiving affection, companionship, satisfactory interpersonal relationships, and identification with a group
   d. Self-esteem: seeks self-respect and respect from others, works to achieve success and recognition within the group, and desires prestige from accomplishments
   e. Self-actualization: possesses a feeling of self-fulfillment and the realization of one's highest potential

E. Elisabeth Kübler-Ross

1. Identified stages of dealing with death or loss
2. Can also apply to the grieving process
3. Stages
   a. Denial: direct denial or periods of disbelief
   b. Anger: realization of what is happening; may display rage
   c. Bargaining: attempts to make deals with a deity
   d. Depression: may show signs and symptoms such as withdrawal, lethargy, and periods of crying
   e. Acceptance: comes to accept the facts and fate

II. Stages of Life Cycle

A. Basic Principles of Growth and Development

1. Each person is unique from the time of conception
2. Growth is continuous
3. Skills increase as physical size increases
4. Development depends on a balance among physical, mental, and psychosocial changes
5. If basic needs are not met, growth pattern is altered

B. Basic Categories of Growth and Development Through the Life Span

1. Physical growth
   a. Physical size
   b. Motor and sensory skills
2. Mental growth
   a. Cognitive development
   b. Thinking
   c. Understanding
3. Psychosocial growth
   a. Emotional development
   b. Social development

C. Newborn to 1 Year

1. Physical characteristics
   a. Head is larger in proportion to the rest of the body at birth; fontanels close between 12 and 18 months
   b. Birth weight doubles by 5–6 months and triples by the first year
   c. Teething begins at approximately 5–6 months
   d. Senses are present at birth and develop more fully during the first year
   e. Blood pressure increases and pulse and respiration decrease as the child ages
2. Developmental milestones
   a. Gross motor skills (involve large muscles of the arms and legs)
      1) 2 months: controls head
      2) 3 months: sits without support
      3) 7 months: sits alone
      4) 10 months: creeps
      5) 9–11 months: stands without support
      6) 12–15 months: walks alone
   b. Fine motor skills (refined use of hands and fingers)
   c. Psychosocial (Erikson's stages of growth and development)
   d. Cognitive (mostly sensorimotor; heightened use of touch, taste, sight, hearing, and smell)

D. Toddlerhood (1–3 Years)

1. Physical characteristics
   a. Grows up to 3 inches each year
   b. Gains 4–6 pounds each year
   c. Extremities grow faster than the trunk
   d. Face and jaw grow bigger to permit room for more teeth
   e. Bones begin to ossify
   f. Visual acuity developing; hearing is fully developed
2. Developmental milestones
   a. Gross motor skills
      1) Depends on growth and maturation of muscles, bones, and nerves
      2) Can usually run and can walk up steps using both feet
   b. Fine motor skills
      1) Puts simple puzzles together
      2) Can turn knobs and open jar lids

    c. Psychosocial
       1) Attached to mother; tolerates short separation
       2) Dresses and undresses self
       3) Nearly toilet trained
    d. Cognitive
       1) Searches for and finds toys
       2) Locates body parts
       3) Gives full name on request
    e. Language
       1) Uses words and gestures to indicate needs
       2) Uses two-word sentences
       3) Initiates sounds and words
       4) Can sing simple songs
       5) Vocabulary of approximately 1000 words

E. Preschool (3–6 Years)

1. Physical characteristics
    a. Trunk and body lengthen in proportion to rest of body
    b. Gains 5–7 pounds each year
    c. Grows 2½– 3 inches each year
    d. Deciduous teeth may begin to fall out; dental health is important
    e. Visual acuity improves to 20/20; frequent ear infections
2. Developmental milestones
    a. Gross motor skills
       1) Able to walk and run on tiptoes
       2) Able to hop and to balance on one foot
       3) May begin sports such as soccer, baseball, skating, and dance
    b. Fine motor skills
       1) Manages self-care activities
       2) Manipulates clothing and clothing fasteners with ease
       3) Handles eating utensils; can begin to learn table manners
       4) Can draw faces, copy letters, and print own name
    c. Psychosocial
       1) Learns to trust
       2) Aware of genital organs and sexual identity
       3) Needs discipline and limits
    d. Cognitive
       1) Longer attention span than as toddler
       2) Develops memory
       3) Can pretend
    e. Language
       1) Becomes talkative
       2) May show some difficulty with pronunciation
       3) Can recite full name, address, and telephone number
       4) Imitates others

F. School Age (6–11 Years)

1. Physical characteristics
    a. Growth is steady but slows
    b. Permanent teeth appear
    c. Weight increases by 4½–6½ pounds each year
    d. Height increases by 2–3 inches each year
    e. Visual maturity achieved; peripheral vision and depth perception improve
    f. Immune system matures

2. Developmental milestones
    a. Gross motor skills
       1) Increase in muscle mass improves skills
       2) Gender differences exist in motor skills
    b. Fine motor skills
       1) Can print and begin to master script writing
       2) Can throw and catch
       3) Can begin to learn to play musical instruments
    c. Psychosocial
       1) Outgoing, talkative, and enthusiastic
       2) Fearlessness puts child at risk for injury
       3) Sexual curiosity continues
       4) Initiates a task and able to see it through to completion
       5) Sibling rivalry can occur
       6) Peers are more important than family
       7) Privacy becomes important
       8) Emotions have wide range of expression
    d. Cognitive
       1) Has collections of stickers, books, and sports cards
       2) Breaks things down into small parts and reassembles them
       3) Takes views of others into consideration
       4) Understands concepts of time, space, and dimension
       5) Starts and continues formal education
    e. Language
       1) Use of language and communication techniques improve
       2) Language becomes important for socialization
       3) Can use proper parts of speech and proper tense of words

G. Adolescence (11–19 Years)

1. Puberty (ages 11–14); puberty ends and adolescence begins with the onset of menses (menarche) in girls and sperm production in boys
    a. Rapid physical growth
    b. Changes in body proportions; trunk and limbs grow swiftly
    c. Development of primary sexual characteristics
    d. Development of secondary sexual characteristics
2. Physical characteristics
    a. Puberty is the period of the greatest amount of rapid growth; growth slows after puberty
    b. Muscular strength increases greatly
    c. Epiphyseal line closes in long bones; growth nearly complete
    d. Trunk broadens at the hips and shoulders
    e. Posture may be poor from the fast growth; slouching
    f. Sexual growth and development are completed
    g. Shows great concern about one's changing body
    h. Sebaceous glands produce more oil and become larger
    i. Changes in fat distribution
3. Developmental milestones
    a. Motor development
       1) Comparable with adult
       2) Hand-eye coordination improves
    b. Sexual development
       1) Heightened emotions
       2) Increased worries

3) Lack of self-confidence
4) Sex is given high priority; girls set limits on interactions
5) Good sex education enables responsible choices
c. Psychosocial
   1) Rebelliousness, argumentative, or rude
   2) Egocentric
   3) Need for privacy
   4) Dishonesty
   5) Responsibility
   6) Curfews
   7) Friends
   8) Self-absorbed
   9) Society places many demands
   10) Discipline is important
d. Cognitive
   1) Maturation of central nervous system leads to formal operational thought processes (logical thought)
   2) School is at the center of development
   3) Moral reasoning and spiritual awareness develop
e. Communication
   1) Vocabulary increases
   2) Verbal communication allows thoughts and beliefs to be known
   3) Development of common language typical to a group, time, and culture (slang)

H. Early Adulthood (20–40 Years)

1. Physical characteristics
  a. Physical growth is completed
  b. Men usually have more muscle mass
  c. Wisdom teeth erupt; may need to be removed
  d. Other body systems begin to decline at the end of this period
2. Developmental milestones
  a. Major milestones include choosing and establishing a career, fulfilling sexual needs, establishing a family and a home, expanding social circles, and developing maturity
   1) Motor development
    a) Peak physical efficiency reached
    b) Physical efficiency declines toward the end of this period
   2) Sexual development
    a) Sexuality established
    b) Ability to experience and share love
   3) Psychosocial development
    a) Strong sense of identity
    b) Sharing of innermost thoughts
    c) Career and work roles understood
   4) Cognitive development
    a) No longer egocentric, as a rule
    b) Can solve problems and process information
    c) Attends college or vocational school
   5) Health concerns
    a) Pap smear
    b) Mammography and breast self-examination

    c) Testicular self-examination
    d) Cholesterol
    e) Obesity
    f) Stress
    g) Family planning

I. Middle Adulthood (40s to Early 60s)

1. Physical characteristics
  a. May lose height
  b. Body contour changes; higher percentage of body fat
  c. Visual and aural acuity decline
  d. Skin becomes less elastic; wrinkles form
  e. Gradual loss of taste
2. Developmental milestones
  a. Sexual development
   1) Menopause and loss of reproductive capacity
   2) Options, opportunities, and means of sexual expression may change
  b. Psychosocial development
   1) Achievement of goals
   2) Desire to serve the larger community
   3) Family roles may change from child-centered to couple-centered roles
   4) Grandparenting
   5) Change in relationship with parents
   6) Peak earning capacity
  c. Cognitive development: capable of thinking in a concrete manner

J. Late Adulthood (Age 65 to Death)

1. Physical characteristics
  a. Quality of life depends on the person's ability to perform activities of daily living
  b. Formation and composition of body changes
  c. Body systems begin to decline
  d. Sensory systems become less efficient
  e. Problems with memory loss and learning difficulty develop
2. Developmental milestones
  a. Motor development
   1) Movement slows
   2) Fine motor skills affected by stiffening of the joints
  b. Sexual development: capable of enjoying a satisfying sexual relationship
  c. Psychosocial development
   1) Ego integrity achieved
   2) Life review reassures about accomplishments and worth
   3) Body image changes
   4) Fear of loss of independence
   5) Death of a spouse produces change of roles
   6) Work and leisure activities change
   7) Concept of death takes on a different meaning
  d. Cognitive development
   1) Healthy persons retain cognitive abilities
   2) Memory changes; short-term stores less than long-term

Communication

I. Communication

A. Definition of Communication

1. Process of sharing meaning
2. Involves two or more individuals
3. Process can involve sending and receiving messages even when not consciously aware

B. Communication Process (Fig. 5.1)

1. Source
   a. Sender of the message
   b. What is sent varies and is affected by the sender's experiences
   c. Sender encodes (creates) message
   d. Sender needs to know the receiver to the create message
2. Message
   a. What is sent by the source
   b. Message has three parts
      1) Meaning: usually ideas or feelings
      2) Symbols: words or actions that represent the meaning; the process of turning words or actions into symbols is encoding
      3) Organization or form: syntax and grammar of the message; putting the symbols in order
   c. Must be understood by the receiver
3. Channel
   a. Mode of communication
   b. Can be visual, audio, print, or touch
4. Receiver
   a. Where the message is being sent
   b. Receiver processes into meaning (decoding)
5. Feedback
   a. Response of the receiver
   b. Can be verbal or nonverbal

c. Tells the source if the message was heard, seen, or understood
6. Noise
   a. Anything that interferes with the communication process
   b. Can be
      1) External: stimuli that draw attention away from the message
      2) Internal: personal thoughts and feelings that draw a person away from the message
      3) Semantic: message symbols that prevent the meaning from being understood (accents, dialect, and grammar)
7. Listening
   a. Important part of feedback
   b. Must be aware of verbal and nonverbal messages
   c. Goals of listening
      1) Hear patient accurately
      2) Listen for what is not being said
      3) Determine how accurately message was received

C. Types of Communication

1. Verbal communication
   a. Message is spoken
   b. Words must be understood by all parties
2. Nonverbal communication
   a. Messages conveyed without the use of words
   b. Body language
   c. Involves grooming, dress, eye contact, facial expressions, hand gestures, space, tone of voice, and posture

D. Personal Space

1. Distance that is comfortable in which to communicate with others
2. Handled differently by various cultures

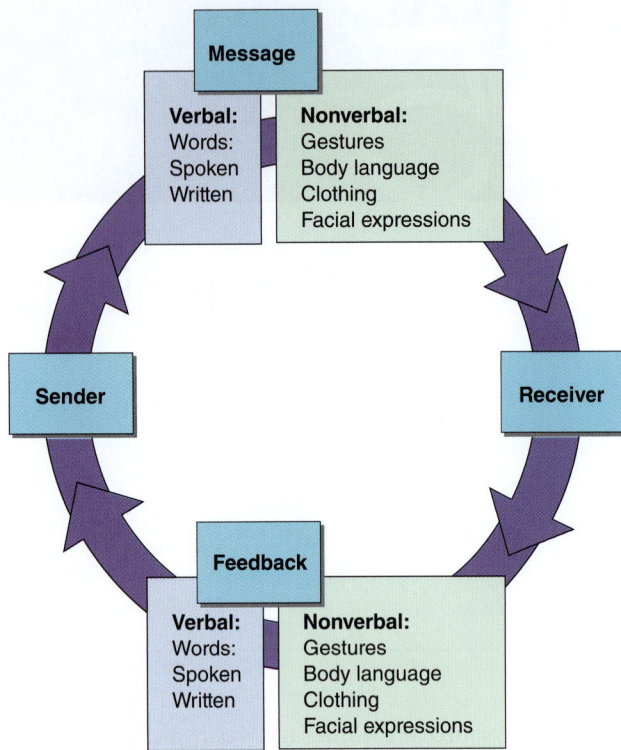

Fig. 5.1 Model of communication. Modified from Bonewit-West K, Hunt S: *Today's medical assistant*, ed 4, 2021, Elsevier.

3. Patients may feel threatened when others invade personal space without permission
   a. Should explain invasive procedures before performing
4. Personal space for the US culture
   a. Intimate/personal: 0–1.5 ft
   b. Casual person: 1.5–4 ft
   c. Social: 4–12 ft
   d. Public: >12 ft

E. Therapeutic Communication

1. Process of relaying information from health care provider to patient
2. Can be through verbal disclosure, touch, or gesture
3. Techniques
   a. Acknowledgment: emphasizes the importance of the patient in the communication process
   b. Establishing guidelines: helps the patient know what is expected of him or her
   c. Focusing: directs the communication toward important topics
   d. Listening: communicates interest in the topics raised by the patient
   e. Open-ended comments: helps the patient to decide what is relevant; encourages discussion ("Describe what you think is going to happen.")
   f. Reflecting: shows the importance of the patient's ideas and feelings
   g. Restating: lets the patient know how the health care provider interpreted the message the patient sent ("I hear you saying…"); paraphrasing

   h. Clarification: demonstrates the desire to understand what the patient is communicating (may ask who, what, where, and when)
   i. Silence: communicates acceptance
4. Ineffective techniques
   a. Advising: telling what the patient should do
   b. Minimizing: health care provider making light of the patient's situation
   c. Defending: health care provider protecting self from criticism
   d. Stereotyping: health care provider using clichés when responding
   e. Probing: health care provider discussing, or trying to discuss, topics the patient does not want to discuss
   f. Approval and disapproval: health care provider overly approving or disapproving of the patient's behavior
   g. Agreeing and disagreeing: health care provider overly agreeing or disagreeing with the patient's perceptions, thoughts, or feelings
5. Barriers to communication
   a. Embarrassment: patient may be in awe of the health care provider and embarrassed to ask questions of the health care provider
   b. Discomfort: patient may be uncomfortable or ashamed to discuss his or her private body parts or symptoms
   c. Communication difficulties: patient can see disabilities as making the patient intellectually inferior
   d. Withdrawal: patient does not respond to health care provider's communication
   e. Ineffective techniques by health care provider may raise barriers
   f. Physical impairment: physical impairments that may limit the ability to communicate
   g. Language: non–English-speaking patients may require more gestures and body language and may also need an interpreter
   h. Prejudice: unfair treatment of a person because of race, age, gender, religion, handicap, or for any other reason
   i. Stereotyping: application of a standardized mental picture
   j. Perception: capacity for comprehension

F. Multicultural Communication

1. Ability to communicate with persons of other cultures
2. Must recognize own personal bias and prejudices and put them aside
3. Trust must be established for the patient to be comfortable with sharing information
4. Staff may need to educate themselves on the culture for better understanding
5. May need an interpreter (family member or employee)
6. Potential barriers
   a. Religious beliefs
   b. Values
   c. Habits
   d. Attitude toward Western medicine

II. Patient Relationships

A. General

1. Medical assistant needs to understand the patient's concerns, needs, and reactions
2. Stress and anxiety are common patient responses
3. First impressions are lasting impressions

B. Unconscious Defense Mechanisms

1. Compensation: overemphasizing a trait to make up for a failure
2. Denial: avoiding reality
3. Displacement: shifting an impulse from a threatening to a nonthreatening one
4. Dissociation: disconnecting the significance from an event
5. Identification: mimicking the behavior of another
6. Introjection: adopting the feelings of others
7. Projection: assigning the person's own feelings to another as if these feelings had originated with the other person
8. Rationalization: justifying the person's thoughts, feelings, or behavior
9. Regression: returning to a former behavior or more immature behavior
10. Repression: putting unpleasant thoughts or events out of the person's mind
11. Sarcasm: biting edge added to words that are said; can be hostile and cruel
12. Sublimation: diverting unacceptable thoughts or feelings into acceptable behaviors
13. Substitution: making up for a deficiency by concentrating on another
14. Suppression: deliberately forgetting or avoiding dealing with an unpleasantness
15. Verbal aggression: attacking another without addressing the original complaint or disregarding it; loudly lashing out verbally

C. Interaction With Patients

1. Interaction is a therapeutic relationship
2. Assists patients to resolve problems and achieve goals
3. Maximizes patient comfort
   a. Children
      1) Establish a friendly relationship
      2) Be aware of your own feelings toward children in general
      3) Speak in quiet tones; speak at the child's physical level (not looking down at the child)
      4) Use language appropriate for the child's age
      5) Allow the child to assist in his or her treatment
      6) Keep the child patient from experiencing long waits
      7) Understand that the child may regress when ill
      8) Be truthful with the child, which fosters trust
      9) Offer rewards for proper behavior
      10) Allow the child to play with the health care provider's equipment if doing so is safe and appropriate
      11) Infants should be held and comforted before any treatment procedures
   b. Adolescents
      1) Patient demands independence yet requires comfort
      2) Permit patient's privacy
      3) Health care provider must allow examinations without the patient's parent present
      4) Treat the patient with respect and dignity
      5) Set fair limits for the patient
      6) Answer the patient's questions openly and honestly
      7) Explain the procedures to the patient in terms he or she will understand
   c. Elderly adults
      1) Allow additional time with the patient; this circumstance may be a social interaction for a lonely patient
      2) Keep the patient physically and environmentally comfortable
      3) Patient may find comfort in a health care provider's routine
      4) Allow as much independence as possible
      5) Do not overprotect or be overattentive
      6) Speak slowly and precisely, but do not patronize
   d. Terminally ill patients
      1) Help both the patient and the patient's family adjust to the patient's loss in strength, sensation, mobility, and endurance
      2) Give support to the patient's family members
      3) Be willing to listen
      4) Patient will likely experience some, or all, of the stages of dying
   e. Angry patients
      1) Patient's anger may be caused by the patient's medical condition
      2) Health care provider's goal is to calm the patient
      3) Health care provider must remain calm, firm, and direct
      4) Health care provider must not take the anger personally
      5) Health care provider must listen closely to the patient's concerns
      6) Health care provider must keep his or her speaking tone calm and in control
      7) Keep the angry patient out of public areas of the office; escort the angry patient to a private room
   f. Sensory-impaired patients
      1) Patient may need an interpreter (if hearing impaired or if speaks only a foreign language) to assist in communication
      2) Health care provider should be positioned directly in front of the patient and should speak slowly
      3) For a sight-impaired patient, the health care provider should ask how best to assist the patient
      4) Health care provider should be flexible, open, and supportive
   g. Frightened patients
      1) A frightened patient may be uncooperative
      2) Health care provider should recognize fear and assist the patient in dealing with the fright
      3) Health care provider should maintain control of the situation

h. Depressed patients
   1) A depressed patient experiences feelings of gloom, hopelessness, and dread and may have feelings of no self-worth
   2) Health care provider should provide sympathy, support, and a friendly ear
   3) Health care provider should demonstrate an interest in the patient's needs
   4) Health care provider should keep the environment secure and nonthreatening
i. Suicidal patients
   1) Suicidal feelings can be the patient's final response to his or her depression
   2) Suicidal patient may disclose intentions to the health care provider
   3) All suicidal threats or attempts must be taken seriously
   4) Health care provider must listen closely to the suicidal patient
   5) Health care provider should demonstrate empathy
   6) Health care provider should seek professional advice or actions for the suicidal patient
j. Mentally impaired patients
   1) Patient may be confused and disoriented
   2) By correcting the patient's confusion, the health care provider may make the patient less frightened
   3) Health care provider must treat the patient kindly but must not be condescending

k. Intellectually challenged
   1) Use "functioning age"
   2) Provide information also to caregiver/guardian
l. Abused patients
   1) Health care provider must treat an abused patient's physical injuries first
   2) Health care provider must focus on the patient as a victim; health care provider should express assurances of the patient's self-worth
   3) Refer the abused patient to existing social agencies
m. Drug-dependent patients
   1) Health care provider should not belittle the patient for the patient's behavior
   2) Health care provider should be compassionate, empathetic, and patient
   3) Health care provider should involve the patient's family in the patient's treatment
n. Significant others
   1) Part of the patient's emotional support group
   2) Health care provider should respect the wishes of the patient concerning the patient's loved ones
   3) Health care provider should keep any waiting relatives notified of progress and keep them informed of any delays
   4) Health care provider should address the concerns of the patient's family and friends
   5) Health care provider must be aware of confidentiality issues

6

Law, Ethics, and Health Insurance Portability and Accountability Act

I. Introduction to the Law

A. Definition of Law

1. System by which society gives order to our lives

B. Functions of Law

1. Regulate: control rules and standards
2. Punish: enforce penalties for infractions of rules and standards
3. Remedy: make wrongs that are committed right
4. Benefit: help society

C. Sources of Law

1. Common law: derived from the customs of society and court decisions
2. Administrative law: derived from agencies that enact state and federal law
3. Constitutional law: derived from the US Constitution
4. Statutory law: derived from the state and federal legislation

D. Types of Law

1. Civil law: a wrong, or perceived wrong, committed against a person or to property; civil laws that affect the practice of medicine include
   a. Contract law: governs enforceable promises
   b. Tort law: governs intentional or accidental acts that bring harm to a person or that damage property
   c. Administrative law: governs regulations set forth by governmental agencies
2. Criminal law: a wrong committed against a person or to property in violation of a statute or ordinance; criminal laws that may affect the practice of medicine include
   a. Infraction: a minor offense that usually results only in a fine
   b. Misdemeanor: violation of a law that includes, as a punishment, a maximum imprisonment of no more than 1 year
   c. Felony: a major crime that includes, as a punishment, an imprisonment of more than 1 year

II. Licensure, Registration, and Certification

A. Licensure

1. Strongest form of administrative regulation
2. Mandatory credential to practice medicine
3. Granted by a state board; verifies that the person holding the license has met minimum standards; for physicians, defined by the Medical Practice Act; for licensed nurses, defined and governed by the Nurse Practice Act
   a. State statute that defines what is included in the practice of medicine within that state
   b. Governs the methods and requirements of licensure and establishes grounds for suspension and revocation of the license
4. Physicians can be licensed through
   a. Examination: passing a written or oral examination
   b. Endorsement: acceptance of a national examination score
   c. Reciprocity: one state accepts another state's license
5. Licenses may be revoked or suspended for
   a. Conviction of a misdemeanor or a felony
   b. Unprofessional conduct
   c. Personal or professional incapacity
6. License must be periodically renewed (if not renewed, the physician will be suspended from practice)

B. Registration

1. Medical assistants can be registered
2. Voluntary process
3. Professional listed on a state or national registry
4. Process similar to certification
5. Usually accomplished by a written examination

C. Certification

1. Medical assistants can be certified
2. Voluntary process
3. Identifies a professional as meeting the minimum standards to be able to practice
4. Usually accomplished by a written examination
5. Governed by a professional organization

III. Regulating Issues for the Medical Office

A. Clinical Laboratory Improvement Act of 1988 (CLIA '88)

1. Identifies standards for laboratory testing
2. Any facility performing laboratory testing is subject to CLIA regulations

B. Certificate of Need (CON)

1. Process of acquiring approval, based on need to the community, to expand service

C. The Joint Commission (TJC)

1. Formerly the Joint Commission on Accreditation of Healthcare Organizations
2. Accreditation of health care facilities

D. Occupational Safety and Health Administration (OSHA)

1. Regulation of safety in the workplace

E. Americans With Disabilities Act (ADA)

1. Sets up rules protecting people with physical or mental disabilities from discrimination

F. American With Disabilities Act Amendments Act (ADAAA)

1. Expanded the definition of disabilities established in the ADA
2. Included people with cancer, diabetes, learning disabilities, and epilepsy

G. Title VII of the Civil Rights Act

1. Protects employees from sexual harassment and hostile work environment
2. Employer liable

H. Federal Discrimination Act

1. Employers with 15 or more employees must not discriminate based on age, gender, sexual orientation, race, creed, marital status, color, national origin, or disabilities

I. Regulation Z of the Consumer Protection Act

1. Truth in Lending Act
2. Requires agreement between patient and provider for payment of bills in more than four installments; must be in writing

J. Controlled Substances Act

1. Administered by the Drug Enforcement Administration (DEA)
2. Regulates any individual who prescribes, administers, or dispenses controlled substances

K. Family Medical Leave Act (FMLA)

1. Requires an employer of 50 or more employees to provide up to 12 weeks of unpaid, job-protected leave each year for care of the employee's own health, care of an immediate family member with a serious health condition, and birth or adoption of a child

L. Health Insurance Portability and Accountability Act (HIPAA)

1. Requires privacy and security standards to protect patient's identifiable health information

IV. Risk Management

A. Definition

1. Techniques that keep the practice, its environment, and procedures as safe for the patient as possible
2. Proper risk management reduces the possibility of negligence and lawsuits
3. Techniques
   a. Perform within the scope of practice
   b. Comply with federal and state statutes
   c. Keep office or clinic areas safe
   d. Keep all patient information confidential
   e. Follow all established office policies
   f. Document completely

g. Log telephone calls and return calls in a reasonable time frame
h. Follow up canceled or missed appointments
i. Never guarantee a cure or diagnosis; never advise without provider's order
j. Secure informed consent
k. Explain appointment delays
l. Be watchful of patients with special needs
m. Report any error to the employer

V. Consent

A. Definition of Consent

1. Voluntary permission given by a capable person to receive medical care

B. Types

1. Express: oral or written expression of consent
2. Implied: actions or behavior that can be reasonably presumed to express consent

C. Informed Consent

1. Provider or other caregiver has an affirmative duty to explain to the patient information necessary to allow the patient to evaluate the medical care and make decisions on that information before having the medical care performed; implies an understanding of
   a. What procedure is to be done
   b. Why the procedure should be done
   c. Risks involved in performing the procedure
   d. Expected benefits of having the procedure performed
   e. Any alternative treatments that can be performed
   f. Risks involved in performing the alternative treatment
2. Form signed and put in the chart before the invasive procedure is performed
3. Medical assistant may witness the signature of the patient

D. Who May and May Not Give Consent

1. Persons who are mentally competent and of the age of majority can give consent
2. A parent, legal guardian, or someone legally charged with standing in place of the parent or guardian can give consent for a minor (a minor is a person not yet of legal age, which is often 18 years old); consent can legally be given by a minor under the following circumstances
   a. Minor serving in the armed forces
   b. Emancipated minor
   c. Testing for sexually transmitted diseases
   d. Seeking contraception or abortion, *depending on state law*
3. Living will
   a. Also known as an advanced directive
   b. Authorizes in advance the withholding of artificial life-support methods in case of terminal illness or accident
   c. Encouraged by the Patient Self-Determination Act of 1990

4. Uniform Anatomical Gift Act of 1968: allows for competent adults to give their body or body parts in the event of their death for research, transplantation, or placement in a tissue bank
5. Persons who are *non compos mentis* ("not of sound mind") cannot give consent; these persons require some form of guardianship to give consent
6. In emergencies, consent to treatment is implied only as long as the emergency exists; the Good Samaritan Act provides immunity from liability to nonnegligent volunteers at the scene of an accident
7. Mentally competent persons have the right to refuse medical treatment (refused consent)
   a. Patient's refusal must be documented
   b. Patient must sign a document (release) absolving the caregiver of liability for not giving treatment
   c. Patient's refused consent can be overruled by a court of competent jurisdiction
8. Consent obtained by fraudulent means or misrepresentations is not binding
9. Without proper consent for treatment, a caregiver may be charged with
   a. Assault: intentional, unlawful attempt of bodily injury to another by force
   b. Battery: willful and unlawful use of force or violence (or touching) on another person

VI. Contracts

A. General

1. An agreement creating an obligation
2. Can be oral or written, expressed, or implied

B. Express Contract

1. Agreement between two or more parties
2. Contains the explicit terms of the agreement, either orally or in writing

C. Implied Contract

1. Conclusion drawn from the actions of two or more parties
2. Patient-physician contract is implied

D. Necessary Elements of a Contract

1. Offer: one party makes an offer
2. Acceptance: another party agrees to the offer made
3. Consideration: mutual exchange of something of value between the parties
4. Capacity: all parties must be legally able to make the offer and accept the terms
5. Legality: legal in nature and not against public policy

E. Patient and Provider Contract May Be Terminated by

1. Patient: circumstances need to be fully documented in the chart

2. Physician
   a. Must give patient notice (abandonment)
   b. Physician writes a certified letter with return receipt; copy in patient's record
   c. Letter should include
      1) Reasons why care is being discontinued
      2) Assurance that the physician will turn over patient records as directed
      3) Notice that the patient should seek alternative care as soon as possible

F. Reasons for Terminating a Contract

1. Provider retirement or moving
2. Patient not paying for services
3. Patient not following/noncompliant with the provider's plan
4. Patient behavior (needy, drug seeking, not showing for appointments, etc.)

VII. Torts

A. Definition of a Tort

1. An act, intentional or accidental, that brings harm against another person or damage to another person's property

B. Negligence

1. Unintentional (accidental) tort
2. Characterized by commission of an act that an ordinary, reasonable, and prudent person would not have done or omission of an act that an ordinary, reasonable, and prudent person would have done
   a. Forms of negligence
      1) Nonfeasance: failure to act when there was a duty to act, causing or resulting in harm
      2) Misfeasance: improper performance of an act causing or resulting in harm
      3) Malfeasance: performance of an improper or unlawful act causing or resulting in harm
      4) Malpractice: negligence of a professional person, with the action or inaction compared with an ordinary, reasonable, and prudent professional
   b. Four Ds of negligence
      1) Duty: exists when a patient-physician relationship has been established
      2) Derelict: neglect of professional obligation
      3) Direct cause: injury was directly caused by the physician's poor actions or by the physician's failure to act
      4) Damages: harm resulting to the patient; three types
         a) Nominal: damage exists in name only; token compensation
         b) Compensatory: actual damages sustained by the patient because of the physician's negligence
         c) Punitive: damages above the actual damage sustained by the patient; to punish the physician for the negligent act

C. Res Ipsa Loquitur

1. Meaning: "the thing speaks for itself"
2. Describes a situation in which the nature of the injury implicates negligence

D. Intentional Torts

1. Assault: deliberate threat to make bodily contact
2. Battery: intentional physical contact
3. Abandonment: one-sided termination of the patient-physician relationship by the physician without proper notice to the patient
4. Invasion of privacy: giving out patient information without patient consent
5. Defamation: injury to a person's reputation caused by a false statement by another person
6. Libel: false or malicious writing against another person
7. Slander: false or malicious oral statement against another person
8. False imprisonment: unlawful restraint, or holding, of an individual against his or her will
9. Fraud: intentional misrepresentation that might cause harm

E. Product Liability

1. Liability of a manufacturer of products for injuries caused by a defect in those products

F. Vicarious Liability

1. *Respondeat superior* (meaning: "let the master answer")
2. Employers are liable for the conduct of their employees while the employees are performing within the scope of their employment

VIII. Advance Directives

A. Advance Directives and Living Wills

1. Advance directive: person's desire to make known in advance his or her choices related to health care
2. Living will: document allowing a person to make choices related to treatment in a life-threatening illness
3. Directives are legal documents
4. Copies kept in the chart

B. Durable Power of Attorney

1. Allows the patient to name another person as the official spokesperson should the patient become unable to make health care decisions

C. Patient Self-Determination Act

1. Gives patients the right to be involved in their health care decisions

IX. Business Law

A. Employment Practices

1. National Labor Relations Act of 1935 (NLRA): defines unfair labor practices and provides hearing or mediation of complaints
2. Fair Labor Standards Act of 1938 (FLSA): defines minimum wage, equal pay for equal work, and child labor restrictions
3. Equal Pay Act of 1963 (EPA): amendment of FLSA that addresses wage disparities based on sex
4. Equal Employment Opportunity Act of 1972 (EEOA): prohibits employment discrimination based on age, race, color, religion, sex, or national origin
5. Age Discrimination in Employment Act of 1967 (ADEA): prohibits discrimination based on age
6. ADA of 1990: prohibits discrimination against persons with physical or mental disabilities
7. Workers' compensation laws: state-mandated programs to provide wage continuation and medical treatment compensation for persons with work-related injuries or illnesses

B. Sexual Harassment

1. *Quid pro quo* ("something for something"); conditions of employment (raise, promotion) are based on a person's acceptance or rejection of unwelcome sexual conduct
2. Hostile work environment: creation of an intimidating, offensive, or hostile workplace resulting from unwelcome sexual conduct; interferes with a person's ability to perform job functions

C. Payroll

1. FLSA requires all employee records of hours worked to be continuously maintained
2. Federal Insurance Contributions Act (FICA): Social Security Tax; applied toward old-age benefits
3. Federal Unemployment Tax Act (FUTA): tax to provide income during unemployment
4. Payroll reports and forms
   a. Form 944: Employer's Quarterly Federal Tax Return; filed every 3 months, with payment of quarterly tax due
   b. Form 8109: Federal Tax Deposit Book; used to pay FICA and federal income tax
   c. Form W-2: Wage and Tax Statement; given to employees yearly, itemizing the wages earned and all taxes deducted from wages for that year
   d. Form W-3: Transmittal of Income and Tax Statement; submitted to Social Security Administration; compares W-2 forms with Form 941
   e. Form W-4: Employee's Withholding Allowance Certificate; employee decides the number of withholding allowances for the company to take out of wages earned, based on the number of dependents claimed

X. Public Health Duties

A. General

1. States require physicians to report certain information
2. Reported information helps to provide for the health, safety, and welfare of the public

B. Births

1. Birth certificate completed by birth attendant

C. Deaths

1. Death certificate completed by physician in attendance
2. Medical examiner must be called in cases of
   a. Violent death or death related to criminal activity
   b. Death without a physician present
   c. Death from an undetermined cause
   d. Death within 24 hours of admission to a hospital or health care facility
   e. Death without a prior medical care

D. Communicable Diseases

1. Communicated to the county health department
2. Includes smallpox, scarlet fever, rubella, measles, tuberculosis, plague, cholera, and sexually transmitted diseases

E. National Childhood Vaccine Injury Act

1. Requires providers who administer vaccines to report the following information to public health agencies
   a. Date the vaccine was administered
   b. Lot number and manufacturer of the vaccine
   c. Any adverse reactions to the vaccine
   d. Name, title, and address of the person administering the vaccine

F. Newborn Diseases

1. Inborn errors of metabolism (e.g., phenylketonuria)

G. Abuse

1. The provider has the legal duty to report suspected abuse to the authorities; varies from state to state
2. Medical assistants are also considered mandatory reporters
3. Types of abuse to be reported
   a. Child abuse
   b. Spouse or domestic abuse
   c. Elder abuse
   d. Drug abuse
   e. Patient abuse in hospitals and nursing homes

H. Criminal Acts

1. The provider has the legal duty to report suspected criminal acts to authorities
2. Types of criminal acts to be reported
   a. Injuries by weapons
   b. Assault
   c. Attempted suicide
   d. Rape (may require a release by the victim because of confidentiality)

XI. Introduction to Ethics

A. General

1. Set of moral principles or values
2. Concerns thoughts, judgments, and actions on issues that have greater implications of moral right and wrong
3. Etiquette: courtesy, customs, and manners; not ethics
4. Contains three main elements: duty, rights, and virtues

B. Duties

1. Obligations or commitments to act in certain ways
2. Includes
   a. Nonmalfeasance: not doing any harm
   b. Beneficence: acting to create good
   c. Fidelity: meeting the patient's expectations through respect, competence, adherence to laws, and honoring agreements
   d. Veracity: telling the truth
   e. Justice: sharing of benefits and burdens
   f. Reparation: making a wrong right

C. Rights

1. Claims made on a person or society
2. Correlated with duties
3. Applies to all persons within a group without prejudice

D. Virtues

1. Character traits that make a person act in a certain way
2. Principles are written in the form of a Code of Ethics

XII. American Association of Medical Assistants (AAMA) Code of Ethics

A. General

1. As an agent of the physician, a medical assistant is governed by ethical standards
2. Decisions made in practice should be based on the professional nature and scope of practice of the professional
3. Code of Ethics is a standard for all medical assistants to honor

4. Patterned after the American Medical Association (AMA) Code of Ethics
5. *Never* practice medicine; a medical assistant should not identify himself or herself as a "nurse"

XIII. AMA Code of Ethics

A. General

1. Written code of conduct for medical practice
2. Includes four components
   a. Principles of medical ethics
   b. Fundamental elements of the patient-physician relationship
   c. Current opinions with annotation
   d. Reports of the Council of Ethical and Judicial Affairs; includes opinions on
      1) Abortion: not prohibited by ethical standards
      2) Abuse: legal and ethical requirement to report
      3) Allocation of health resources: the physician must remain a patient advocate and allow institutional procedures to determine allocation
      4) Artificial insemination: requires informed consent; deals with who has parental rights
      5) Clinical investigation: the patient-physician relationship does not exist in clinical investigation
      6) Cost: quality of patient care should be the physician's first consideration, not cost
      7) Provision of adequate health care: an adequate level of health care for all persons
      8) Genetic counseling: concerns for the quality of life
      9) Organ donation: the donor should not receive payment for organ donation; involves protection of the right to privacy for both the donor and recipient
      10) Quality of life: primary consideration of what is best for the patient
      11) Withholding or withdrawing life-prolonging treatment: the physician must be committed to saving life and relieving suffering; the patient may have his or her wishes known
      12) Euthanasia: incompatible with the physician's role

XIV. Professional Relationships

A. Hospital Relations

1. Privileges granted based on competence and experience, not fees

B. Advertising

1. Only restrictions are restrictions that protect the public from deceptive practices; physicians can advertise fees, identification of educational background, and specialty, but physicians cannot include any statements regarding the quality of their services

C. Communication With the Media

1. Physician may not discuss a patient's condition with the press (unless a release has been granted); may release only authorized information that is in the public domain (births, deaths, accidents, and police cases)

D. Computers

1. AMA has developed guidelines for the use and sharing of computerized information

E. Fees and Charges

1. Physician may not split patient fees with another physician for patient referral (fee splitting)
2. Physician's staff should assist in completing insurance forms without charge
3. Physician may request that the patient make payment at the time treatment is rendered
4. Insurance copayments may be waived or written off if access to care is threatened by inability to pay the copayment
5. Professional courtesy is a tradition

F. Physician's Records

1. Physician owns the notes prepared by him or her while treating a patient
2. Original medical records may not be released; records can be reproduced only on the physician's death, retirement, or sale of the physician's practice

XV. Professional Rights and Responsibilities

A. Discipline

1. Physician should expose dishonest, corrupt, incompetent, or unethical colleagues

B. Free Choice

1. Physician in private practice may decline to accept any individual as a patient

C. Patent

1. Physician may patent any device that he or she discovers or invents

D. Patient-Physician Relationship

1. Both parties are free to enter into, or decline to enter into, the relationship

E. Infectious Disease

1. Physician who is infected with an infectious disease should not engage in any patient contact or activity that may create a risk for the patient

F. Substance Abuse

1. Physician should not practice under the influence of any controlled substance, alcohol, or chemical agents that impair the ability to render treatment

XVI. HIPAA

A. HIPAA

1. Involved with privacy, security, and claims issues in the health care system
2. Standards for the privacy of individually identifiable health information
3. Allows the flow of health information while protecting the privacy of patients
4. Issues identified by state and federal agencies
5. Failure to comply with mandates can lead to sanctions and fines
6. Enacted in 1996
7. Two provisions
   a. Title I: Insurance Reform
   b. Title II: Administrative Simplification
8. Long-term benefits of HIPAA
   a. Lower administrative costs
   b. Increased accuracy of data
   c. Increased patient and customer satisfaction

B. Title I: Health Insurance Reform

1. General
   a. Provision of continuous insurance coverage for workers and their insured family members when the worker changes or loses a job
   b. Limits the use of preexisting condition exclusions
   c. Prohibits discrimination for past or present poor health
   d. Guarantees individuals the right to purchase gap health insurance coverage after losing a job
   e. Allows renewal of health insurance coverage regardless of an individual's health condition

C. Title II: Administrative Simplification

1. General
   a. Focuses on the health care setting
   b. Intended to reduce administrative costs
   c. Accomplished by standardizing the exchange of health care data
   d. Includes provisions to ensure the privacy and security of an individual's health data
   e. Standardization of electronic transmissions to reduce the number of forms and methods used in claims processing
   f. Two parts to provision
      1) Development and implementation of standardized electronic transactions using common sets of descriptors (code sets)
      2) Implementation of privacy and security procedures to prevent the misuse of health information and ensure confidentiality

D. Roles and Relationships

1. General
   a. Department of Health and Human Services (HHS): establishes and implements standards
   b. Centers for Medicare and Medicaid (CMS): enforces insurance portability and code set requirements of HIPAA
   c. Office of Civil Rights (OCR): enforces privacy standards
   d. Covered entity: may be a health plan (e.g., Blue Cross/Blue Shield), health care clearing house, or health care provider
   e. Electronic media: mode of electronic transmission; may include the Internet, extranet, telephone lines, fax modems, or disks or magnetic tape
   f. Transaction: transmission of information between two parties; can include
      1) Health care claims
      2) Health care payments
      3) Coordination of benefits
      4) Claim status
      5) Enrollment and disenrollment in a health plan
      6) Eligibility for a health plan
      7) Premium payments
      8) Referral certification or authorization
      9) First report of injury

E. Privacy Rule

1. General
   a. Privacy: condition of being secluded from the view or presence of others
   b. Confidentiality: use of discretion in keeping information private
   c. Disclosure: release, transfer, access to, or divulgence of information
   d. Individually identifiable health information (IIHI): any part of an individual's health information collected from an individual (e.g., demographic information, date of birth)
   e. Protected health information (PHI): IIHI that is transmitted by electronic media, maintained in electronic form, or transmitted or maintained in any other form or medium; all patient information is protected regardless of the way it is maintained; includes paper records, computerized practice management or billing systems, spoken words, and x-ray films
   f. Use: sharing, application, use, examination, or analysis of IIHI; PHI is protected both inside and outside of the organization unless the use is specifically required or permitted

F. Patient Rights Under HIPAA

1. Right to notice of privacy practices
   a. Patients are entitled to receive written notice of privacy practices (Notice of Privacy Protection [NPP]) from the provider at the first appointment
   b. NPP outlines patients' rights
   c. Must be written in plain language; staff should obtain a signature acknowledging receipt
   d. Can be done at the front desk
2. Right to request restrictions on certain uses and disclosures of PHI
   a. Patient has the right to ask for restrictions on how the office will use and disclose PHI
   b. Restrictions must be agreed on by the office; if agreed, restrictions must be documented and followed
   c. Practice may disclose confidential information without written authorization, such as communicable diseases, victims of abuse, and law enforcement purposes
   d. Patient may identify any other person to whom information may be disclosed or not disclosed
3. Right to request confidential information
   a. Patient can request to receive confidential communication by alternative means or alternative location (call patient at work instead of home; test results sent in writing instead of over the telephone)
   b. Office must accommodate reasonable requests
   c. Requests may be required in writing
4. Right to access PHI
   a. Patient has the right to access, inspect, and obtain a copy of his or her PHI
   b. Request must be made in writing
   c. Request must be acted on within 30 days
   d. Reasonable fee for copies and postage may be applied
   e. Patients do not have the right to access psychotherapy notes, information compiled for use in legal proceedings, or information exempted under CLIA '88
   f. If health care provider has determined that the patient may be endangered by accessing information, access may be denied
   g. State law may take precedence
5. Right to request amendment of PHI
   a. Patient has the right to request that his or her PHI be changed
   b. Request should be made in writing
   c. Must be done in a timely manner
6. Right to receive an accounting of disclosures of PHI
   a. Providers should keep a log of disclosures
   b. Patients may request an accounting or tracking of their disclosures once a year without charge; additional accountings may be charged a fee
7. Organization and staff responsibilities
   a. General
      1) Organization must implement written policies and procedures
      2) Guidelines tailored to each practice
      3) Documentation must be maintained in written or electronic form and maintained for 6 years
   b. Verification of identity
      1) Office must verify the identity of person requesting PHI
      2) Identification may be by date of birth, Social Security number, or password
   c. Validation of patient permission
      1) Office must have appropriate permission
      2) Permission is maintained in the practice management system or patient chart

d. Training
   1) Office must train all staff
   2) Must include the practice's policies and procedures that deal with PHI
   3) Each person's role should be addressed
e. Safeguards
   1) Ensure that information is secure
   2) Include administrative, technical, and physical measures that safeguard PHI from any intentional or accidental disclosure
f. Complaints
   1) Process must be in place for complaints
   2) Staff members are subject to appropriate sanctions for failure to comply (warning to termination)

8. Code set regulations
   a. General
      1) Transaction and code set (TCS): developed to streamline electronic data transactions
      2) Makes data processing transactions more efficient and reduces costs
      3) Single standard similar to a bank's automatic teller machine or grocery self-checkout
      4) Can be used by anyone to enter into a specific space on a form
      5) Electronic, not paper
      6) Documents why patients are seen (diagnosis, *International Classification of Diseases*, 10th Edition, Clinical Modification [ICD-10CM]) and what is done to them at the encounter (procedure, *Current Procedural Terminology [CPT-4]*, 4th Edition, Health Care Financing Administration Common Procedure Coding System [HCPCS])

9. Guidelines for HIPAA privacy compliance
   a. Reasonable and appropriate safeguards must be taken to ensure that all confidential information is protected
      1) Conversations can be overheard; consider privacy glass at the front desk and moving conversations away from populated settings; move dictation stations away from patient areas; telephone conversations in front of patients should be avoided
      2) Check medical record to see if any special instructions for contacting the patient are noted
      3) Limit the information (reason for visit) on patient sign-in sheets; change sign-in sheets throughout the day
      4) Patient must sign a form acknowledging receipt of the NPP
      5) Formal policies for transferring and accepting PHI must be in place; these include couriers, billing services, transcription services, and e-mail
      6) Computers should be turned so the screen is not visible to others; screensavers may be used; computer should automatically log off a user after a period of being idle
      7) Keep user names and passwords confidential and change them often
      8) Safeguard the work area by keeping confidential information from patient view; keep PHI from cleaning services that may have access after business hours
      9) Medical records should be placed face down at the reception area; when placing a medical record on the door of the examination room, turn the chart so that the identifying information faces the door
      10) Do not post the provider's daily schedule in areas accessible to patients
      11) Fax machines should not be placed in patient rooms or the reception area where incoming documents may be viewed
      12) Direct mail and telephone calls to the appropriate persons
      13) For coding and billing purposes, recognize, learn, and use HIPAA TCS
      14) Send all privacy-related concerns and questions to the appropriate staff member
      15) Immediately report any suspected or known improper behavior to the supervisor
      16) Privacy rule allows parents to see a child's medical record unless the parent is not the child's personal representative

XVII. HITECH Act

A. Health Information Technology for Economic and Clinical Health Act

1. Part of the American Recovery and Reinvestment Act (ARRA) of 2009
2. Contains specific incentives designed to accelerate the adoption of electronic health records (EHR) systems
3. Widens the scope of privacy and security available under HIPAA
4. Increases potential for legal liability for noncompliance
5. Provides for more enforcement

B. Meaningful Use

1. Providers must show that they are using EHR technology in ways that can be measured in quality and quantity
2. If providers meet requirements, they qualify for incentive payments
3. Three main components:
   a. Use of EHR in a meaningful manner (e.g., e-prescribing)
   b. Use of EHR technology for electronic exchange of health information, thus improving the quality of care
   c. Use of EHR to submit clinical quality reports, diagnosis and procedure codes, and other measures
   d. Licensed health care professionals and credentialed medical assistants can enter orders into the medical records. Credentialing for a medical assistant must come from an organization other than the organization employing the medical assistant
   e. Necessary for payment from Medicare and Medicaid

7

Professionalism and Career Development

I. Customer Service

A. Definition

1. What is done for a customer to improve his/her experience in the healthcare facility

B. Customer

1. One who purchases goods or services
2. Patients are customers

C. Customer Service Closely Relates to Professional Behavior

1. Patient's base confidence, trust, and satisfaction in those who show professionalism

II. Professionalism

A. Definition

1. Acting in a courteous, conscientious, and businesslike manner in the workplace
2. Conforming to the technical and ethical standards of a profession
3. Keeping calm in stressful situations
4. Not responding in anger when patients or coworkers are rude
5. Includes both appearance and attitude

B. Characteristics of Professional Behavior

1. Competence: ability to perform one's job to standards
2. Dependability: being punctual, efficient, and reliable
3. Integrity: honest and straightforward
4. Compassion: using empathy to sense someone else's concerns or feelings
5. Respect for others: treating others with dignity
6. Responsibility: taking ownership of one's actions
7. Professional demeanor: acting in a thoughtful way; respect for self and others
8. Loyalty: devotion to another
9. Positive attitude: state of mind; way of carrying one's self; reflected in tone of voice and body language
10. Teamwork: working together
11. Ability to prioritize: determining which task must be completed before another
12. Flexibility: ability to adapt to a variety of situations
13. Courtesy: use of kind words, compassion, and consideration

C. Professional Abilities

1. Competence: ability to get things done on time and correctly; understanding implications of actions; knowing when to ask for help
2. Dexterity: ability to move with skill or ease
3. Effective communication: ability to communicate on many levels with different types of people; includes English skills and facial expression
4. Empathy: putting oneself into the patient's place
5. Attitude: pleasant and courteous; patient never treated with disrespect or in an unfriendly manner

6. Initiative: ability and willingness to work independently
7. Flexibility: ability to adapt
8. Desire to learn: willing to grow and learn in the profession
9. Ability to communicate: verbally and nonverbally
10. Ethical behavior: perception of right and wrong

D. Professional Image

1. Personal appearance
   a. Bathe or shower daily; brush teeth
   b. Hair away from face, styled neatly
   c. Clean nails; practical length; no artificial nails
   d. Minimal makeup; very little fragrance
   e. Minimal jewelry
   f. Uniform or scrubs clean and pressed; proper fit; worn with undergarments that should not be visible
   g. Socks or stockings should be worn
   h. Shoes should fit properly; no open-toe shoes or sandals; no canvas shoes
   i. No gum chewing; no tobacco odor
   j. Do not use cell phones or personal computer

E. Barriers to Professionalism

1. Bringing personal problems into the workplace
2. Taking care of personal business while at work
3. Inappropriate discussions in front of patients
4. Procrastination of duties

F. Maintaining a Professional Image

1. Leave personal problems at home.
2. Avoid office gossip.
3. Do not conduct personal business during office hours.
4. Stay out of office politics.
5. Do not procrastinate.

III. The Professional Medical Assistant

A. Professional Duties

1. Administrative: having to do with the "front office".
2. Clinical: having to do with the "back office"; patient care.
3. Transdisciplinary: general knowledge.
4. Medical assistant works under the direct supervision of healthcare provider.
5. Duties may vary from state to state.

B. Training Programs

1. Accredited programs: voluntary process to help programs set, achieve, and maintain educational goals to meet guidelines and standards of the profession
2. Commission on Accreditation of Allied Health Education Programs (CAAHEP)
3. Accrediting Bureau of Health Education Schools (ABHES)

C. Credentials

1. Promotes the profession
2. American Association of Medical Assistants (AAMA): Certified Medical Assistant (CMA)
3. American Medical Technologists (AMT): Registered Medical Assistant (RMA); Certified Medical Administrative Assistant (CMAA)
4. National Healthcareer Association (NHA): Certified Clinical Medical Assistant (CCMA); CMAA
5. Clinical Medical Assistant Certification (CMAC): American Medical Certification Association
6. National Center for Competency Testing (NCCT)
7. Credentials awarded after passing exam
8. Continuing education required to maintain credential, keep up with knowledge, and reinforce areas related to job responsibilities

D. Continuing Education

1. Credits for courses, classes, or seminars related to a person's profession
2. Designed to promote education and keep individuals up to date on current trends in their field
3. Often required for licensing or certification

IV. Scope of Practice

A. Definition

1. Performance of delegated duties within the supervising provider's scope of practice consistent with the medical assistant's education, training, and experience.
2. Duties performed by the medical assistant do not constitute the practice of medicine.
3. *A medical assistant is not a nurse and should not refer to himself or herself as a nurse.*

B. Provider Responsible for the Medical Assistant

1. Duties vary from state to state.
2. A medical assistant performs as an agent of the provider under supervision.
3. A medical assistant performs duties that he or she is told to perform; provider responsible for actions.
4. Duties can be relayed to the medical assistant verbally, through a supervisor, or by way of office policy or procedure manual.
5. *Respondeat superior.*

C. Websites

1. AAMA: www.aama-ntl.org
2. AMT: www.amt1.com
3. NHA: http://www.nhanow.com
4. CMAC: www.amcaexams.com

8

Computer Concepts, Written Communications, and Mail Processing

I. Computer Basics

A. General

1. Electronic device that accepts, processes, exports, and stores data
2. Used to schedule appointments, process patient statements and insurance statements, order supplies, maintain computerized patient medical records, prescribe patient medications, enter and receive e-mail, and create reports

B. Data Processing Cycle

1. Input
   a. Allow communication between the user and the computer hardware
   b. Allow data to be entered into the computer
   c. Keyboard: allows input of alphanumeric data
   d. Mouse: handheld pointing device; contains a ball that is moved when the mouse is rolled on a flat surface; movement of the mouse and the ball moves the cursor on the computer screen; can also use light-emitting diode (LED) and lasers to detect movement; may be wireless
   e. Scanner: device that reads, or converts, printed matter directly into a computer-readable format
   f. Voice recognition: device that reads voices and creates a computer-readable format
   g. Tablets (e.g., iPad), smartphones, and touchscreen technology
2. Processing
   a. Handling and arranging of data by the computer
   b. Can include classifying, calculating, sorting, or listing of data entered
3. Output
   a. Allow data to be displayed or recorded
   b. Monitor: device that resembles a television set; displays computer-generated information
   c. Printer: device that records computer-generated information onto paper (hard copy)
4. Storage
   a. Methods of saving information input for future reference or for printing
   b. Hard drive: part of the computer hardware inside the computer box; contains the computer-operating information
   c. Portable disk drives: zip drive; flash drive; jump drive; external hard drives; attached externally to the computer; contains a very high storage capacity; usually used as backup; can be stored somewhere other than the facility

C. Software

1. Typically referred to as a program; provides processing instructions to the computer
2. Systems software: manages the overall operations of the computer system; program instructions that control, interface with, and communicate between the applications software and the workstation
3. Applications software: mainly commercially prepared programs that perform specific data-processing functions

D. System Security

1. Necessary to protect system from unauthorized access
2. Operating system: select system with few flaws
3. Firewall: limits access to the system from the outside
4. Antivirus software: protection from viruses, worms, and malware

5. Password: password required to access medical and financial data
6. Training: train personnel not to open e-mail or visit websites from unknown sources
7. Inventory control: keep track of all devices
8. Data management: purge, archive, or destroy inactive files
9. Data backup: backup systems on regular basis

II. Input Devices

A. General

1. Use of computer to produce documents
2. Software programs that allow the preparation of written documents

B. Keyboard Keys

1. Alphanumeric: keys that represent letters, numbers, and symbols
2. Backspace: allows the cursor to be moved to the left; erases character over which it is backspaced
3. Caps Lock: keeps the alphabet keys in uppercase
4. Ctrl and Alt (control and alternate keys): used in combination with other keys to increase the number of functions on the keyboard
5. Cursor control arrows: allow the cursor (the blinking arrow [or dash] on the screen that identifies where the data will be placed on the screen) to be moved up, down, to the left, or to the right
6. Del (delete): erases characters to the right of the cursor
7. End: moves the cursor to the end of a line of print
8. Enter (or Return): returns the cursor to the beginning of the next blank line
9. Esc (escape): allows the exit of a program or window
10. F1 through F12 (function keys): perform special program-directed actions
11. Home: moves the cursor to the upper, lower, left, or right margin
12. Page Up, Page Down: moves the cursor one page up or down
13. Print Screen: allows only the displayed screen to be printed (if allowed by the program)
14. Shift: places the alphabet key in uppercase when the Shift key is pressed simultaneously
15. Space bar: allows blank spaces to be placed between letters or words
16. Tab: moves the cursor a predetermined number of blank spaces; used to indent

C. Formatting

1. Determines the physical layout of the document
   a. Margins: amount of blank space at the edges of the document
   b. Tab set: sets a specific number of blank spaces to be used in each tab
   c. Line spacing: sets a specific number of blank lines between each line of input text (usually set for single or double spacing)
   d. Pitch: number of characters per inch of type
   e. Justification: alignment of text to the left or right margin, or both
   f. Header and footer: information to be included at the top (header) or bottom (footer) of each page
   g. Pagination: positions and prints the page numbers on each page
   h. Widows and orphans: eliminates a last paragraph line that appears alone at the top of the next page (widow) or eliminates a first paragraph line that appears at the bottom of the previous page (orphan)
   i. Font: style and size of print used

D. Editing

1. Allows changes to be made within a document
   a. Highlight and block: text can be highlighted for manipulation by using the cursor
   b. Delete: erases the highlighted text block
   c. Copy and paste: copies the highlighted text block for placement (paste) elsewhere in the document, at the new cursor location, without erasing
   d. Cut and paste: takes (cuts) the highlighted text block and places (pastes) it elsewhere in the document, at the new cursor location
   e. Print: allows the document to be recorded (printed) on paper (hard copy)
   f. Save: allows data to be placed in storage on a CD, a flash drive, or on the hard drive
   g. Retrieve (open): allows stored data to be brought onto the screen

E. Word Processing Terminology

1. Default: predefined settings automatically loaded by the program used, unless changed by the user
2. Directory: index of files on a hard drive
3. Grammar check: application that identifies input grammar or punctuation errors
4. Help screen: provides explanations or instructions about a particular task within a particular program
5. Menu: display on the screen that gives a list of options for word processing
6. Page break: places the beginning of a new page where the cursor is positioned
7. Prompt: message displayed on the screen that gives the user helpful information or instructions
8. Reveal codes: normally invisible word processing codes are made visible for quick editing
9. Sort: organizes a list in alphabetical or numerical order
10. Spell check: application that checks for misspelled words (medical spell check programs are available)
11. Thesaurus: identifies synonyms and antonyms for the word on which the cursor sits
12. Window: application that allows more than one program to be in use at the same time
13. Word wrap: automatically moves the beginning of a line to the next line without having to press Enter (or Return)

III. Computers in the Medical Office

A. Use of the Computer

1. Perform administrative procedures
2. Must know computer concepts to operate system effectively

B. Advantages of Computerization

1. Speed and productivity: process a large amount of data quickly
2. Efficiency: can transfer information that is used over and over again (e.g., patient name)
3. Accessibility: information is easy to retrieve when needed
4. Reduced costs: reduces operating costs by reducing amount of time needed to perform front office tasks

C. Disadvantages of Computerization

1. Initial cost: purchase of hardware and software is costly
2. Time investment: considerable time to learn programs
3. Start-up tasks: tasks that must be performed before a program can be operational

D. Medical Practice Management Program

1. Provides instructions to computer for performing front office procedures
2. Can be specialized to fit practice
3. Functions
   a. Patient registration system: sets up record for each patient
   b. Appointment system: makes, cancels, reschedules, finds, and prints log and patient reminder cards; keep written record in case system goes down
   c. Posting transactions system: post charges and payments
   d. Patient billing system: prepares bills and prints statements
   e. Insurance billing system: prepares and generates insurance claims
   f. Reports system: generates reports for the practice
   g. File maintenance system: adds additional information to the system

IV. Computers and Health Insurance Portability and Accountability Act

A. Information That May Be Used and Shared

1. Patient care and treatment coordination
2. To pay physicians and facilities for health care
3. With family members whom the patient has identified as being involved in his or her care
4. To make certain good care is provided
5. To protect public health
6. To make required reports to law enforcement

B. Information That Cannot Be Shared or Used Without Patient Consent

1. Cannot give health information to an employer
2. Cannot use or share information for marketing
3. Cannot share mental health information obtained in counseling

C. Health Care Facility Must Train Anyone Using the System Regarding What Information Can and Cannot Be Shared

1. Individual logins and passwords
2. Patient information should not be accessed unless the user needs to know content for patient care
3. Care must be taken when releasing any kind of information

V. Written Communication Skills

A. Types of Written Communication Within the Medical Office

1. Formal handwritten consultation and surgical reports
2. Composition of letters to patients, consulting physicians, and suppliers
3. Replies to inquiries
4. Responses to requests for information
5. Written collection letters
6. Supply orders
7. Documentation of treatment instructions for patients
8. Other types of office communication

B. Letters

1. Parts of a letter
   a. Heading
      1) Printed letterhead at the top of the page
      2) Dateline: three blank lines below the letterhead; name of the month written in full, followed by the day and year
   b. Opening
      1) Inside address
         a) Four blank lines below the dateline
         b) Title, name, and address of receiver
         c) Street, avenue, or boulevard and east, west, north, and south all are spelled out
         d) Numbered street names 1 through 10 are spelled out
         e) Numbered street names 11 and above are identified by numerals
         f) City is spelled out, followed by a comma
         g) Standard two-letter US postal service abbreviation without any period is used for state
         h) Zip code uses the five, or nine if available, numerals one space after the state
      2) Attention line (optional)
         a) Placed two blank lines below the inside address

b) Directs the letter to a particular department or person when the letter is addressed to an organization

3) Salutation
  a) Opening greeting to the letter
  b) Two blank lines below the inside address
  c) Recipient's title and name followed by a colon (personal correspondence allows use of a comma)
  d) Use the courtesy title ("Dr.," "Mr.," "Mrs.," and "Ms.") when the letter is addressed to a specific individual
  e) Use the phrase "To Whom It May Concern:" or "Dear Sir or Madam:" when the letter is addressed to an unidentified individual within an organization

c. Body
  1) Placed two blank lines below the salutation
  2) Contains the message of the letter
  3) Each line is single spaced; a double space is placed between paragraphs

d. Closing
  1) Complimentary closing
    a) Placed two blank lines below the body of the letter
    b) Only the first letter of the first word in the closing is capitalized
    c) Comma follows the complimentary closing
    d) May be formal ("Truly yours," or "Very truly yours,") or common ("Sincerely," or "Sincerely yours,")
  2) Signature line
    a) Placed four or five blank lines below the complimentary closing
    b) Typed name of the person authoring the letter
    c) Author's title follows author's name, separated by a comma
    d) Author signs name above the signature line
  3) Reference notation
    a) Placed two lines below the signature line
    b) Identifies the letter's author and the transcriber ("DH:lb" or "DH/lb"), with the author's initials in uppercase letters and the transcriber's initials in lowercase letters
    c) If the author types his or her own letter, no reference notation is necessary
  4) Enclosure notation
    a) Placed one or two blank lines below the reference notation (or signature line)
    b) Identifies any printed material accompanying the correspondence ("Enc:," "Enclosure:," "Enclosures:")
  5) Copy notation
    a) Placed one or two lines below enclosure notation
    b) Indicates that a copy of the correspondence, with any enclosures, was also forwarded to a third party ("cc: Rob David")
    c) If more than one third-party recipient exists, the recipients are listed alphabetically or in order of authority

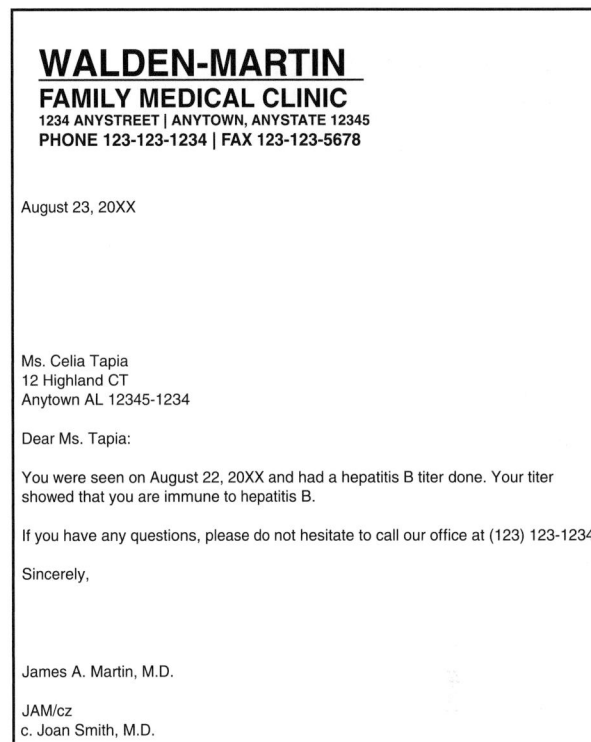

WALDEN-MARTIN
FAMILY MEDICAL CLINIC
1234 ANYSTREET | ANYTOWN, ANYSTATE 12345
PHONE 123-123-1234 | FAX 123-123-5678

August 23, 20XX

Ms. Celia Tapia
12 Highland CT
Anytown AL 12345-1234

Dear Ms. Tapia:

You were seen on August 22, 20XX and had a hepatitis B titer done. Your titer showed that you are immune to hepatitis B.

If you have any questions, please do not hesitate to call our office at (123) 123-1234.

Sincerely,

James A. Martin, M.D.

JAM/cz
c. Joan Smith, M.D.

Fig. 8.1 Block letter style. (From B. Niedzwiecki et al: *Kinn's The administrative medical assistant: an applied learning approach*, ed 14, 2020, Elsevier.)

d) Blind carbon copy ("bcc: Rob David") allows a short note to be typed on the copy to be sent to one-third party; the short note is placed only on the one copy of the letter that is sent to the blind carbon copy recipient

2. Letter styles
  a. Full block (Fig. 8.1)
    1) All lines begin flush at the left margin
    2) Most efficient style, although the least attractive on paper
  b. Modified block (Fig. 8.2): all lines begin flush at the left margin except for the dateline and the complimentary close (these two lines begin at the center of the page)
  c. Semiblock (Fig. 8.3): same as modified block except the beginning of each new paragraph of the body of the letter is indented five blank spaces
  d. Hanging indentation: same as the modified block except the first line of each new paragraph of the body of the letter is indented five blank spaces
  e. Simplified: same as the full block except that no salutation and no complimentary close are inserted

3. Margins
  a. Short letter (<100 words in the body): 2-inch margins
  b. Medium letter (100–200 words): 1½-inch margins
  c. Long letter (>200 words): 1-inch margins

4. Multiple pages
  a. Use plain paper in same stock (weight) as letterhead
  b. Type the recipient's name seven blank lines from the top of the page; type the page number one line below the recipient's name; type the current date one line below the page number

WALDEN-MARTIN
FAMILY MEDICAL CLINIC
1234 ANYSTREET | ANYTOWN, ANYSTATE 12345
PHONE 123-123-1234 | FAX 123-123-5678

August 23, 20XX

Ms. Celia Tapia
12 Highland CT
Anytown AL 12345-1234

Dear Ms. Tapia:

You were seen on August 22, 20XX and had a hepatitis B titer done. Your titer showed that you are immune to hepatitis B.

If you have any questions, please do not hesitate to call our office at (123) 123-1234.

Sincerely,

James A. Martin, M.D.

JAM/cz
c. Joan Smith, M.D.

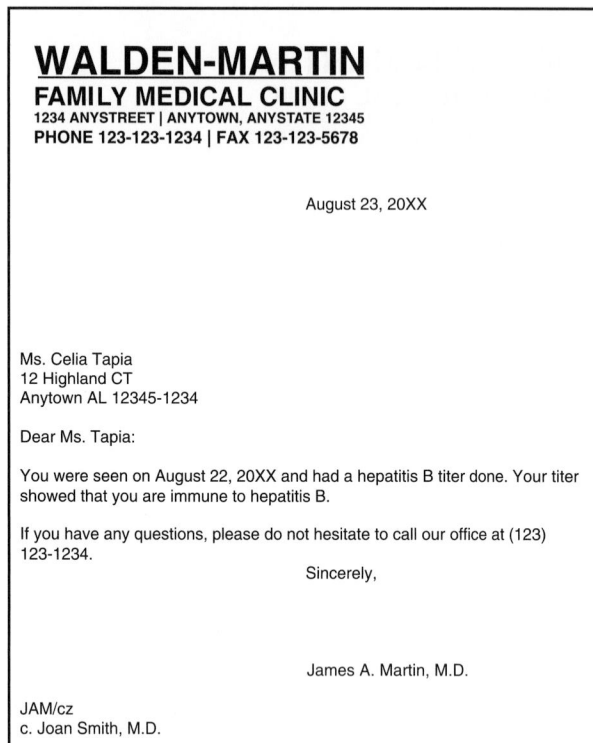

Fig. 8.2 Modified block letter style. (From Niedzwiecki B, et al: *Kinn's The administrative medical assistant: an applied learning approach*, ed 14, 2020, Elsevier.)

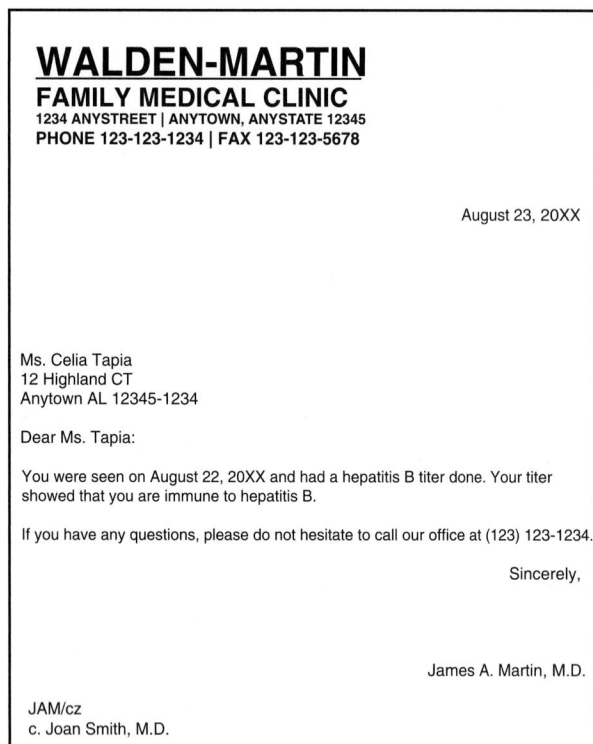

WALDEN-MARTIN
FAMILY MEDICAL CLINIC
1234 ANYSTREET | ANYTOWN, ANYSTATE 12345
PHONE 123-123-1234 | FAX 123-123-5678

August 23, 20XX

Ms. Celia Tapia
12 Highland CT
Anytown AL 12345-1234

Dear Ms. Tapia:

You were seen on August 22, 20XX and had a hepatitis B titer done. Your titer showed that you are immune to hepatitis B.

If you have any questions, please do not hesitate to call our office at (123) 123-1234.

Sincerely,

James A. Martin, M.D.

JAM/cz
c. Joan Smith, M.D.

Fig. 8.3 Modified block letter style with indented paragraphs. (From Niedzwiecki B, et al: *Kinn's The administrative medical assistant: an applied learning approach*, ed 14, St Louis, 2020, Elsevier.)

c. The body of the letter continues three blank lines below the page heading
d. The same page heading (with corresponding page number) on all subsequent pages

C. Envelopes

1. Sizes
   a. #6¾: 6½ × 3⅜ inches
   b. #10: 9½ × 4⅛ inches
2. Folding letters for insertion (Fig. 8.4)
   a. #6¾ envelope
      1) Fold the page in half, bottom up, and crease
      2) Fold the right one-third over the left and crease
      3) Fold the left one-third over the right and crease
      4) Insert the last-creased edge into the envelope first
   b. #10 envelope
      1) Fold the bottom one-third, bottom up, and crease
      2) Fold the top one-third, top down, and crease
      3) Insert the last-creased edge into the envelope first
3. Return address
   a. Place three blank lines from the top edge and five spaces from the left edge (if the return address is not preprinted on the envelope)
   b. Always place the complete return address on the envelope
4. Mailing address (Fig. 8.5)
   a. #6¾ envelope: place 2 inches down from the top edge and 2 inches to the right of the left edge
   b. #10 envelope: place 2 inches down from the top edge and 4 inches to the right of the left edge
   c. Type the address in block format; capitalize all letters; no punctuation used (copy the inside address from the letter to insert onto the envelope)
   d. Use standard two-letter state abbreviation
5. Notations
   a. Directed to the recipient ("Personal and Confidential"): place two blank lines below the return address
   b. Directed to the post office ("Special Delivery" or "Certified Mail"): capitalize all letters in upper-right side, below the area of stamp placement

D. Memoranda (Fig. 8.6)

1. Written communication within an office or organization
2. Use headings including TO, FROM, DATE, and SUBJECT; each office has a template to be used in all memoranda
3. Information pertaining to the headings should be on the same line and two or three spaces after the heading, separated by a colon
4. Message should begin three blank lines below the last line of the headings
5. Can have a reference notation and a copy notation (use the same format as for letters)

E. Meeting Agendas

1. Lists the specific items that will be discussed
2. Follows *Robert's Rules of Order*
3. Copies should be sent to all group members before the date

F. Meeting Minutes

1. Written record of what happened during a meeting
2. Should include
   a. What actions were taken
   b. Who made and seconded the motion

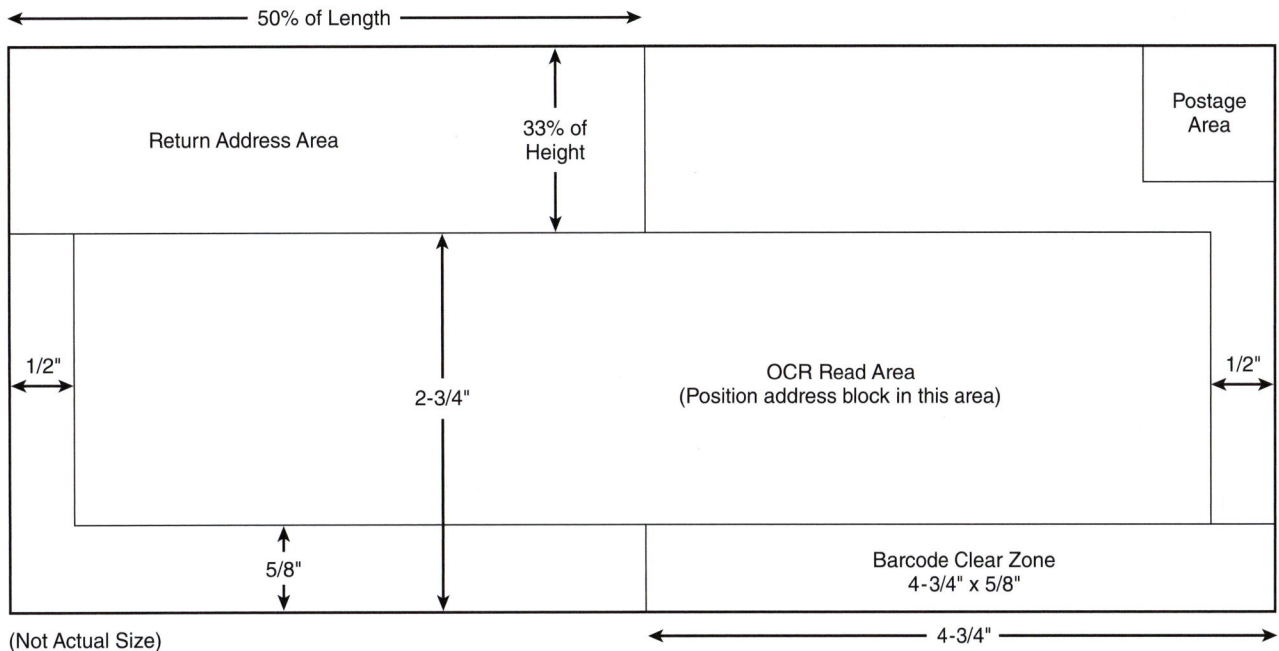

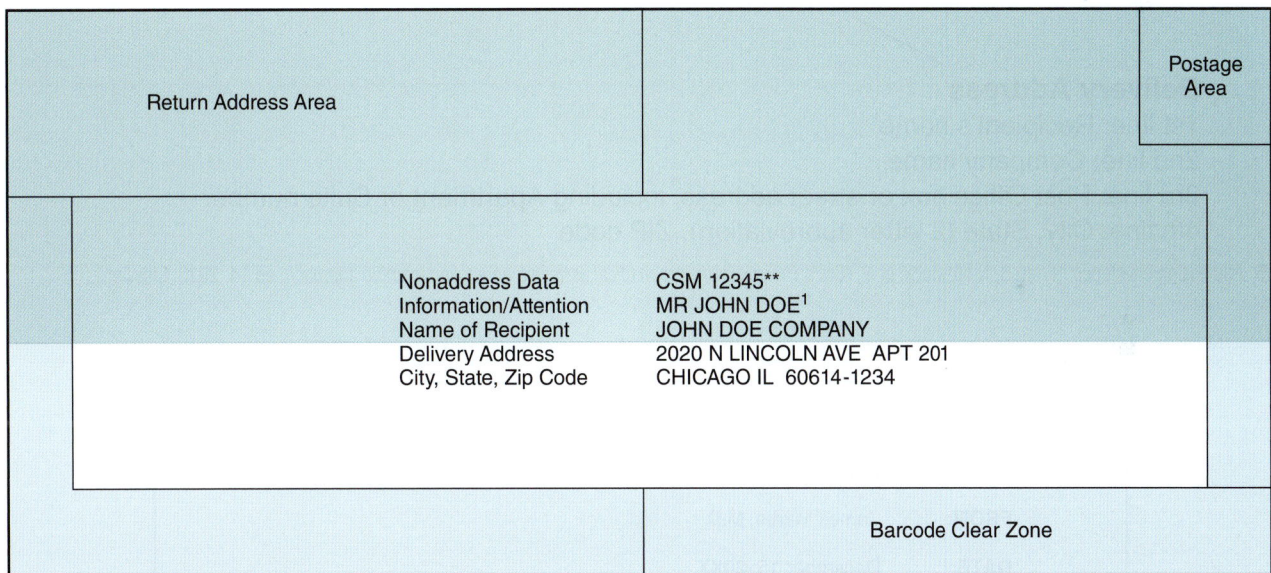

Fig. 8.4 Correct methods of folding letters.

c. Any discussion
d. Whether the motion was passed
3. Signed copies kept in a notebook

G. Manuscripts

1. Written document submitted for publication
2. Different professional organizations require different standard formats (template) for manuscript preparation and submission (each will forward its template on request)
3. Parts of a manuscript
    a. Title page
      1) Identifies the title or theme of the manuscript
      2) Title, author, and author's credentials are normally centered horizontally and vertically on the title page
    b. Acknowledgments
      1) Identifies persons who have assisted the author in research or preparation
      2) Placed on a separate page following the title page
    c. Abstract
      1) Summary of the manuscript, normally in 100–200 words
      2) Placed on the third page
    d. Text
      1) Title is typed, in capital letters, 13 lines from the top of page
      2) Body of the manuscript begins three blank lines below the title
      3) Text of the manuscript is double spaced
    e. References
      1) Identifies published works of others referenced within the text

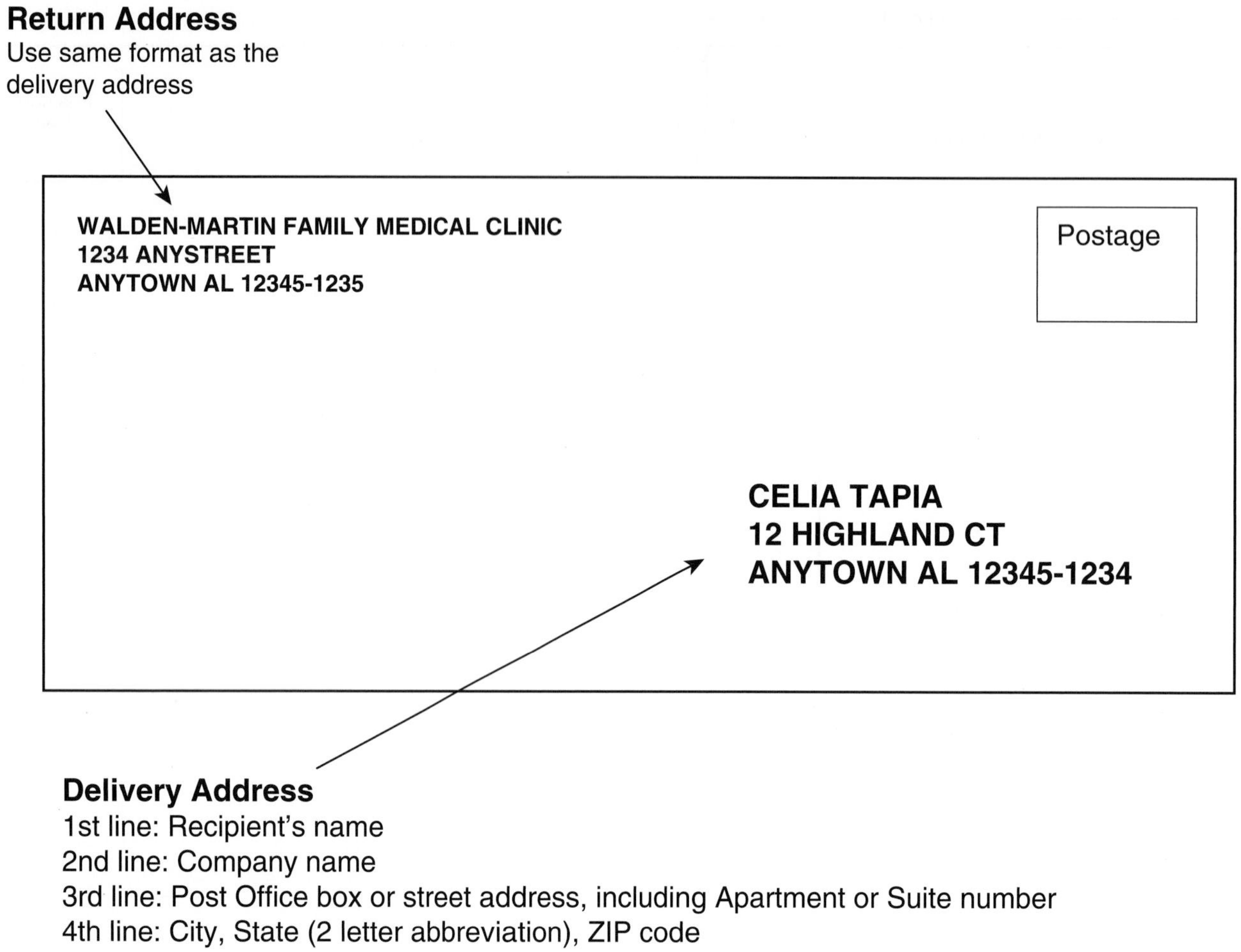

Return Address
Use same format as the
delivery address

WALDEN-MARTIN FAMILY MEDICAL CLINIC
1234 ANYSTREET
ANYTOWN AL 12345-1235

Postage

CELIA TAPIA
12 HIGHLAND CT
ANYTOWN AL 12345-1234

Delivery Address
1st line: Recipient's name
2nd line: Company name
3rd line: Post Office box or street address, including Apartment or Suite number
4th line: City, State (2 letter abbreviation), ZIP code

Fig. 8.5 Addressing envelopes. (From B. Niedzwiecki et al: *Kinn's The administrative medical assistant: an applied learning approach*, ed 14, 2020, Elsevier.)

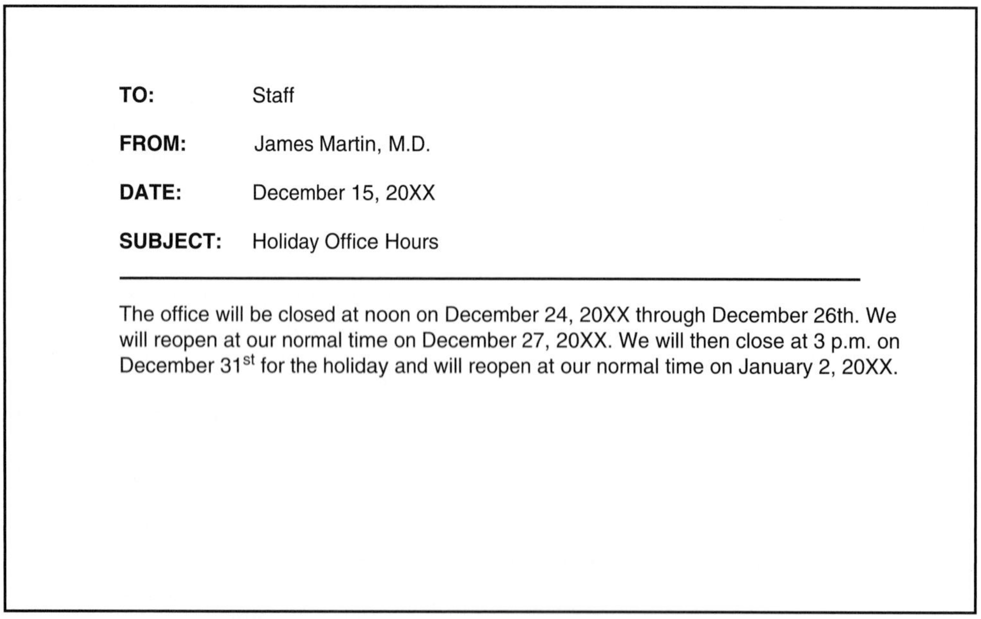

TO:	Staff
FROM:	James Martin, M.D.
DATE:	December 15, 20XX
SUBJECT:	Holiday Office Hours

The office will be closed at noon on December 24, 20XX through December 26th. We will reopen at our normal time on December 27, 20XX. We will then close at 3 p.m. on December 31st for the holiday and will reopen at our normal time on January 2, 20XX.

Fig. 8.6 Format for a memorandum. (From B. Niedzwiecki et al: *Kinn's The administrative medical assistant: an applied learning approach*, ed 14, 2020, Elsevier.)

2) In the final version, each reference is indicated by numerical superscripts or numbers in parentheses after each citation (depending on the style of the journal to which the manuscript is being submitted); references are listed in numerical order at the end of the manuscript

   f. Footnote: cites references and their explanations near the bottom of the page on which the referenced material is written

   g. Bibliography: list of reference books, manuscripts, articles, or other sources that were used to prepare the manuscript; listed in alphabetical order by name of document or by last name of document author

   h. Illustrations and tables: placed on separate sheets at the end of the manuscript and assigned consecutive numbers

H. E-mail

1. Electronic mail used for communication
2. Can be sent to more than one person at the same time
3. Should follow a format style; brief subject line; body contains short, clear sentences
4. Can be used to communicate with patients
   a. Used for communication that is not urgent
   b. Used to schedule appointments, send reminder notices, provide follow-up instructions, answer billing questions, refilling prescriptions
   c. E-mails from and to patients should be printed and filed in chart
   d. Used with patient permission
5. Not the most secure form of communication
   a. Confidentiality must be considered; privacy disclaimer

VI. Processing Mail

A. Mail Classifications

1. Priority Express mail, next-day service
   a. Available 7 days a week, 365 days a year
   b. Cost is normally one standard price per item
2. First class
   a. Sealed or unsealed material
   b. Includes letters, postcards, and business-reply mail
   c. Cost is based on weight (in 1-oz increments)
3. Priority mail
   a. First-class mail weighing more than 11 oz (maximum weight is 70 lb)
   b. Postage calculated on the combined basis of weight and destination
4. Second class
   a. Regular rates
   b. Available to newspapers and periodicals preauthorized by the post office

5. Third class
   a. Includes catalogs, circulars, books, photographs, and other preprinted materials
   b. Must be marked Third Class
6. Fourth class: merchandise, books, and preprinted material (media mail) not included in first or second class and weighing 16 oz or more
7. Registered mail
   a. First-class mail additionally protected by registration
   b. The post office receives an additional fee for this service
   c. The post office verifies delivery of the material
   d. The recipient may be required to sign a form to acknowledge receipt, if the sender requests
   e. The registered mail request form must be filled out before mailing
8. Certified mail
   a. Delivery of mail requiring the recipient's signature as proof of delivery
   b. Certified mail request form must be filled out before mailing
9. USPS Marketing Mail
   a. Used to send large quantities of mail

B. Equipment and Supplies

1. Postage scale: used to weigh mail to determine correct postage
2. Postage meter
   a. Machine used to print prepaid postage directly on the envelope or on an adhesive label, depending on the weight of the material
   b. The date and the amount of postage are set by pressing the appropriate buttons
3. Stationery
   a. Standard size and weight, as determined by the office manager
   b. Normally light-colored paper with darker imprinting
4. Rubber stamps
   a. Can indicate the date of receipt of mail
   b. Can be used to endorse checks for deposit

C. Incoming Mail

1. Schedule a set time during which to sort and distribute received mail
2. Date-stamp the front (or the back) of each piece of paper within each envelope and date-stamp the envelope, depending on the office method (except for checks)
3. "Personal" or "Personal and Confidential" noted mailings are delivered directly to the addressee without being opened
4. Any mail that is opened by mistake must be resealed with tape and noted on the envelope that it was opened by mistake
5. All checks received must be endorsed immediately and forwarded to the accounts receivable clerk

9

Records Management

I. Medical Record

A. General

1. The "chart"
2. Chronologic system used to annotate patient's medical care rendered by the health care provider
3. Ensures competent and necessary (nonredundant) medical care
4. Legal document
5. Two types
   a. Paper
   b. Electronic
      1) Incentive from the government to convert to electronic health record (EHR)

B. Purpose

1. Establishes the patient database
2. Serves as a communication link between the health care provider and the staff
3. Helps with the planning of effective patient care
4. Provides evidence of care given to the patient
5. Can provide data for research or education
6. Support for claims for reimbursement

C. Content

1. Specific to types of practice
2. Usually includes
   a. Chief complaint (CC): main reason for the patient seeking care
   b. Past medical history (PH or PMH): information regarding usual childhood diseases (UCD), past illnesses, surgeries, and current health status; may be prepared by the patient, by the health care provider, or by the medical assistant
   c. Family history (FH): information regarding the patient's parents and siblings; may include health status, age, cause of death, and hereditary diseases
   d. History of present illness: expanded CC
   e. Social history (SH): information on patient's personal habits; may include exercise, sleep, diet, tobacco and alcohol use, drug use, sexual history, sexual preference, and hobbies
   f. Occupational history (OH): information regarding patient's employment
   g. Physical examination (PE): complete physical examination; gives information regarding each body system (review of systems [ROS]); may serve as a baseline against the future
   h. Test results: diagnostic and laboratory tests; arranged with most recent at the top
   i. Consultations: reports on evaluations made by other health care providers
   j. Past medical records: records from other health care providers that have bearing on present treatment
   k. Correspondence: all correspondence related to patient care
   l. Progress notes: notes written in the chart by the health care provider regarding the patient's care, diagnosis, and treatment
   m. Medication and prescription record: record of all medications and prescriptions given or renewed in the office
   n. Immunization record: record of all immunizations administered in the office
   o. Consent forms: outline the details of procedures or treatments to be performed
   p. Release of information form: necessary for release of information for payment or transfer of information
   q. Patient registration record: demographic and billing information; placed in front of chart; may include copy of insurance card and photo identification

D. Organization

1. Source-oriented record
   a. Observations and data are categorized according to their source (health care provider, laboratory, radiography, nurse)
   b. Forms are filed in reverse chronologic order (most recent on top)
   c. Information is filed in separate sections (e.g., laboratory reports section, x-ray reports section, progress notes section, insurance section)
2. Problem-oriented medical record (POMR)
   a. Data are organized according to patient's disease or condition
   b. Divided into four parts
      1) Database: includes CC, HPI, PE findings, and laboratory results; each condition has its own page
      2) Problem list: numbered and titled list of every patient complaint; may include physical, psychological, and social problems related to the patient's condition
      3) Plan: diagnostic and treatment decisions for the condition; each plan is titled and numbered
      4) Progress notes: structured notes that correspond to each problem number; uses the acronyms SOAP, SOAPE, SOAPER, SOAPIE, or CHEDDAR
         a) SOAP
            (1) S (subjective data): signs, symptoms, and feelings that the patient describes in the patient's own words
            (2) O (objective data): clinical evidence that the health care provider determines
            (3) A (assessment = S + O): describes the physical impression and final diagnosis
            (4) P (plan = S + O + A): action needed to resolve the problem; may include treatment, medications, consultations, and surgery
         b) SOAPE: S + O + A + P + E (E: evaluation)
         c) SOAPER: S + O + A + P + E (education: any patient education presented) + R (response: how the patient is responding to care and education given)
         d) SOAPIE: S + O + A + P + I (intervention: what was done) + E (evaluation)
         e) CHEDDAR
            (1) C: chief complaint
            (2) H: history
            (3) E: examination
            (4) D: details (of problems and complaints)
            (5) D: drugs and dosages
            (6) A: assessment
            (7) R: return visit, if applicable

E. Documentation (Charting)

1. Process of making written entries into the medical record
2. Check the name on the chart before making an entry
3. Chart in black ink
4. Write in legible handwriting
5. Entry should be brief but contain all pertinent information
6. Spell and abbreviate correctly
7. All entries must be dated and initialed, or signed, by the health care provider making the entry
8. All patient visits and telephone calls must be documented
9. No-shows must be recorded
10. Patient's name should appear on each page
11. Corrections are made by using the SLIDE rule (Fig. 9.1)
    a. SL: single line through the error
    b. I: initials of the person correcting the error
    c. D: date and correct the error
    d. E: write the word *error*
12. Correspondence sent to the patient requires a note in the chart
13. Patient education noted in chart
14. Six "Cs" of charting
    a. Current
    b. Complete
    c. Concise
    d. Correct
    e. Confidential
    f. Clean
15. "If it was not charted, it was not done"

F. Legalities and the Medical Record

1. The chart is a legal document
2. The chart belongs to the health care provider or the clinic, but the patient controls the information found on the chart
3. Records that patients or third parties request may be released only if the health care provider and the patient give consent, usually by a written medical records release form
4. Records can be withheld from patients if the information can reasonably be expected to cause harm to the patient (doctrine of professional discretion)
5. Patient information is confidential and privileged (this patient confidentiality can be waived in writing by the patient or overruled in a courtroom)
6. Release of confidential patient information without the patient's written consent could lead to a charge of invasion of privacy by the patient

| 10/15/XX | error 10/15/XX ----- D. Bennett, CMA(AAMA)
9:30 a.m. T- 98.6, P-84 ~~and irregular~~, R-12, BP 118/80 Ⓛarm sitting, |
| | pulse is regular ---------------------------------- D. Bennett, CMA (AAMA) |

Fig. 9.1 Proper method of correcting an error in a patient's medical record (the SLIDE rule). (From Bonewit-West K, Hunt S: *Today's medical assistant: clinical and administrative procedures*, ed 4, 2021, Elsevier.)

7. Medical records must be kept up to date, complete, and accurate
8. Entries into medical records should be keyed into electronic record or written in black ink

G. Retention and Destruction of Medical Records

1. Records are filed according to three classifications
   a. Active: patients who are currently receiving treatment or have been seen within a time frame specified by the office
   b. Inactive: patients who have not been seen for 6 months or longer; become active when patient returns for care
   c. Closed: patients who have died, moved away, or terminated relationship with the practice
2. Purging
   a. Process of moving a file from active to inactive
   b. Ongoing process determined by date
3. Records are retained according to the requirements of each state's statutes; medical records are usually retained until the patient's death; records of Medicare and Medicaid patients are retained for 10 years
4. Before old records are destroyed, patients should be given opportunity to claim a copy
5. Medical records are destroyed by shredding or burning
6. Facility should keep a master list of all records that have been destroyed

H. Medical Transcription

1. Transforming written or dictated medical information into a permanent, accurate document
2. Document describes encounter between patient and provider
3. New technology has brought changes in medical transcription profession
4. Electronic medical record (EMR) allows recording directly into the record
5. Transcription may be outsourced at lower cost and with faster turnaround
6. Voice recognition software converts voice to text
7. Process divided into three stages
   a. Dictating into a dictation unit
   b. Listening to what has been dictated
   c. Keying dictated text to a printed document using correct format and required punctuation

II. Management of Paper Records

1. To classify, arrange, and store documents in an efficient, orderly, and accessible manner
   a. Records to be stored
      1) Medical records (charts)
      2) Financial records
      3) Patient correspondence
      4) Business records
      5) Research records
   b. Records can be stored as
      1) Hard (printed) copies of the records

2) Computer documents
3) Microfiche and microfilm

A. Equipment and Supplies for Records Management

1. Storage cabinet
   a. Vertical: file cabinet style
   b. Lateral: chest of drawers style
   c. Shelf: open or closed storage
2. Guides
   a. Plastic or cardboard dividers; permit grouping of similar type files
   b. Outguide: guide used to replace a file taken from the cabinet; enables technician to replace the file in the proper place when ready
3. Folders
   a. Cardboard or plastic holders that contain the patients' medical records
   b. Have tabs within them for separating contents
4. Labels
   a. Small stickers placed onto folders to identify the contents or folder identity

B. Filing Process

1. Condition
   a. Check for damage and, if found, repair it before refiling the record
   b. Remove all pins, paper clip, and brads
   c. Staple related papers together; attach small items to a regular size sheet with tape or rubber cement
   d. Date your work on the record, if required
2. Inspect and release
   a. Documents cannot be filed until the responsible parties have seen the document and have taken action on the record
   b. Release mark of some sort (office protocol) must be noted on the file
3. Index and code
   a. Determine where the document should be filed
   b. Identify the caption to be used in filing the document
   c. Every paper placed in the patient's record should have the date and patient's name on it
4. Sort
   a. Arrange the documents according to the office protocol (system) used
5. Store
   a. Place the documents in the appropriate file folder and place in the filing cabinet

C. Filing Methods

1. Alphabetical
   a. Used with names of persons, businesses, or organizations; oldest, simplest, and most commonly used method
   b. Indexing rules
      1) Names are divided into units and filed left to right
      2) Surname is unit 1, given name is unit 2, and middle name (initial) is unit 3

3) Names are alphabetized according to first unit letter; second unit considered if first units are the same; third unit considered if first two units are the same
4) Initials filed before complete names starting with the same letter
5) Units having no name filed before those that do (nothing before something)
6) Hyphenated name is considered a single unit; if business name, each name is a separate unit
7) Apostrophes are disregarded
8) Abbreviations are indexed as if written in full
9) Numbers as part of a name are indexed as if written out
10) Titles and degrees are indexed last
11) Married women are indexed by their own given name (first name)
12) If two names are identical, patient's address is used as an index unit
13) For names of organizations
   a) Index in order as written except when organization name includes a person's name (surname first, then given name)
   b) Numbers are indexed as if written out
   c) Disregard punctuation
   d) Directional terms are indexed as separate units
   e) Articles, conjunctions, and prepositions are disregarded unless *the* is the first word (if so, *the* is indexed as the last unit)

2. Numerical
   a. Used when each patient is assigned a number that is used on the patient's chart
   b. Patient number is cross-referenced with the patient's name and filed alphabetically
   c. Numerical filing is used in large clinics, group practices, and hospitals
   d. Types
      1) Consecutive numerical system
         a) Simplest system
         b) Patients are assigned consecutive numbers in the order of the date of their first visit to the facility
      2) Terminal digit system
         a) Patients assigned consecutive numbers as they visit the facility
         b) Digits in the patient number are separated into groups of two or three
         c) Read in groups from right to left, instead of left to right, and filed backward in groups

3. Subject
   a. Documents indexed by subject matter and filed alphabetically, numerically, or both
   b. Generally not used for medical records

4. Color coding
   a. Colored tabs are used to represent patient information at a glance
   b. Used on letters of the patient's surname
   c. Can help keep files from being misfiled
   d. Selection of colors and division of the alphabet are determined by the needs of the practice
   e. Can be used as colored folders, adhesive labels, or a combination
   f. Can be filed alphabetically or numerically

5. Tickler file
   a. System that organizes items chronologically for follow-up
   b. Can be notations on the daily calendar or a card file divided into months, with months divided into days
   c. To be effective, must be checked daily

III. The Electronic Medical Record

A. General

1. Computerized record of important health information of a patient
2. Provides interaction with all divisions of the medical office (Fig. 9.2)
3. Complete record is stored on hard drive of the computer
4. EMR software allows for creation, storage, organization, editing, and retrieval of medical records on a computer
5. Linked to practice management software to facilitate administrative tasks (billing and insurance)
6. Mandated by President George W. Bush to promote interoperability of health records: American Recovery and Reinvestment Act of 2009 (ARRA) signed into law in 2009; sections that pertain to health care are known as the Health Information Technology for Economic and Clinical Health Act (HITECH Act)
7. Interoperable: able to work with another system
8. End goal: provide high-quality and efficient care to patients
9. Information is entered during or immediately after each patient interaction
10. Paper reports or records are scanned into the record as soon as possible; originals are shredded
11. Password protected; access should be limited to the information a staff member needs to view
12. Signatures are taken electronically (electronic signature)
13. EMRs should be backed up regularly and securely

B. Terminology Related to Electronic Records

1. EHR
   a. Electronic record of health-related information about a patient
   b. Conforms to recognized standards for interoperability
   c. Created and managed by authorized staff from more than one health care organization
2. EMR
   a. Electronic record of health-related information about a patient
   b. Created, gathered, and managed by authorized staff within a single health care organization
3. Personal health record (PHR)
   a. Electronic record of health-related information about a patient
   b. Conforms to national standards for interoperability
   c. Managed, shared, and controlled by the individual

C. Advantages of EMRs

1. Speed and productivity
   a. Documents can be retrieved quickly

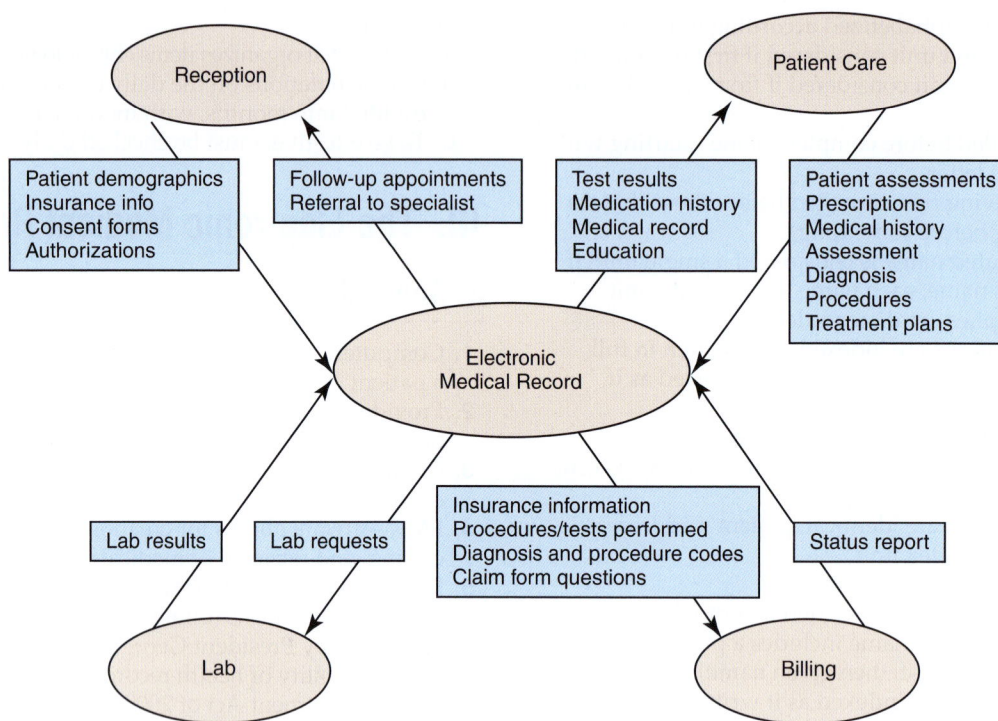

Fig. 9.2 Electronic medical record interacts with every part of the medical office.

b. Documents do not need to be filed
c. Frees up space
   1) Saves paper costs
2. Efficiency
   a. Facilitates entry of data
   b. Uses checkboxes and drop-down lists
   c. Can scan handouts and forms
   d. Can generate prescriptions
   e. Allows various statistical information to be recalled
3. Accessibility
   a. Ready access to the record
   b. Available at any workstation
   c. Information can be accessed through smartphone or personal digital assistant (PDA)
4. Reduction in errors
   a. Keeps prescriptions, allergies, and other information organized
5. Legibility
   a. Computer keyboard used to enter information
6. Security
   a. User names and passwords required for entrance into the system

D. Disadvantages of EMRs

1. Initial and maintenance costs
   a. Cost of hardware and software
   b. Upgrade of EMR software
2. Time investment for training
3. Operational tasks
   a. Older records need to be scanned into electronic record
4. Extensive training
5. Space for equipment
6. Security and confidentiality

IV. Capabilities of EMR Systems

A. Specialty Software

1. Terminology and patient care treatments compatible to provider's specialty

B. Appointment Scheduler

1. Allows staff to schedule and track appointments (Fig. 9.3)
2. Matrix the schedule

C. Appointment Reminder

1. System can be programmed to initiate reminder and confirmation calls to patient

D. Prescription Writer

1. Produce electronic prescriptions
2. Lists can be created with provider's medication choices and dosages
3. Allergy function can block what a patient cannot take

E. Billing System

1. Program can interface with clearing houses for electronic claims submission

F. Charges

1. Can store lists of billing codes (International Classification of Diseases [ICD] and Current Procedural Terminology [CPT])

	Sun 5/31	Mon 6/1	Tue 6/2	Wed 6/3	Thu 6/4	Fri 6/5	Sat 6/6
8am	**Other** All Staff						**Other** All Staff
9am						**Staff Meeting** All Staff	
10am				**Willis, Erma I** Jean Burke, NP Physical Exam			
11am				**Tran, Truong K** Jean Burke NP **Siever, Mora V** Jean Burke, NP High blood p **Rodriguez, N** Jean Burke NP **Yan, Tail** Jean Burke NP			
12pm		**Lunch** All Staff	**Lunch** All Staff	**Lunch** All Staff	**Lunch** All Staff **Pharmaceutic** All Staff	**Lunch** All Staff	
1pm							

Fig. 9.3 Appointment schedule form SimChart for the Medical Office.

G. Insurance Eligibility Verification

1. Allows provider to confirm patient's insurance benefits
2. Facilitates communication between provider and insurance company

H. Referral Management

1. Coordinate and automate patient information with another physician
2. Allows for records to be sent to referral

I. Laboratory Order Integration

1. Allows for interaction with outside laboratories to order tests and post results

J. Patient Portal

1. Allows patients to access medical records, make appointments, print immunization records, review billing statement, and complete new patient registration
2. Allows patients to communicate with health care team
3. Allows patients to request medication refills

V. EMR Documents

A. Administrative Documents: Efficient Management of the Office

1. Patient registration record
   a. Demographic and billing information
   b. Patient completes paper form; data are entered into record; paper form is shredded
   c. Patient may be asked to enter information
2. Privacy policy (Notice of Privacy Practices [NPP]) acknowledgment form
   a. Written document that explains how protected health information (PHI) will be used and protected by the office
   b. Patient signs form acknowledging receipt of form
   c. Form scanned into record

3. Correspondence
   a. Transferred directly into record if in digital format
   b. Must be scanned into record if in paper format

B. Clinical Documents: Assist the Provider in Care and Treatment of Patient

1. Health history report
   a. Patient may complete paper form; data are entered into record; form is shredded
   b. Medical assistant may enter data directly into the record while interviewing patient
2. PE report
   a. Provider may enter data by free-text entry, drop-down lists, or checkboxes
   b. EMR program generates PE report from information entered
3. Progress notes
   a. Provider or medical assistant enters information directly into the record by free-text entry, drop-down lists, or checkboxes
   b. Updated at every visit

4. Medication record
   a. Medical assistant enters information into the record at each visit (Fig. 9.4)
   b. EMR program includes prescription program, which can generate and print prescriptions or transmit prescriptions electronically to patient's pharmacy
5. Consultation report
   a. Electronic letters are transferred into record
   b. Paper format is scanned into record and then shredded
6. Laboratory documents
   a. Requisitions are completed on the computer screen using fill-in boxes, drop-down lists, or checkboxes; transmitted electronically to laboratory
   b. When tests are completed, results sent electronically to office; EMR program receives the information and puts it in patient's chart
   c. Copy of laboratory results sent to provider's "review bin" for electronic signature
   d. Abnormal values are highlighted
7. Diagnostic procedures
   a. Procedures reports from outside facility sent electronically to office and stored in patient's record

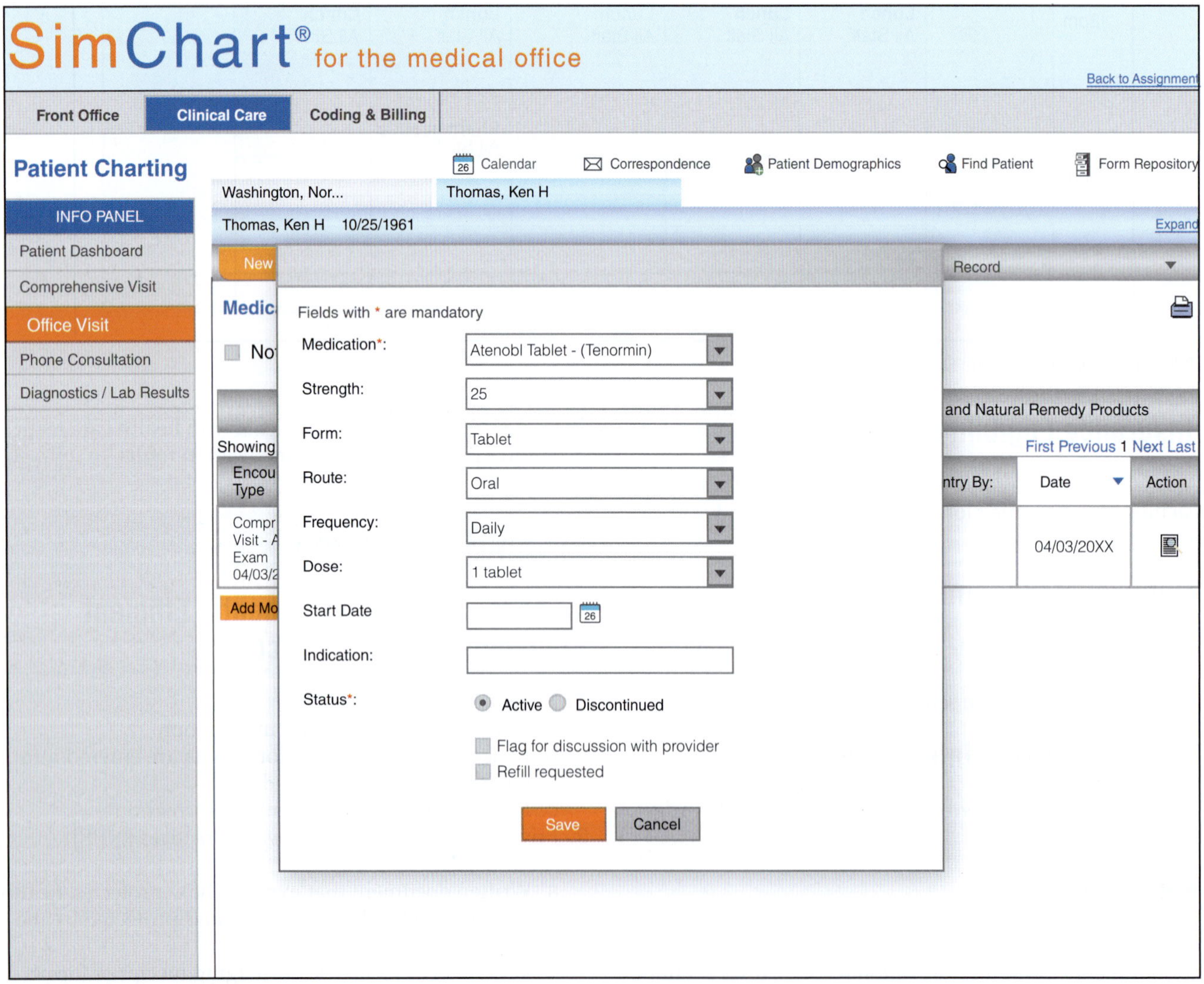

Fig. 9.4 Adding a medication in SimChart for the Medical Office.

b. Paper forms must be scanned and transferred into record
c. Images of procedure (x-ray, MRI, ECG, CT scan) can be stored in record as a digital image
d. If procedure is performed in office, diagnostic equipment must be linked to office computer system

8. Hospital document
   a. Includes any care of patient at a hospital including emergency department
   b. Electronic format is transferred into record
   c. Paper records must be scanned and shredded

9. Consent forms
   a. Legal documents required for care and to release information
   b. Patient signs paper form; scanned into record

VI. Use of EMR by Medical Assistant

A. General

1. Select patient being seen and enter information
2. Functions
   a. Access of daily schedule
   b. Patient selection
   c. Time of check-in
   d. Examination room number
   e. Chief complaint
   f. Review of patient history
   g. Enter or review allergies
   h. Enter or review current medications
   i. Enter vital signs
   j. Enter height and weight
   k. Enter test results (vision screening, hearing screening)
   l. Enter results of laboratory tests performed in office (e.g., urinalysis, strep throat)
   m. Enter administration of medications, immunizations (Fig. 9.5)
3. Making corrections and additions
   a. Additions require new entry
   b. Never delete a previous entry or change it; new entry must be made to correct it
4. Nonverbal communication
   a. Medical assistant must ensure nonverbal communication sends the right message when using the EMR

b. Eye contact is important; patient may feel alienated if medical assistant is looking at computer screen
c. Do not hide information from patient
d. Modify position at computer screen so patient feels like he or she is a part of the process

VII. Security of Network

A. Authentication

1. Each worker must have password to log in to access

B. Levels of Authorization

1. Certain functions are available only to users with the correct level of authorization

C. Automatic Logoff

1. All users should log off if workstation unattended
2. Software feature automatically logs off use after predetermined period of no activity

D. Antivirus Software

1. After installation, operates in background and monitors all files for viruses

E. Firewall

1. System that protects network from unauthorized access by users on its own network or another network

F. Backup

1. Allows office to function if system goes down
2. Duplicate copy of data
3. Should be done daily
4. Several methods
   a. External hard drive: connects to main computer; stores information on CD, DVD, or thumb drive
   b. Full server backup: large capacity server used only for EMR systems
   c. Online backup: subscription fee

| Zoster (Shingles) ⓘ | 1 | HZV ▼ | 0.65mL | 04/25/201 📅 26 | Willis | LA subcu | 656858/0 | 06/16 | None | 📝 |

Fig. 9.5 Administration of immunization in SimChart for the Medical Office.

10

Patient Reception and Appointment Scheduling

I. Reception

A. General

1. Patient's first impression of the health care provider's office
2. Influences patient's perception of the office
3. Receptionist's attitude and appearance are important to set the tone of the office

II. Reception Area

A. General

1. Place to receive patients
2. Planned for patient comfort
3. Should be clean and uncluttered
4. Receptionist should be behind a counter that is high enough for health care provider privacy (e.g., of hard records, of patient information on computer screens, of patient financial records)
5. Colors should be calming and restful
6. Lighting should be adequate for reading and safety
7. Adequate ventilation is essential
8. Temperature should be regulated for patient comfort (average 72°F)
9. Play area for children, if appropriate
10. Spacious coat rack to store patients' outerwear
11. Furniture arranged for patient comfort, movement, and safety
12. Periodicals should be up to date and appropriate
13. Accessibility to all patients under Americans with Disabilities Act

III. Receptionist

A. General

1. First professional person with whom the patient comes in contact, either in person or by telephone
2. Medical assistant should display pride in himself or herself and the job
3. Communication skills should demonstrate competence and a positive attitude
4. Clothing, hair, and makeup should be appropriate; follow office policies
5. Should have friendly, cheerful, caring, courteous, and respectful demeanor
6. Should be professional at all times
7. Try to greet every patient on arrival by name (using correct pronunciation); if not, a smile
8. A friendly farewell can show caring and courtesy
9. Duties may include
   a. Answering telephones
   b. Scheduling appointments
   c. Registering patient and taking history
   d. Handling complaints
   e. Preparing charts
   f. Handling nonpatient visitors (vendors, sales representatives, pharmaceutical representatives)

B. Opening the Office

1. Turn lights on; unlock and open doors; turn on equipment
2. Check telephone messages, office email messages; check for received faxes
3. Make sure charts are prepared for current day's patients
4. Check offices and waiting area for cleanliness

C. Closing the Office

1. Reverse morning activities
2. Prepare bank deposit slip
3. Back up a copy of the computer system's hard drive
4. Turn on telephone answering machine
5. Close and lock exterior doors

IV. Telecommunications

A. General

1. Most of receptionist's communication occurs through the telephone
2. Telephone is a crucial component of a successful health care provider's practice
3. Communication and listening skills are important
4. Incoming telephone calls may include
   a. Established patients calling for appointments or advice
   b. Patient emergencies
   c. Other physicians making patient referrals
   d. Laboratories reporting information regarding a patient
   e. New patients making a first contact
5. Telecommunication devices for the deaf

B. Equipment

1. Multiline telephone
   a. Several incoming lines
   b. Office intercom line
   c. Hold button
   d. Lights flash slowly for incoming calls, flash rapidly for reminder for calls on hold
2. Two-line speakerphone
   a. Allows conversation without using the handset
   b. Last number redial
   c. Volume control
   d. Speed dial and memory for frequent calls
   e. Intercom paging
   f. May have liquid crystal display (LCD) screen
3. Headset
   a. Lightweight plastic earphone and microphone combination
   b. Allows hands-free telephone use
4. Cellular telephone, smartphone
   a. Mobile, transportable telephone
   b. Permits communication outside an office or within a vehicle
5. Pager
   a. Activated by calling the pager number
   b. Can leave a voice message or digital message
6. Laptop, tablet, smartphone, scanner
   a. Used for the transmission of electronic health records
7. Email
   a. Method of composing, sending, and receiving messages over the Internet
   b. Files can be attached
8. Facsimile (fax) machine
   a. Transmits print material over telephone lines to other facilities that have fax capability
   b. Can send and receive copies of printed documents
   c. If sending sensitive patient information, call ahead to ensure that only the appropriate person receives the fax
9. Directories
   a. White pages: alphabetical listing by last name, includes last name, first name, sometimes middle initial, address, and telephone number
   b. Yellow pages: alphabetical listing by category of commercial business; in each category, alphabetical listing by company name (or businessperson's last name), includes company name (or businessperson's name), company address, and company telephone number or numbers
   c. Online directories: directory services available on the computer
   d. Personal office directory: collection of frequently called telephone numbers within an office; can be stored in a Rolodex or in a 3 × 5 index card file
   e. Computerized directory: program that can hold names, information, and telephone numbers to access patients, providers, vendors, laboratories, and referrals; many programs available

C. Incoming Calls

1. Answer promptly (ideally on the first ring, always by the third ring)
2. Hold the telephone instrument correctly (with the mouthpiece approximately 1 inch from your mouth)
3. Develop a pleasing telephone voice
4. Identify the health care provider's office; identify yourself
5. Obtain the identity of the caller (ask to whom you are speaking if the caller does not first identify himself or herself)
6. Offer assistance (using proper words and proper tone)
7. Screen incoming calls (follow any office policies about how incoming calls are to be handled and categorized)
8. Minimize caller waiting time (caller should experience a wait of no more than 1 minute without voice contact of some type)
9. When answering a second call, ask the first caller to please hold, transfer to the second incoming line, identify the second caller, ask the second caller to please hold, and return to the first caller
10. End each call pleasantly and graciously (say "thank you" and some form of "good-bye")

D. Telephone Messages

1. May be recorded on message sheet or in an office telephone log
2. Message should include the following information
   a. Name of the person to whom the call is directed
   b. Name of the person calling
   c. Caller's daytime telephone number (include pager and cellular telephone numbers as appropriate)
   d. Reason for the call, giving specific details
   e. Action to be taken by the recipient
   f. Date and time call was received
   g. Initials of the person taking the call

E. Calls Referred to the Provider

1. Other providers
2. STAT reports
3. Provider's family

F. Outgoing Telephone Calls

1. Know what needs to be said and how it is to be said, and have all pertinent information on hand before placing the call
2. Voice should convey warmth, friendliness, confidence, and intelligence
3. Address the person by name
4. Use "please" and "thank you"
5. Do not rush call
6. Use discretion when conveying personal or confidential patient or medical information
7. Long distance (check with office manager to verify this procedure because different long-distance carriers have different calling requirements)
   a. Direct dial: 1 + area code + 7-digit telephone number
   b. Long-distance directory assistance: 1 + area code + 555-1212
   c. Operator assisted: 0 + area code + 7-digit telephone number
      1) Person to person (operator will not connect the line until the person to whom you requested answers the telephone)
      2) Station to station (operator will connect the line as soon as anyone at the receiving telephone number answers the telephone)
      3) Collect call (operator will not connect the line until a recipient agrees to be billed for the long-distance telephone call)
      4) Bill to third party (operator verifies that a third party [someone not a party to this long-distance telephone call] will accept the charges for the call)
      5) Request for time and charges (the operator, if asked before connecting the long-distance line, will call you back after the call is ended and will tell you the time of the long-distance call as well as the cost of the call; you will then be able to verify the long-distance charge against the next telephone bill)
   d. Time zones
      1) Pacific Standard Time: 1:00 (WA, OR, NV, CA)
      2) Mountain Standard Time: 2:00 (MT, UT, ID, WY, CO, NM, AZ; parts of ND, SD, NE, KS)
      3) Central Standard Time: 3:00 (MN, WI, IA, MO, AR, OK, TX, LA, MS, IL, AL; parts of TN, KY, ND, SD, NE, KS)
      4) Eastern Standard Time: 4:00 (all other states, except for HI and AK)
   e. Wrong number dialed
      1) Verify the telephone number with the person answering
      2) Apologize
      3) If long distance, call the operator to credit the office account

G. Answering Services

1. Health care provider must be able to be contacted at all times to respond to emergencies (to prevent abandonment charges)
2. Answering services
   a. Provides coverage when the office is closed
   b. Answering services answer and screen incoming telephone calls
3. Electronic answering devices
   a. Recorded message that tells the caller how to reach the health care provider (or health care provider's colleague) or invites the caller to leave a voice message
   b. Messages can be retrieved directly from the machine or can be remotely accessed
   c. Answering message may be changed as necessary
4. Voice mail: computerized system used to record, send, or retrieve voice message from the telephone system
5. Automatic routing
   a. Telephone calls answered by automated operator that announces a list of options from which the caller selects one
   b. This system is impersonal but may be good for the larger clinic

V. Appointment Scheduling

A. General

1. Process that determines which patients will be seen by the health care provider (appointment), the dates and times for the appointments, and the allotted time for each appointment
2. Allotted time for each appointment is based on the patient's complaint and the health care provider's availability
3. Important factor in the success of health care provider's practice
4. Can be done manually (appointment book) or electronically (practice software)

B. Guidelines

1. Understand the nature of the practice
2. Know the personalities and habits of the medical staff
3. Be aware of the time needed to assess each patient complaint type
4. Plan realistically

C. Materials Needed (Manual)

1. Appointment book (Fig. 10.1)
   a. May be for one or several health care providers
   b. May show day, week, or month per page
   c. May be blank or preprinted
   d. May be loose leaf or spiral bound
   e. Each block of time must have sufficient space to record the patient's name, the patient's telephone numbers, and the purpose of patient's visit to the health care provider

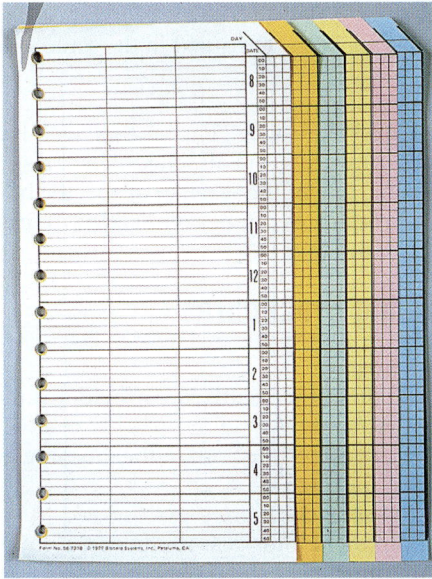

Fig. 10.1 Appointment matrix. (From Niedzwiecki B, et al: *Kinn's The administrative medical assistant: an applied learning approach*, ed 14, 2020, Elsevier.)

f. Entire book must fit comfortably on the receptionist's desk and be easily accessible to all who are responsible for scheduling; the book must always be left in place

g. Appointment book is a legal document and must be preserved as such

2. Pencil

  a. Use of a pencil is more practical than a pen in anticipation of any appointment changes or cancellations

  b. Colored ink (or pencil) may be used to denote new or special patient

3. Appointment card

  a. Given to each patient after the follow-up appointment is made in the office

  b. Often preprinted with the clinic name, address, and telephone number, with space on the card for date, day, and time of appointment and patient name

D. Computer Scheduling (Fig. 10.2)

1. Appointment intervals can be programmed in, depending on practice needs

WALDEN-MARTIN Family Medical Clinic

James Martin, MD
Schedule for May 30, 20XX

Time	Name	Reason	Home Phone	Work Phone
9:00 AM	ROBERT RICIGLIANO	Physical exam	(123) 459-2811	(123) 459-7218
9:15 AM	*****************************			
9:30 AM	*****************************			
9:45 AM	JUNE ST. JAMES	BP & ECG	(123) 123-5807	(123) 123-9222
10:00 AM	DARLA SISSLE	Influenza vaccine	(123) 268-1156	
10:15 AM	NORMA WASHINGTON	Recheck	(123) 754-4685	
10:30 AM	Catch-up			
10:45 AM	ESTELLE JORDAN	New patient	(123) 459-8249	(123) 459-0419
11:00 AM	*****************************			
11:15 AM	*****************************			
11:30 AM	ROBIN SOTO	Well-baby check	(123) 459-1349	
11:45 AM	*****************************			
12:00 PM	Lunch			
12:15 PM	*****************************			
12:30 PM	*****************************			
12:45 PM	*****************************			
1:00 PM	CELIA TAPIA	Recheck	(123) 858-1545	(123) 858-6603
1:15 PM	THOMAS MAXWELL	Recheck	(123) 459-4123	(123) 459-1062
1:30 PM	LUCILLE MORENA	School physical exam	(123) 268-6677	
1:45 PM	*****************************			
2:00 PM	LLOYD RIDLON	Recheck	(123) 220-4242	(123) 220-0419

Fig. 10.2 Sample computer appointment schedule. (From Bonewit-West K, Hunt S: *Today's medical assistant: clinical and administrative procedures*, ed 4, 2021, Elsevier.)

2. Ability to add, delete, or change appointments easily
3. Patient appointment entered into the data entry screen
4. Daily schedule can be printed out

E. Daily Appointment Schedule

1. List of patients to be seen for the day
2. Contains patient's name, telephone number, and reason for visit
3. Following Health Insurance Portability and Accountability Act (HIPAA) guidelines, daily schedule must be posted in an area inaccessible to patients
4. Legal document

F. Types of Scheduling

1. Open-office hours (open booking)
   a. Clinic is open only for a specified time period
   b. Patients are seen in the order of their arrival in the clinic (patients sign into a logbook on arrival), with provision that emergency treatment is given priority
   c. Least efficient method of scheduling
   d. Common among urgent care centers
   e. Triage: used to screen and classify sick or injured patients for priority
2. Flexible office hours
   a. Clinic is open additional hours besides normal office hours (e.g., early morning or evening hours on certain days of the week)
   b. Accommodates various work schedules of patients
   c. Usually used in group practices
3. Time-specified (stream) scheduling
   a. Most common system
   b. Each patient is given a specific time on a specific day for the appointment; time allotted depends on the reason for the visit
   c. Does not easily accommodate sudden illnesses or accidents and does not allow any buffer time (unless one or two open appointments each day are kept for such use)
4. Wave scheduling
   a. Gives short-term flexibility within each hour
   b. Assumes that the time needed for each appointment will average out over the course of the day
   c. Each hour is divided into the average time the health care provider should spend with each patient (i.e., hour divided into 10-minute, 15-minute, or 20-minute blocks)
   d. Patients are scheduled on the hour (e.g., 6 per hour for 10-minute block, 4 per hour for 15-minute block) and are seen by the health care provider in the order in which they sign in with the receptionist
   e. This system allows for late arrivals, patients whose accident or illness needs more (or less) time than the average, failed appointments ("no-shows"), and unscheduled interruptions of the health care provider
   f. Variable waiting times may result from this method of scheduling
5. Modified wave: appointments are staggered throughout the health care provider's hour
6. Double booking
   a. Scheduling two patients at the same time
   b. Not an efficient way to schedule
   c. Can be wave like if two patients each needing 5 minutes are both scheduled in the same 15-minute block
7. Grouping (clustering)
   a. Similar procedures (e.g., Pap smears, well-baby checks, complete physicals) are all scheduled at a specific time of a specific day of the week or at specific hours
   b. Similar procedures can be color coded for ease of viewing

G. Scheduling Procedures

1. Establish a matrix
   a. Block out times the health care provider is unavailable for appointments
   b. Establish a buffer time both in the morning and in the afternoon for catch-up
   c. Takes into consideration
      1) Appointment intervals: 10-minute, 15-minute, or 20-minute blocks
      2) Physician needs: time out of office, lunch, meetings, or rounds
      3) Facility or equipment requirements: availability of rooms or equipment for procedures
2. Chief complaint
   a. Identify the reason for the patient visit
   b. Identify the level of urgency of the patient visit
   c. Identify the health care provider resources available
3. Referral: determine whether the patient has been referred by another health care provider
4. Locate the first available time to see the patient and one alternative time; offer the dates and times to the patient
5. Enter the patient's name, telephone numbers, and complaint in the appointment book in the corresponding date and time block agreed to by the patient
6. Explain the pertinent office policies and instructions to the patient
7. Repeat the date and time to the patient for double-check before ending the call

H. Appointment Problems

1. Patient habitually late: schedule this patient near the end of the day
2. Consecutive appointments: schedule at the same time and day (different dates) for ease of remembering
3. Cancellations: offer the patient an alternative appointment
4. Missed appointment and no-show
   a. Prevent with a reminder telephone call the day before the appointment
   b. Patient may legally be charged for the missed appointment
   c. Patient may be discharged from health care provider's care for habitual no-shows
   d. Note all missed appointments in both the patient's chart and the appointment book
5. Emergencies
   a. Follow office protocol
   b. Emergencies take precedence over all other appointments
   c. Call 911 if the emergency is outside of the office protocol

6. Acute needs
   a. Provide the first available appointment to patient
   b. Double booking may be necessary
7. Referrals
   a. Process of sending patient to another health care provider (a specialist) for diagnosis and treatment
   b. Appointment may be made by the patient or by the referring health care provider
   c. Make sure all appropriate documents are provided to the referred health care provider (i.e., necessary patient records, x-rays, insurance referral letter)
8. Delays
   a. Attempt to call affected patients about health care provider delays, and request that they come later that day or reschedule for another date and time
   b. Explain courteously if the health care provider is called out of the office on an emergency
   c. Waiting patients should be given an explanation, an estimated time of the current delay, and the option to wait on the health care provider or reschedule

I. Computerized Appointments

1. Software varies from simple to complex
2. Offer great flexibility
3. System searches provider's schedule to locate available time
4. Schedule can be printed
5. More than one person can access the system at one time
6. Backup system should be in place (appointment book)

J. Self-Scheduling

1. Method by which a patient can log on to the Internet, view a facility's schedule, and make an appointment
2. Confidentiality is provided by showing only times available, not names
3. Can reduce number of calls to office
4. Available 24 hours a day
5. Best used for uncomplicated appointments
6. Allowances must be made for patients who do not have a computer, are computer illiterate, or do not want their name posted on the Internet

K. Scheduling Other Types of Appointments

1. Inpatient surgery
   a. Call facility where procedure will be performed as soon as the operation is planned
   b. Provide all necessary information, including special requests of the surgeon
   c. Provide patient's insurance information and telephone number
2. Outpatient and inpatient procedures
   a. Include laboratory, radiography, magnetic resonance imaging, computed tomography scans, and ultrasonography appointments
   b. Make sure all necessary information is available
   c. Inform the patient of time, place, and any instructions; note this information in the chart
   d. Must coordinate with the hospital instead of an outside facility

11

Office Management

I. Ambulatory Healthcare Settings

A. Individual Practices

1. One primary provider sees and treats all patients
2. Provider pays for everything: space, equipment, supplies, and personnel

B. Group Practices

1. Two or more providers share costs
2. Patients may see the same provider

C. Urgent Care Centers

1. Provide primary care, services for routine injuries and illnesses, and minor surgery
2. Expanded hours

D. Managed Care Operations

1. Health insurance organization
   a. Emphasizes preventive care, patient education, and patient compliance
   b. Health maintenance organization (HMO)
   c. Can be under one roof or a network of providers within a geographic area

E. "Concierge" or "Boutique" Practice

1. Providers may be discouraged by managed care plans dictating what tests and procedures they can perform
2. Patients pay a set fee per year for care; patients also expected to have major medical insurance
3. Care may include priority access to provider, unlimited office visits, preventive care, annual physicals, and wellness screenings

II. Types of Medical Practice Management

A. Sole Proprietorship

1. Entitles the solo practitioner all rights to all aspects of the practice

B. Partnerships

1. Two or more practitioners join together to share in all aspects of the practice
2. Partners liable for own actions

C. Corporations

1. Formed by partners
2. Defined as "body that is granted a charter recognizing it as a separate legal entity having its own rights, privileges, and liabilities distinct from those of its members"
3. Regulated by the state

III. Healthcare Team

A. Doctor of Medicine

1. Requires medical degree and license to practice

B. Nurse Practitioner

1. Requires advanced education (master's level)

C. Nurse

1. Requires at least 2-year course of study and license

D. Physician Assistant

1. Requires formal training and certifying exam

E. Doctor of Osteopathy

1. Training and education similar to medical doctor; requires license to practice

F. Alternative Healthcare Providers

1. Doctor of chiropractic
   a. Branch of healing arts that is based on the physiologic and biochemical aspects of the body's structure
2. Doctor of naturopathy
   a. Based on the belief that the cause of disease is based on a violation of nature's laws
3. Oriental medicine and acupuncture
   a. Based on the body's energy instead of biochemistry
   b. Includes acupuncture (very fine needles inserted into energy points on the body)

G. Integrative Medicine

1. Western medicine + alternative therapies

IV. Introduction to Medical Practice Management

A. General

1. Process of developing, implementing, and achieving organizational goals
2. Administration (nonhuman resources) and leadership (human resources) work together to achieve goals
3. Chain of command is the line of authority in clinics

B. Process of Management

1. Planning: development of goals
2. Organizing: assembling resources needed to achieve goals
3. Coordinating: bringing various resources together to achieve goals
4. Directing: supervising the use of resources to achieve goals
5. Controlling: making necessary adjustments to achieve goals

C. Supervision

1. Begins with leadership
2. Leadership is the process of working with and through employees to achieve goals
3. Leadership requires two types of behavior:
   a. Task behavior: leader tells what, when, how, where, and who is to perform a specific task
   b. Relationship behavior: the way the leader communicates, listens, supports, and facilitates in assisting employees in performing a specific task
4. Leadership styles
   a. Telling: makes decisions and supervises employee performance
   b. Selling: makes and explains decisions to employees
   c. Participating: shares ideas and facilitates employee decision making
   d. Delegating: turns responsibility for making and implementing decisions over to employees

D. Human Resources

1. Hiring process
   a. Recruiting: potential candidates are notified of an available position through advertisement
   b. Interviewing: face-to-face meeting and discussion with employee candidate
   c. Checking references: calling the references indicated by the employee candidate to verify the candidate's information
   d. Selection: choosing the best employee candidate based on the candidate's education, experience, references, and "fit"
   e. Offer: formally offering the position to the employee candidate, including wage and benefit information
   f. Negotiation: negotiating the specific terms of the employment offered
   g. Acceptance or rejection: employee candidate accepts the job offer and begins employment, or the candidate rejects the offer, and the employer begins the process again (or offers the position to the next-best candidate)
2. Job description should include the following:
   a. Job title
   b. Job summary
   c. Supervisor's title
   d. Job duties and employee responsibilities
   e. Job specifications
3. Orientation: transition from candidate to employee
4. Probation
   a. Time needed to determine whether the newly hired employee is a good "fit"
   b. Usually 60 to 90 days
5. Performance appraisal
   a. Objective employee performance assessment
   b. Should assess the employee's work, dependability, teamwork, appearance, and attitude
   c. Should be done regularly
   d. Result must be discussed with the employee
6. Discipline: all actions related to employee performance should be recorded in the employee's personnel file
7. Professional development
   a. Encourage and subsidize professional development
   b. Encourage membership in professional organizations
   c. Promote the employee's attendance at seminars, workshops, and conventions
   d. Enable the employee to obtain continuing education units (CEUs) or continuing medical education units (CMEs)

V. Meetings

A. General

1. Keep a calendar of all scheduled meetings (with date, time, place, and topic)
2. Meetings conducted in accordance with *Robert's Rules of Order*
3. Person chairing the meeting is responsible for all portions of the meeting process to ensure that objectives are met
4. Agenda should be typed and distributed to meeting members
5. Minutes are the record of the meeting; should include the date, time, place, and topic of the meeting; persons in attendance and absent persons; issues discussed; and time of adjournment

VI. Employer Travel

A. General

1. Travel arrangements may be made by the medical assistant, a travel agent, or both
2. Itinerary should be typed; must include departure and arrival times and locations, contact telephone numbers, destination ground transportation, hotel accommodations, and a schedule of events and activities involved in the travel function; a copy of the travel itinerary must be kept in the office; a copy of the itinerary is given to the traveler
3. If the travel function is a speaking arrangement, confirm the time, place, and topic; also confirm the honorarium (payment)
4. Check with the airlines before leaving for the airport in case of flight delays
5. Confirm ground transportation at the destination location (courtesy car, taxi service, hotel shuttle, rental car)
6. Confirm hotel accommodations; copy the reservation confirmation number onto the travel itinerary

VII. Resource Management

A. Facility

1. Temperature: 68°F to 74°F, with proper ventilation
2. Lighting: fluorescent lighting in all examination and working areas
3. Floor covering: carpeting in waiting room, office, and hallways; sheet vinyl flooring in all examination, bathroom, and laboratory areas
4. Walls: soft or pastel colors, paint, or wallpaper
5. Storage: locked space for supplies, equipment, and patient charts; locked and secure cabinets for drugs
6. Noise control: examination rooms and physician offices should be arranged to keep sounds at a minimum
7. Patient rooms: arranged so that the patient cannot be seen by others when the door is opened
8. Offices: separate from the patient examination areas

9. Clinical areas: checked between patients to maintain cleanliness and to keep neat and well stocked with supplies
10. Laboratory area: well ventilated; ensure that contamination is well controlled
11. Bathrooms: clean and well stocked; patient bathrooms should be separate from staff facilities
12. Janitorial services: staff should keep all areas neat, clean, and repaired; staff should schedule janitorial services for the remainder of cleaning duties
13. Safety: continually monitor the office for hazards; smoke alarms and fire extinguishers should be strategically placed and checked often to ensure they are properly functioning; fire exits should be clearly marked and kept free of obstacles
14. Security: an adequate number of security personnel should be readily available
15. Regulated waste disposal: schedule regular removal of regulated waste and sharps biohazard waste

B. Office Equipment

1. Keep warranties filed for future reference
2. Maintain a file for service agreements
3. Maintain a file with service technician telephone numbers
4. Keep inventory reports on file, with a physical inventory completed at least once a year; inventory should include the following:
    a. Name of item
    b. Model and serial number
    c. Date of purchase or lease (and price)
5. Inventory should be made of the following properties:
    a. Laboratory equipment
    b. Clinical equipment
    c. Clinical instruments
    d. Office equipment
    e. Office furniture
    f. Anything of value that is not consumed in the treatment of patients

C. Supplies

1. Includes consumable items that are needed to operate the office, housekeeping supplies, and medical supplies
2. Ordered on an ongoing basis
3. One person within the office should be designated to order supplies and to maintain and inventory supplies
4. Supply inventory (separate from office equipment inventory) should be kept up to date so that supplies never run out
5. Contents of supply deliveries should be checked in and verified against the purchase order and packing slip
6. Supplies must be stored in a neat and orderly fashion

VIII. Resources for Staff and Patients

A. Policy and Procedure Manuals

1. Information about the office for employees
    a. Office or clinic mission statement
    b. Orientation information

c. Dress code
d. Job descriptions
e. Holidays, leaves, vacations, and sick days
f. Payroll and benefits
g. Disciplinary actions
2. Procedure manual
   a. Description of steps taken to handle a situation or perform a certain task
   b. Regular review of procedures is necessary to ensure they are up to date and conform to legal regulations
   c. May be separate manuals for clinical and administrative procedures
   d. All personnel should be encouraged to use manuals as a reference

B. Emergency Preparedness and Evacuation Plan

1. Plan needs to be in place to respond to a fire, natural disaster, or emergency situation that affects the entire office
2. Occupational Safety and Health Administration (OSHA) requires businesses to have a written plan to guide employees during an emergency
3. Written plan must include the following:
   a. Protection of safety of patients, visitors, and staff
   b. Provision of prompt, efficient medical care
   c. A clear chain of command

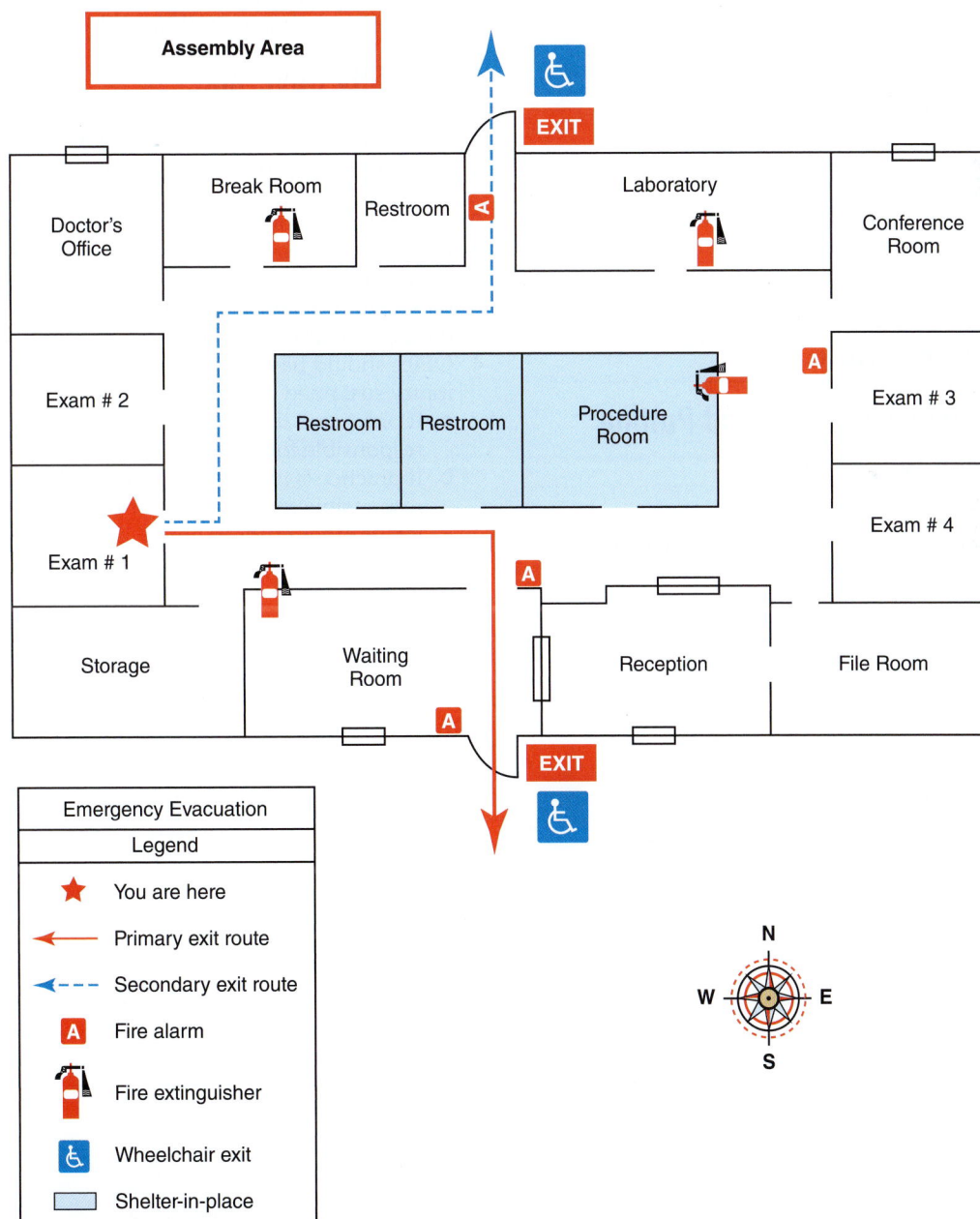

Fig. 11.1 Evacuation floor plans should be posted in the medical office. (From Bonewit-West K, Hunt S: *Today's medical assistant: clinical and administrative procedures*, ed 4, 2021, Elsevier.)

d. Protection of clinic property
e. Means of reporting emergencies
f. Evacuation procedures and emergency escape routes
g. Procedures to account for all employees
h. Specific assignments for employees to follow
4. Map of the floor plan clearly showing marked escape routes should be posted (Fig. 11.1)

C. Community Resources

1. Help for patients who require community services to meet health needs
2. Office may keep a list of local organizations in the following areas:
   a. Support for alcoholism or addiction
   b. Support for caregivers of individuals with decreased mental or physical disability
   c. Visiting nurse and homemaker services
   d. Legal aid
   e. Local organizations to help children, families, older adults, and homeless people
   f. Local health department
   g. Cardiopulmonary resuscitation and first aid training
   h. Immunization clinics
   i. Weight control and smoking cessation programs
3. Medical assistant may also assist patient in Internet search for resources

IX. Risk Management

A. Process of Assessing Risk and Putting Policies in Place to Minimize It

1. Office manager can be responsible
2. Policies are designed by provider, working with an attorney and insurance company
3. When new policies are adopted, a copy is given to each employee

B. Incident Reports

1. Report filed whenever anything happens in the office that could be considered liable
2. Initiated by staff member who is injured or closest to patient when injured
3. Reports vary, but usually ask for the following information:
   a. Date and time of incident
   b. Name of individual involved
   c. Address where incident occurred
   d. Description of how the incident occurred and exactly what happened
   e. Complete description of any injury
   f. Name of witness
   g. Name and contact information of person to whom the incident was reported
   h. Date of receipt and follow-up by supervisor

C. Liability Coverage

1. Adequate insurance protection against professional liability (malpractice) and accidents that may occur in the office
2. Medical assistant can purchase professional liability through a professional organization or may be covered by provider
3. Office should have adequate insurance to cover property damage to the office in case of fire, storm, or flooding
4. Office should have adequate coverage against personal injury sustained on the office's property
   a. If practice is in an office building, landlord is responsible for public areas
   b. If practice is in a free-standing building, the practice is responsible for any occurrences on walkways, parking lot, or other outdoor areas

Finances

I. Accounting

A. General

1. Process of recording, classifying, summarizing, reporting, analyzing, and interpreting financial data
2. Provides financial information about the business operation

B. Accounting Elements

1. Asset
   a. Property owned or controlled by a business
   b. Includes the following:
      1) Land, buildings, fixtures, and furnishings
      2) Medical and office equipment
      3) Money
      4) Accounts receivable
      5) Stocks, bonds, and investments
2. Liability
   a. Debt obligation of the business
   b. Includes the following:
      1) Accounts payable
      2) Bank debts
3. Owner's equity
   a. Amount by which assets exceed liabilities; net worth
   b. Includes the following:
      1) Revenue (assets in)
      2) Expense (assets out)
      3) Drawing (personal use of assets)
4. Accounting equations
   a. Assets = liabilities + owner's equity
   b. Liabilities = assets − owner's equity
   c. Owner's equity = assets − liabilities

II. Bookkeeping

A. Systems

1. Single-entry system
   a. Oldest and simplest method
   b. Simple to use, inexpensive, and requires little training
   c. Includes three basic records:
      1) Journal: also called the daily log, daybook, day sheet, or charge journal; records of charges and receipts are entered daily
      2) Cash payment journal: simple form of a checkbook
      3) Accounts receivable ledger: record of the amounts that patients owe the office; each patient has his or her own card; statements are prepared manually from these cards
   d. Lacks methods for cross-checking to prevent errors
2. Pegboard (write-it-once) system
   a. Most common manual method used in the physician's office
   b. All transactions are recorded at one time
   c. Uses charge slips, paper ledger cards, and paper day to keep track of individual accounts
   d. Bookkeeping entries are made and recorded simultaneously on all forms on the pegboard
3. Double-entry system
   a. Inexpensive method but requires some training
   b. Transactions may be recorded manually or by computer
   c. Each transaction is recorded in a way that keeps a balance of accounting equation
   d. Each transaction affects two accounts: one is debited, and the other is credited
4. Total practice management system (Fig. 12.1)

WALDEN-MARTIN
FAMILY MEDICAL CLINIC
1234 ANYSTREET ANYTOWN, ANYSTATE 1234
PHONE 123-123-1234   FAX 123-123-5678

Ledger for Guarantor: Mora Siever

Home phone: 123-914-3584

Address: 1 Trinity Lane
Anytown
AL 12345

Account #:   72534

DOB: 01/24/1964

Date	Patient	Service	Charges	Payment	ADJUSTMENT	Balance
12/02/20XX	Mora Siever	99396	$ 105.00	$ 20.00	$ 0.00	$ 85.00
12/02/20XX	Mora Siever	99300	$ 89.00	$ 0.00	$ 0.00	$ 89.00
10/22/20XX	Mora Siever	Ins payment	$ 0.00	$ 35.00	$ 15.00	$ −50.00
10/07/20XX	Mora Siever	99203	$ 70.00	$ 20.00	$ 0.00	$ 50.00
					Total:	$ 174.00

Fig. 12.1 Patient ledger from SimChart for the Medical Office.

a. Accounting software package
b. Based on principles of pegboard or double-entry system
c. Can be customized for the needs of the practice
d. Software can be used to
   1) Prepare statements
   2) Prepare insurance forms
   3) Compose collection letters
   4) Manage practice's finances

B. Accounts Receivable

1. Fees that patients owe for services performed
2. Most receipts come from third-party payments (e.g., insurance carrier); payments might not be received for 30 to 90 days after service
3. Accounts are classified, aged, according to the amount of time that the balance remains unpaid (i.e., current, 30 days, 60 days, >90 days, past due)

C. Accounts Payable

1. Money owed to vendors
2. Payments to vendors for purchases and services
3. Invoice normally accompanies purchase
4. Record of payments kept by making an entry into the appropriate accounts payable record

D. Petty Cash

1. Cash kept within the office to cover minor purchases
2. Usual amount is small and in small denominations
3. Eliminates the need to write a check for minor purchases
4. Fund is established by writing a check on the office account; this check is cashed by the bank, and the cash is placed in a safe place within the office

5. One person is designated to make disbursements from the petty cash fund
6. A voucher is normally required to draw cash out of the fund; the voucher should show the name of the person taking the cash, the amount of cash taken, and the purpose of the petty cash draw; this voucher is used to balance the account
7. A register should be maintained to track the vouchers
8. The petty cash fund is replenished by again writing and cashing a check

E. Purchasing Supplies and Equipment

1. Purchase order: form used to request the purchase of needed supplies for the practice
2. Sent to the supplier; copy kept in the office for verification of shipment and payment of invoice
3. When order arrives, verify with purchase order for correctness and completeness

III. Billing

A. Fees

1. Should reflect the revenue necessary to maintain the financial stability of the practice
2. Influenced by the time to be spent and the degree of difficulty in providing the service
3. Set up by a schedule that includes code numbers, detailed description, and cost of each particular service rendered within the practice
4. Fee schedule must be available to all patients
   a. Usual fee: fee most frequently charged for a particular service

b. Customary fee: range of usual fees charged for the particular service by practitioners of similar training and experience

c. Reasonable fee: fee assigned to an unusual service or a service that has complex features; meets the criteria of usual and customary fees

5. May be discussed in advance with patient
6. Adjustment: increase or decrease to patient account not due to charges incurred or payments received; often due to third-party payor agreements
7. Professional courtesy: provider treats another healthcare professional for free or a reduced fee

B. Forms

1. Patient information form
   a. Used to collect and maintain general information about the patient for billing purposes
   b. Includes the patient's name, home address, home telephone number, occupation, business address, business telephone number, Social Security number; name of the insured, insurance carrier, and policy number; spouse's name, occupation, business address, and business telephone number; and emergency contact telephone number
2. Release of information form
   a. Used to request information gathered by other medical providers
   b. Patient's signature authorizes a third party (e.g., insurance company) to be given information about the patient's treatment
3. Assignment of benefits form: patient's signature requests the insurance company to send insurance proceeds directly to the provider

C. Billing Methods

1. Time-of-service
   a. Fee collected when the service is provided
   b. Reduces collection costs
   c. Increases cash flow
2. Monthly billing: a bill is sent to each patient on a monthly basis
3. Cycle billing: a bill is sent to certain segments of the patient population at a consistent time each month, with each segment being sent at a different time during the month
4. Billing service: the office may contract with an outside agency to prepare and send bills to patients

D. Statements

1. Individual: each patient bill is individually prepared
2. Ledger cards: copies are made of the patient's ledger card entries and mailed to the patient
3. Encounter form (superbill, routing slip) (Fig. 12.2)
   a. Presented to the patient at each visit
   b. Can be used as a charge slip for office treatment
   c. Should have all elements required to file an insurance claim or bill the patient

1) Name and address of patient
2) Name of insurance carrier
3) Insurance identification number
4) Procedure and diagnostic codes
5) Fees for each service
6) Place and date of service
7) Provider's name, address, and signature

d. Payment is made at the time of the office visit or mailed in at a later date

4. Computerized: data are keyed into an accounting computer program; statements are automatically generated by accounting software

IV. Collections

A. General

1. Revenue from services rendered must be collected to cover expenses
2. Harassing debtors is illegal
3. Aging accounts: determined by the date of the first bill; schedule is 30 days past due, 60 days past due, 90 days past due, and 120 days past due

B. Telephone Collections

1. Making threatening or abusive calls when attempting to collect a debt is illegal
2. Call between 8:00 a.m. and 8:00 p.m. and only to the patient's home telephone when attempting to collect a debt
3. Determine the identity of the person with whom you are discussing debt collection by using the debtor's full name
4. Be positive and assertive
5. State the purpose of your call
6. Attempt to obtain a commitment by the debtor before ending the debt collection call; attempt to get the debtor to promise to deliver a certain sum by a certain date
7. After this initial debt collection contact, follow up with another confirmation call

C. Mailings

1. Use letters within opaque envelopes for debt collection; never use postcards
2. Prepare correspondence to meet the situation (begin debt collection process with a friendly tone, progressing to a more assertive tone as debt collection lags)
3. Inform the patient by Certified Mail or Return Receipt Requested of possible collection agency action or legal action to collect the debt

D. Progressive Collection Process

1. Office should have developed a color-coded or written stage-by-stage process by which the office can keep track of debt collection efforts (with the process identified first by friendly tones, progressing to more assertive tones as debt collection lags)

Tri-State Medical Group

008112

400 North 4th Street • Anytown, Iowa 50622
Phone: 319-555-5734 • Fax: 319-555-5758
Fed. Tax I.D. # 42-1435XXX

ACCOUNT NO.		DOB			DATE OF SERVICE	
PATIENT NAME				PROVIDER		
INSURANCE ID #-PRIMARY				SECONDARY		

DESCRIPTION	CODE		FEE	DESCRIPTION	CODE	FEE	DESCRIPTION	CODE	FEE
OFFICE VISIT	NEW	ESTAB.		DT, Pediatric	90702		Removal Skin Tags up to 15 Lesions	*11200	
Minimum	99201	99211		MMR	90707		Exc. Malignant Lesion, Trunk, Arm or Leg		
Brief	99202	99212		Oral Polio	90712		Exc. Malignant Lesion, Face, Ear, Eyelid, Nose		
Limited	99203	99213		IVP Polio	90713		Exc. Malignant Lesion, Scalp, Hand, Neck, Feet		
Extended	99204	99214		Varicella	90716		Lacer, Repair 2.5cm or Less/Location:	*12001	
Comprehensive	99205	99215		Td, Adult	90718		Scalp, Nk, Axille, Ext. Genitalia, Trk, Hands/Feet		
Prenatal Care	59400			DTP & HIB	90720		Lacer, Repair 2.5cm or Less/Location:	*12011	
Global		99024		Influenza	90659		Face, Ears, Eyelids, Nose, Lips & Mucous Mem.		
PREVENTIVE	NEW	ESTAB.		Hepatitis B, Newborn to 11 Years	90744		Burn w/Dressing, w/o Anesth. Small	16020	
Infant	99381	99391		Hepatitis B, 11-19 Years	90747		Wart Removal	*17110	
Age 1-4	99382	99392		Hepatitis B, 20 Years & Above	90746		Removal FB Conjunct. Ext. Eye	*65205	
Age 5-11	99383	99393		Pneumococcal	90732		Removal FB Ext. Auditory Canal	69200	
Age 12-17	99384	99394		Hemophilus Infl. B	90645		Ear Lavage	69210	
Age 18-39	99385	99395		Therapeutic:	90782		Tympanometry	92567	
Age 40-64	99386	99396		Allergy Inject Single	95115		EKG Tracing Only w/o Interp. & Rept	93005	
Age 65 & Over	99387	99397		Allergy Inject Multiple	95117		Nebulizer Therapy (x)	94640	
OFFICE CONSULTATION				B-12	J3420		Pulse Oximetry	94760	
Limited		99241		Injection / Aspiration	20600		Cryosurgery		
Intermediate		99242		Small joint-Finger, Toes, Ganglion			Debridement	11041	
Extended		99243		Injection / Aspiration	20605		Excise Ingrown Toenail	11730	
Comprehensive		99244		Intermediate jt-Wrist, Elbow, Ankle			Colposcopy w/Biopsy	57454	
Complex		99245		Injection / Aspiration	20610		Leep	57460	
LABORATORY PROCEDURES				Major jt. - Shoulder, Hip, Knee			Endometrial Bx	58100	
Venipuncture		36415		Inject Tendon/Ligament	20550		Cryotherapy	57511	
Routine Urinalysis w/o Microscopy		81002		Aristocort	J3302		Peak Flow Measurement	94160-52	
Hemoccult		82270		Depo Provera	J1055		Intradermal Tests CMI # Doses =	95025	
Glucose Blood Reagent Strip		82948		Rocephin	J0696		Intradermal Tests/Allergens	95024	
Wet Mount		87210		OFFICE PROCEDURE / MINOR SURGERY			Intravenous Access	36000	
PAP Smear		88155		I & D Abscess	10060		Immunotherapy/Single Injection	95120	
Urine Pregnancy		81025		Removal FB Subcutaneous	*10120		Immunotherapy/Double Injection	95125	
Other:		99000		I & D Hematoma	10140		Regular Spirometry	94010	
X-RAY				Puncture Aspiration Abscess	10160		Spirometry Read by Physician	94010-26	
X-ray Cervical Spine		75052		Exc. Ben. Lesion #:			Spirometry w/pre & Post Bronchodilator	94060	
X-ray Thoracic Spine		72070		Location:			Spirometry/Bronchodilator read by Doctor	94060-26	
X-ray Lumbar Spine (2)		72100		Exc. Ben. Lesion #:			Skin Prick Test: # of Tests =	95004	
X-ray Lumbar Spine (Comp)		72110		Location:			Vial Preparation	95165	
X-ray Pelvis (1 view)		72170							
X-ray Sacrum & Coccyx		72220							
X-ray Clavicle (Complete)		73000							
X-ray Shoulder (2) or		73030							
X-ray Humerus (2 views)		73060							
X-ray Elbow (AP & LATE)		73070							
X-ray Forearm (AP & LA)		73090							
X-ray Wrist (AP & LATE)		73100							
X-ray Wrist (3 Views)		73110							
X-ray Hand (2 Views)		73120							
X-ray Hand (3 Views)		73130							
X-ray Finger (2 Views)		73140							
X-ray Hip (2 Views)		73510							
X-ray Hips (Bilateral)		73520							
X-ray Scoliosis (2 AP & LA)		72069							
X-ray Femur (AP & LATE)		73550							
X-ray Knee (AP & LATE)		73560							
X-ray Knee (3 Views)		73564							
X-ray Tibia & Fibula		73590							
X-ray Ankle (3 Views)		73610							
X-ray Foot (AP & LATER)		73620							
X-ray Foot (AP. LA.,)		73630							
X-ray Calcaneus (2 Views)		73650							
X-ray Toes		73660							
X-ray Pelvis & Hip Inf		73540							
Elbow, Minimum of 3 Views		73080							
IMMUNIZATIONS & INJECTIONS									
PPD Intradermal TB Tine		86580							
DTaP		90700							

HOSPITAL ORDERS

OB Non-Stress Test	Cystogram	Physical Therapy
OB Ultrasound-Diagnostic	MRI	
OB Ultrasound-Routine	CT Scan _____	
Biophysical Profile	Chest X-ray	Diet Consultation
Mammogram-Diagnostic	X-ray _____	
Mammogram-Routine	Bone Densitometry	
	EKG	Laboratory
Ultrasound _____	Holter Monitor	
Gallbladder Ultrasound	Echocardiogram	_____
Pelvic Ultrasound	Treadmill	_____
Doppler Studies _____	Thallium Stress Test	_____
	Doppler Studies _____	_____
IVP	PFT-Partial	_____
Upper GI	PFT-Complete	_____
Lower GI	Cardiac Rehab	_____
Barium Enema		
Barium Swallow		

AUTHORIZATION TO PAY BENEFITS AND RELEASE INFORMATION TO TRI-STATE MEDICAL GROUP: I hereby authorize payment directly to the undersigned Physician of all Surgical and / or Medical Benefits, if any, otherwise payable to me for his / her services as described above. I have read and understand the Financial Policy and that I am financially responsible for charges not covered by this insurance. I also authorize the undersigned Physician to release any information acquired in the course of my examination or treatment.

Signed: _____

Date: _____

Provider's Signature   Date

PREVIOUS BALANCE	
CHARGES TODAY	
TOTAL	
AMOUNT PAID	
BALANCE DUE	

DX or Other Information   Samples:

Your next appointment is:

BILLING COPY

Fig. 12.2 Sample encounter form. (From Beik JI: *Health insurance today: a practical approach*, ed 6, 2018, Saunders.)

E. Collection Agency

1. Forward a past due account to a collection agency when the account has been determined uncollectible by office personnel
2. Once the account is given to a collection agency, the clinic may not continue collection efforts on the debt
3. Patients should make payments on their debt only to the collection agency after the account has been turned over to the agency
4. The collection agency keeps a percentage of the amount collected as their fee

V. Payroll

A. General

1. Affected by federal and state laws and regulations
2. Income tax, Federal Insurance Contributions Act (FICA) and Federal Unemployment Tax Act (FUTA) amounts withheld from employee checks must be paid to the Internal Revenue Service (IRS) and to the state tax commissioner at regular intervals
3. Payroll procedures must be explained to all new employees

B. Laws and Regulations

1. Detailed records must be kept in the office for each employee, including
   a. Name, address, and Social Security number
   b. Amount and date of each wage payment and period covered by the payment
   c. Amount of wages subject to taxes
   d. Amount and type of taxes withheld from employee's pay
   e. Date when employee begins work; date when employee leaves the employment
2. Fair Labor Standards Act
   a. Sets minimum wage
   b. Requires employers to pay 1 ½ times employee's regular wage for additional time worked over 40 regular hours per week
3. Title VII, Civil Rights Act of 1964: prohibits discrimination based on employee's race, color, religion, or gender in hiring, firing, or promoting employees
4. Age Discrimination in Employment Act: prohibits unfair practices in employment decisions regarding people older than 40 years of age
5. Americans with Disabilities Act: prohibits unfair practices in employment decisions (and in many other areas) regarding people with physical, mental, or medical disabilities
6. Family Medical Leave Act of 1993
   a. In the case of birth, adoption, or sick or injured family member, an employee is entitled to unpaid leave to care for the child, spouse, parent, or for himself or herself; 12-week limit for full-time employees
   b. The employee is entitled to benefits and job protection while on leave

C. Taxes

1. Income tax
   a. Employers are required by law to withhold employee income tax
   b. Amount withheld from the employee's paycheck is based on a graduated rate table
2. Federal Insurance Contributions Act
   a. Social Security and Medicare tax
   b. Employers are required to withhold (collect) these taxes from employee wages
   c. Employer submits amounts withheld to the IRS when the employer pays the employer's taxes
   d. Taxes are deducted from the employee's earnings each pay period
   e. Every dollar paid by the employee is matched, dollar for dollar, by the employer
3. Federal Unemployment Tax Act
   a. Federal law requires employers to withhold tax to support unemployment insurance programs
   b. Amount of tax withheld is computed on a graduated rate table based on employee earnings

D. Forms and Reports

1. Form SS-4
   a. Federal Tax Identification Number application form
   b. Required for employers who hire employees and who withhold taxes from employee pay
2. Form SS-5
   a. Social Security number application form
   b. All employees are required to have a Social Security number
3. Form W-2
   a. Wages and Tax Statement
   b. Given to all employees
   c. Lists the wages earned (by one employee) and taxes withheld on wages for the preceding year
   d. Used to prepare personal income tax return
   e. Must be provided to employees by January 31 of the following year
   f. Consists of six parts
      1) Copy A: sent to the Social Security Administration
      2) Copy 1: sent to the state tax department
      3) Copy B: filed with the employee's federal tax return
      4) Copy C: kept by the employee
      5) Copy 2: filed with employee's state tax return
      6) Copy D: retained by the employer
4. Form W-3
   a. Transmittal of Income and Tax Statement
   b. Used to report the total amount of income and FICA tax withheld during the year
   c. Filed by the employer with the Social Security Administration
5. Form W-4
   a. Employee's Withholding Allowance Certificate
   b. Identifies the total number of withholding allowances claimed by the employee
6. Form 940: employer's annual federal unemployment tax return

7. Form 941
   a. Employer's quarterly federal tax return
   b. Filed quarterly to report FUTA and income tax amounts to the federal government
8. Form 8109
   a. Federal Tax Deposit Coupon Book
   b. Used to make quarterly federal income tax and FUTA payments
9. Form 1099
   a. IRS form to report income other than wages
   b. A physician-employer's honoraria from speaking engagements would be claimed on this form
10. Form I-9: confirms US citizenship or legality of working papers if a foreign national

E. Payroll Systems

1. Manual
   a. Most common for smaller organizations
   b. Payroll is computed and processed by hand
2. Computerized
   a. Data are entered into accounting management computer program
   b. Payroll calculations automatically prepared by the software
   c. Detailed records and reports are automatically prepared by the software
3. Payroll services
   a. Payroll data are sent to the payroll service
   b. Service prepares the payroll and delivers detailed records, reports, and payroll checks to the office

VI. Checking Accounts

A. General

1. Many money transactions out of the office are conducted by checking account
2. A check is a commercial paper drawn on funds deposited in a bank account
3. Can be handwritten or computer generated
4. A check is a written order for the bank to pay a person a specific amount of money (Fig. 12.3)
5. A check is negotiable; anyone who properly endorses the check is entitled to receive the money
6. Parties involved in a check
   a. Drawer: the person writing the check
   b. Drawee: the bank
   c. Payee: the person who is to receive the money from the check

B. Opening a Checking Account

1. Requires approval from a bank official
2. Requires an initial deposit, in accordance with the bank's rules
3. Requires a signature card: signature card contains the names and signatures of all persons who are authorized to access the checking account

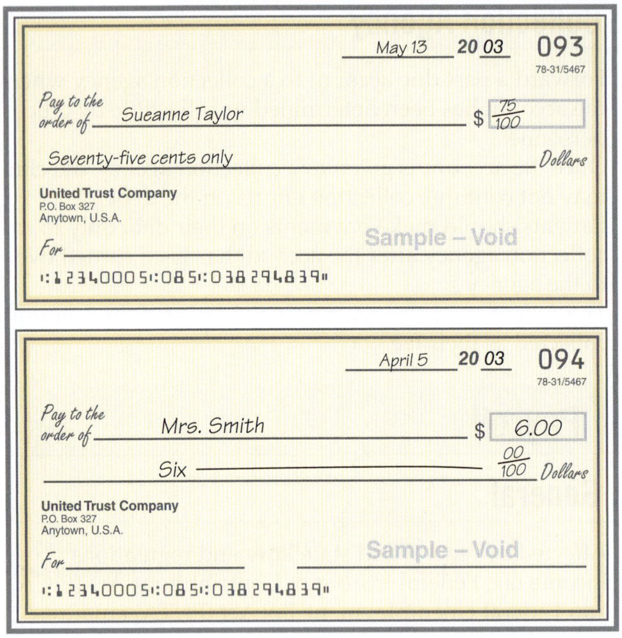

Fig. 12.3 Correct method and incorrect method of writing a check.

C. Deposits

1. Can be made by using
   a. Paper money
      1) Arranged in order of denomination (smallest value bill on top)
      2) All bills should be arranged face up and top up
   b. Coins: a large quantity of coins should be wrapped in coin wrappers before deposit
   c. Checks
      1) Office personnel should verify each check for completeness
      2) Each check must be endorsed (in writing or by stamp) directing how the check is to be applied
   d. Deposit slip: a preprinted form with account information; identifies all items being deposited (Fig. 12.4)
      1) Enter the date of deposit
      2) Enter total amount of coins and currency being deposited
      3) Enter and note separately each check to be deposited
      4) Record the total amount of the deposit
      5) Withdraw cash by entering the amount to be withdrawn on the designated space on the deposit slip and subtracting this amount from the deposit total; if a withdrawal of cash is needed, the deposit slip must be signed

D. Dishonored Checks

1. A check that the bank refuses to pay
2. Usually the result of insufficient funds in the account (not sufficient funds [NSF])
3. If a check is deposited and not accepted by the bank it is written on, the payee's bank returns the dishonored check

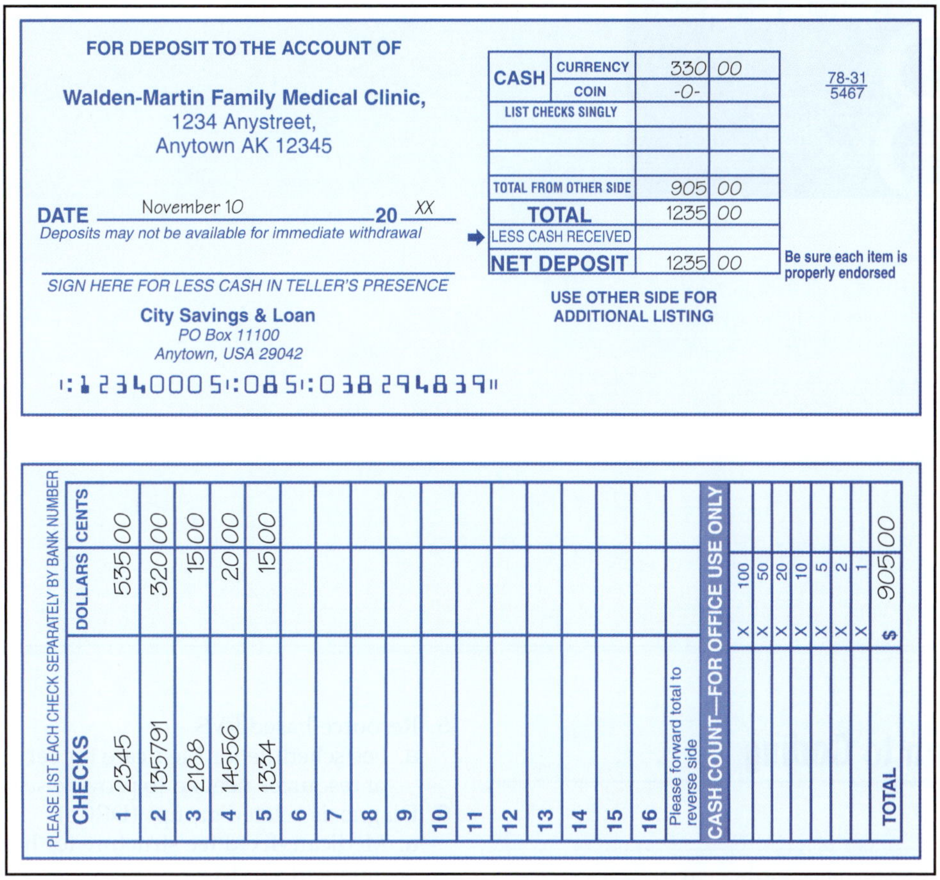
FOR DEPOSIT TO THE ACCOUNT OF

Walden-Martin Family Medical Clinic,
1234 Anystreet,
Anytown AK 12345

DATE November 10 20 XX
Deposits may not be available for immediate withdrawal

SIGN HERE FOR LESS CASH IN TELLER'S PRESENCE

City Savings & Loan
PO Box 11100
Anytown, USA 29042

⑆1234000 5⑆085⑆038 294839⑈

CASH	CURRENCY	330	00
	COIN	-0-	
LIST CHECKS SINGLY			
TOTAL FROM OTHER SIDE		905	00
TOTAL		1235	00
LESS CASH RECEIVED			
NET DEPOSIT		1235	00

78-31/5467

Be sure each item is properly endorsed

USE OTHER SIDE FOR ADDITIONAL LISTING

PLEASE LIST EACH CHECK SEPARATELY BY BANK NUMBER

CHECKS		DOLLARS	CENTS
1	2345	535	00
2	135791	320	00
3	2188	15	00
4	14556	20	00
5	1334	15	00
6			
7			
8			
9			
10			
11			
12			
13			
14			
15			
16			
Please forward total to reverse side			
CASH COUNT—FOR OFFICE USE ONLY			
	X 100		
	X 50		
	X 20		
	X 10		
	X 5		
	X 2		
	X 1		
TOTAL		$ 905	00

Fig. 12.4 Front and back of a deposit slip. (From Niedzwiecki B, et al: *Kinn's the administrative medical assistant: an applied learning approach*, ed 14, 2020, Elsevier.)

back to the payee, deducts the amount of that check from payee's account, and normally assesses the payee a fee for the work caused

a. Overdraft
   1) Issuing check without sufficient funds in the writer's account
   2) Knowingly issuing an NSF check is illegal
b. Postdated check: issuing a check but putting a date in the future on the check; a bank may not honor a check until the date on the check

E. Bank Statements

1. Statement of account sent to each depositor once a month by the bank
2. Gives the account holder the following information:
   a. Account balance at the beginning of the period
   b. Amount of deposits made during the period
   c. Amount of checks paid during the period
   d. Other items paid or credited during the period
   e. Account balance at the end of the period
3. Canceled checks may be enclosed with the statement
4. Statement needs to be reconciled (to ensure that the bank balance agrees with the office balance)
   a. Compare the deposited amounts recorded in the office files with the amounts recorded on the statement
   b. Compare the canceled check amounts with amounts on the statement and on the office check register
   c. Identify all debits and credits to the account between the bank and the office records
   d. Identify any errors found on the bank statement or on the office register
   e. Add and subtract all adjustments made to the bank statement and to the office register; both balances should be equal

13

Coding

I. Introduction to Coding

A. Purpose

1. Coding system translates descriptions of diseases, illnesses, injuries, and procedures into numeric codes
2. Helps insurance company quickly and accurately review what services the patient received and how they are related to the illness or injury
3. Facilitates the use of computers in insurance claim processing
4. Developed for
   a. Tracking disease processes
   b. Classification of medical procedures
   c. Medical research
   d. Evaluation of hospital utilization
   e. Reimbursement

B. Types of Coding Systems

1. International Classification of Diseases, 10th Revision (ICD-10-CM)
   a. Used to code disease conditions or diagnosis
2. Current Procedural Terminology, 4th edition (CPT)
   a. Used to code procedures and medical services provided by practitioner
3. Health Care Financing Administration (HCFA) Common Procedural Coding System (HCPCS)
   a. Used to report services performed to Medicare program
4. Relative value scale (RVS)
   a. Assigned unit value given to commonly performed medical procedures
   b. Based on time, knowledge, and skill required by the practitioner
   c. Point value is multiplied by a dollar factor to find a final fee amount

5. Resource-based RVS
   a. Fee schedule for Medicare for services based on level of resources needed to provide service
6. Diagnosis-related groups (DRGs)
   a. Medicare-fixed fee structure for hospital billing of inpatient services
   b. Based on principal diagnosis

C. Coding Terminology

1. Downcoding: using procedure codes that do not reflect a high enough level of service
2. DRGs: a system for grouping hospital inpatients who utilize similar amount of hospital resources as a basis for Medicare reimbursement
3. Established patient: a patient who has been seen in the practice in the same specialty within the past 3 years
4. Inpatient: a patient who has been formally admitted to a healthcare facility
5. Medical necessity: healthcare that is necessary and reasonable for a patient's health
6. Modifier: an addition to CPT Code that indicates unusual circumstances in relation to the procedure
7. Not elsewhere classified: a diagnosis code used when a more specific code for the condition is not available
8. New patient: a patient who has not received service during the past 3 years from this medical practice
9. Not otherwise specified: used when there is not enough specific information given with which to select a more specific code
10. Outpatient: a patient who has not been admitted to this medical practice
11. Panel: a group of related diagnostic tests
12. Related value unit: a number that quantifies the amount of physician expertise, labor, and resources necessary to provide the service represented by a CPT Code

13. Sequela: any condition that results from a disease, injury, or treatment for a disease or injury
14. Surgical package: surgical services covered by a single-procedure code; includes preoperative visit, postoperative care, and local anesthesia (if applicable)
15. Upcoding: using a code to obtain a higher level of reimbursement than is justified by medical procedures performed as documented in the patient's medical records; can result in serious fines and penalties for the practice.

II. International Classification of Diseases, 10th Revision

A. General

1. Assigns numeric codes to illnesses, diseases, injuries, and health-related conditions
2. Two separate systems
   a. ICD-10-CM: diagnostic coding
      1) Used in physicians' offices and outpatient settings
      2) Used to code diseases, signs, symptoms, abnormal findings, complaints, social circumstances, and external causes of injury or disease
   b. ICD-10-PCS: procedural coding
      1) Used in inpatient hospital setting
      2) Used to repost inpatient procedures only
      3) Helps establish DRGs to determine payment for related services

B. International Classification of Diseases, 10th Revision Manual

1. Alphabetic Index
   a. Contains a list of terms arranged alphabetically along with their corresponding codes
2. Tabular List
   a. List of alphanumeric codes organized by organ systems, etiology, external causes, or other signs/ symptoms
   b. Coding instructions and conventions are listed here
   c. Arranged in 21 chapters

C. International Classification of Diseases, 10th Revision Code Sets

1. Codes are all alphanumeric and all letters except "U"
2. Injury codes expanded and grouped by body parts
3. Incorporation of common fourth- and fifth-digit subclassifications

4. Addition of sixth- and seventh-character subclassifications
5. Codes consist of three to seven characters (Fig. 13.1)
6. First digit is alpha
7. Second and third digits are numeric; fourth, fifth, sixth, and seventh digits may be alpha or numeric
8. Placeholder or dummy "x" concept present
9. Allows for indication of right, left, or both sides of the body

D. Coding Steps for the Tabular List

1. Locate the code in the Tabular List of Diseases and Injuries
2. Read and follow instructional notes
3. Determine whether an additional character must be added
4. Determine laterality
5. Assign the correct code to its greatest specificity

III. Current Procedural Terminology, 4th edition

A. General

1. Lists and codes procedures and services performed by practitioners
2. Each procedure is identified by a five-digit code
3. Simplifies reporting to insurance carriers
4. CPT book is divided into six sections; subsections include anatomic, procedural, conditions, and descriptors
   a. Evaluation and Management (E&M): 99,200–99,499
   b. Anesthesia: 00,100–01,999
   c. Surgery: 10,000–69,999
   d. Radiology, Nuclear Medicine, and Diagnostic Ultrasound: 70,000–79,999
   e. Pathology and Laboratory: 80,000–89,999
   f. Medicine: 90,701–99,199

B. Format and Conventions

1. Main statement followed by a semicolon; subordinate statement describes procedure or extent of services
2. Terms: indented below main statement giving additional statements
3. Guidelines: specific directions at the beginning of each section; necessary to code correctly
4. Modifiers: two-digit, terminal code; represents an alteration of the procedure or circumstances
5. Major headings are boldface

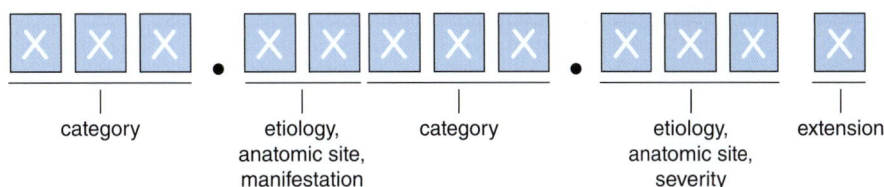

Fig. 13.1 Code structure of the International Classification of Diseases, 10th Revision.

6. Notes: provide coding instructions
7. Descriptive qualifiers: descriptions surrounding a code provide more detailed information; sometimes in parentheses

C. Coding Steps

1. Review the guidelines beginning each section
2. Turn to the index and locate the main term
3. Locate the subterm and follow the cross-references
4. Read the code descriptors of all code numbers
5. Record the proper code

D. Evaluation and Management

1. Includes basic diagnostic and treatment services
2. E&M section divided into broad categories with two or more subdivisions
   a. New patient: patient who is new to the practice or who has not received any professional services by the practitioner for 3 or more years
   b. Established patient: patient who has received professional services from the practitioner within the last 3 years
   c. Concurrent care: rendering of similar services to the same patient by more than one practitioner on the same day
   d. Counseling: discussion with the patient or family regarding diagnosis, treatment, and patient education
3. The following must be determined within each category to select the correct E&M code:
   a. History
      1) Problem focused: chief complaint and brief history of problem
      2) Expanded problem focused: chief complaint, brief history, and review of system affected by the problem
      3) Detailed: chief complaint; expanded history of the problem; expanded review of system affected; and pertinent past, family, and social history
   b. Examination
      1) Problem focused: examination limited to affected body area or system

      2) Expanded problem focused: examination limited to affected body area or system and other closely related systems
      3) Detailed: extended examination of affected body area or system and other closely related systems
      4) Comprehensive: complete single-system specialty examination or complete multisystem examination
   c. Complexity of medical decision making (diagnosis or management or both)
      1) Straightforward: all three criteria are minimal
      2) Low complexity: low degree in each criterion
      3) Moderate complexity: moderate degree in each criterion
      4) High complexity: high degree of complexity in each criterion
4. Criteria to be considered at each complexity level
   a. Number of diagnoses or management options available
   b. Amount and complexity of data
   c. Risk of complication, morbidity, or mortality

IV. Healthcare Common Procedural Coding System

A. General

1. HCFA: government agency that regulates Medicaid and Medicare
2. Coding system that expands CPT system
3. Provides a temporary list of new codes before inclusion in CPT system
4. Three levels
   a. Level I: existing CPT codes
   b. Level II: additional codes that provide greater precision in CPT categories; five-character alphanumeric system (A0000–V5999); includes
      1) Nonphysician services
      2) Codes not found within the existing CPT system

14

Health Insurance

I. Definition

A. General

1. Protection against financial loss by unplanned health-related events

B. Types of Health Insurance Programs

1. Traditional: policies created and sold by private companies
   a. Fee-for-service
   b. Usually have a deductible
   c. Commonly pay for percentage of allowed charges (commonly 80%)
   d. Patient can make appointment with any provider in any specialty; insurance pays designated amount for services
2. Managed care plans: movement to control healthcare costs while improving preventive care
   a. Each patient chooses one provider as a primary care provider
   b. Care may be restricted to providers, laboratories, and hospitals that accept payment
   c. Patient may not have access to providers or services outside the plan
   d. Plan may require referrals from primary care provider (gatekeeper) for consultations, therapy, and testing
   e. Plan usually requires preauthorization for surgery or other procedures
   f. Types of plans include
      1) Health maintenance organization (HMO): organization that provides a comprehensive range of services for a prepaid fee
      2) Preferred provider organization (PPO): agreement between managed care organization and physician to provide services to employee subscribers at a discount
      3) Exclusive provider organization (EPO): members must receive services within the network only
      4) Point-of-service plans: in network combined with out of network
3. Government plans
   a. Medicare (Fig. 14.1)
      1) Federal program administered by Centers for Medicare and Medicaid Services (CMS)
      2) Established in 1965 as Title 18 of the Social Security Act
      3) Eligibility
         a) Age 65 or older
         b) Disabled under Medicare rules
      4) Benefits
         a) Part A: covers inpatient care after applicable deductible is satisfied
         b) Part B: voluntary program; covers certain outpatient services; deductible and coinsurance
         c) Part C: Medicare + choice, Medicare advantage; expanded benefits for a fee through private health insurance programs
         d) Part D: drug and prescription benefits
      5) Supplemental insurance: Medigap; commercial insurance policies available to cover the Medicare deductible, coinsurance, and some specific treatments not covered by Medicare
   b. Medicaid
      1) Federal program administered by each state; funded jointly by state and federal government
      2) Established in 1965 as Title 19 of the Social Security Act
      3) Eligibility
         a) Determined by the state
         b) Available to persons with income levels below the federal poverty level

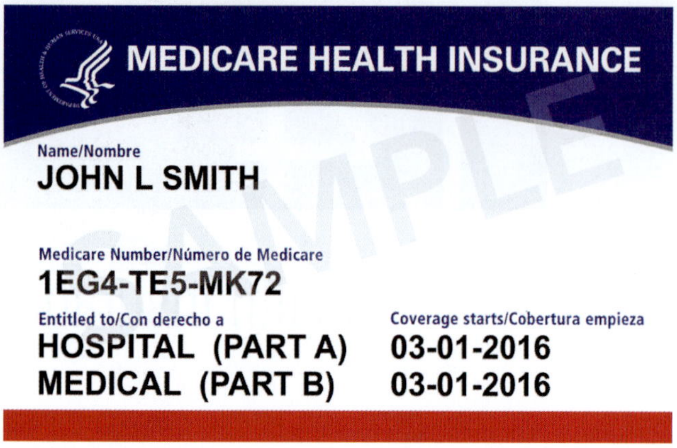

Fig. 14.1 Sample Medicare identification card. (From Smith L: *Fordney's Medical insurance*, ed 15, 2020, Saunders.)

   c) Eligible patients receive an official identification card for their period of eligibility

   d) Persons may be covered by both Medicare and Medicaid (Medi/Medi); Medicare is the primary carrier and is always billed first

  c. State Children's Health Insurance Plan

   1) Federal government funding for states to further assist children whose parents cannot afford insurance for them

   2) Administered by the state

  d. Workers' compensation

   1) State-administered program

   2) Established to help pay the cost of medical care and lost wages associated with work-related injuries or illnesses

   3) Patients are compensated in full for their related medical expenses and for a portion of their lost wages

   4) Eligibility: patients must have sustained an injury or illness while carrying out their job duties

   5) Classification of cases

     a) Claim with no disability: filed for minor injuries or illnesses; patient returns to work in a few days

     b) Temporary disability: filed for injuries and illnesses requiring more than a few days of recuperation before returning to work

     c) Permanent disability: filed for injuries and illnesses resulting in diminished capacity of the patient; ranges from 10% to 100% disability

     d) Vocational rehabilitation: filed for permanently or temporarily disabled persons who require training or education to return to work

  e. Armed Services and Veteran Insurance Plans

   1) TRICARE

     a) Comprehensive health benefits program offering three types of plans for the dependents of men and women in the uniformed services

       (1) TRICARE Standard: fee-for-service

       (2) TRICARE Extra: PPO plan

       (3) TRICARE Prime: HMO plan with point-of-service option

   2) Civilian Health and Medical Program of Veterans' Affairs (CHAMPVA)

     a) Provides inpatient and outpatient benefits for dependent spouses and children of veterans who have suffered total, permanent service-connected disabilities

  f. Affordable Care Act

   1) Attempts to define patients' rights and ensure access to affordable, high-quality healthcare for all Americans

   2) Holds insurance companies accountable

   3) Restricts the use of annual limits on benefits

   4) Prohibits discrimination against preexisting conditions

   5) Includes preventive services such as immunizations, mammograms, colonoscopies, prenatal care, and well-baby care

C. Insurance Terms

1. Assignment of benefits: authorization for reimbursement to be made to the provider rather than the insured
2. Beneficiary: person designated to receive the benefits of the insurance policy
3. Birthday rule: rule stating that when an individual is covered under two insurance policies, the insurance plan of the policyholder whose birthday comes first in the calendar year (month and day) becomes the primary insurance
4. Carrier: insurance company; insurer
5. Coinsurance: percentage of the allowed amount that is the patient's responsibility; policyholder and insurance company share the cost of covered losses in a specified ratio
6. Copayment: portion of the cost of service to be paid by the insured at time of appointment
7. Deductible: annual amount to be paid by the insured toward the cost of service before insurance policy benefits are paid
8. Eligibility: enrollment status related to an insurance plan
9. Exclusion: treatment or conditions not covered by the insurance policy
10. Explanation of benefits: document prepared by the carrier that identifies the services covered by the policy, the amount billed by the provider, the amount paid by the carrier, and the amount for which the insured is responsible
11. Fee-for-service: provider bills for each service rendered
12. Group policy: policy purchased by an organization for the benefit of its members
13. Guarantor: person financially responsible for payment of services
14. Insured: policyholder; subscriber
15. Managed care: integrated system that manages healthcare services for its beneficiaries to provide quality care and contain costs
16. Nonparticipating provider: provider that does not have any contract with a third-party payor (non-PAR)
17. Participating provider: provider that has a contractual agreement with a third-party payor (PAR)
18. Preauthorization: process required by some insurance carriers where the provider obtains permission to perform certain procedures or services or refer a patient to a specialist
19. Precertification: verification from patient's insurance carrier that a test/procedure is covered by patient's health insurance and that the test/procedure is medically appropriate

20. Preexisting condition: medical condition present or being treated at the time a health insurance application is made
21. Premium: fees paid for the health insurance coverage
22. Primary care provider (PCP): a provider chosen by patient to provide general medical care to the patient
23. Primary insurance: the patient's medical insurance company that is billed first
24. Referral: directing a patient to a specialist by the PCP
25. Reimbursement: the amount paid by patient's health insurance carrier for healthcare services
26. Provider: health professional who provides services
27. Secondary insurance: health insurance owned by patient in addition to patient's primary health insurance coverage
28. Signature on file: indication on insurance claim form that patient's signature is maintained on record by the medical office whereby patient has authorized medical office to submit claims to health insurance carrier
29. Rider: clauses to the health insurance policy designating coverage items in addition to the items included within the standard contract
30. Third-party payor: insurance carrier or managed care organization that issues payment on healthcare insurance claims submitted by medical office

D. Plan Options (Traditional Insurance)

1. Basic benefits include
   a. Diagnostic studies
   b. Hospitalization
   c. Surgical treatments
   d. Obstetric care
   e. Intensive care
   f. Chemotherapy
2. Major medical services not normally covered by a basic plan may include
   a. Outpatient visits
   b. Minor surgery
   c. Physical and occupational therapies
   d. Cost of medical equipment
   e. Mental healthcare
   f. Dental care
   g. Prescriptions
3. Companion plan: policy that pays in addition to health insurance policies carried; pays fees not covered by conventional plans

E. Methods of Payment

1. Physician fee profile: usual, customary, and reasonable charges
2. Assignment of benefits
   a. Gives the carrier instructions to send insurance payments directly to the provider
   b. Most commercial carriers reimburse the patient unless instructed not to do so
   c. Assignment of benefits is accomplished by the patient (insured) signing the appropriate box on insurance claim form or completing a separate assignment of benefits form

   d. Patient is responsible for paying the difference between the provider charge and the insurance benefits paid
   e. If the provider accepts the assignment, the carrier makes payment to the provider (in accordance with the policy language); if the claim is a government plan claim, the provider must indicate on the claim form whether the assignment is accepted or rejected
   f. If the provider rejects the assignment of benefits, the provider may bill the patient the difference between the fee charged and the fee reimbursed
3. Medicaid and workers' compensation: provider must accept government reimbursement as payment in full if the provider agrees to treat Medicaid or workers' compensation patients
4. Deductibles and copayments: patients are responsible to pay any deductible or copayment according to the terms of the insurance policy

F. Coordination of Benefits

1. Term for the rules insurance companies use to coordinate payments so that no provider is paid more than 100% for services
2. If patient has more than one insurance policy, claim is first sent to primary insurance
   a. Private insurance must be billed before government insurance; Medicaid is always last insurance billed
3. If both members of a couple have insurance
   a. Patient's insurance is primary, and spouse's is secondary
   b. If a child is the patient, birthday rule applies: parent whose birthday comes first becomes the primary insurance
4. Medicare recipients may also have private insurance: private insurance is primary

II. Insurance Claims

A. CMS-1500 Claim Form (Fig. 14.2)

1. Universal health claim form developed by Healthcare Financing Administration (HCFA)
2. Standardizes data required by most carriers so that claims can be processed
3. Before submitting a claim for payment, make sure patient information release forms are current
4. Can be submitted electronically or manually
5. Key information onto the form using uppercase letters
6. Do not use periods, hyphens, commas, dollar signs, or slashes
7. Use two zeros (00) in the cents column for whole dollar amounts, no decimal points
8. Dates should be filled in using the eight-digit date (mmddyyyy)
9. Boxes that should be checked are filled in with an "X"
10. Type corrections are made by permanent correction methods (correction fluid)
11. Completed forms should be maintained in provider files for 6 years

HEALTH INSURANCE CLAIM FORM

APPROVED BY NATIONAL UNIFORM CLAIM COMMITTEE (NUCC) 02/12

| | | PICA | | | | | | PICA | |

1. MEDICARE ☑ (Medicare#) MEDICAID ☐ (Medicaid#) TRICARE ☐ (ID#/DoD#) CHAMPVA ☐ (Member ID#) GROUP HEALTH PLAN ☐ (ID#) FECA BLK LUNG ☐ (ID#) OTHER ☐ (ID#)

1a. INSURED'S I.D. NUMBER (For Program in Item 1)
123-45-6789A

2. PATIENT'S NAME (Last Name, First Name, Middle Initial)
ROSE DAWSON

3. PATIENT'S BIRTH DATE MM 02 DD 17 YY XXXX SEX M ☐ F ☑

4. INSURED'S NAME (Last Name, First Name, Middle Initial)
ROSE DAWSON

5. PATIENT'S ADDRESS (No., Street)
123 TITANIC PLACE

6. PATIENT RELATIONSHIP TO INSURED
Self ☑ Spouse ☐ Child ☐ Other ☐

7. INSURED'S ADDRESS (No., Street)
123 TITANIC PLACE

CITY NEW YORK STATE NY

8. RESERVED FOR NUCC USE

CITY NEW YORK STATE NY

ZIP CODE 10001 TELEPHONE (Include Area Code) ( )

ZIP CODE 10001 TELEPHONE (Include Area Code) ( )

9. OTHER INSURED'S NAME (Last Name, First Name, Middle Initial)
ROSE DAWSON

10. IS PATIENT'S CONDITION RELATED TO:

11. INSURED'S POLICY GROUP OR FECA NUMBER
123-45-6789A

a. OTHER INSURED'S POLICY OR GROUP NUMBER
123-45-6789

a. EMPLOYMENT? (Current or Previous) YES ☐ NO ☑

a. INSURED'S DATE OF BIRTH MM 02 DD 17 YY XXXX SEX M ☐ F ☑

b. RESERVED FOR NUCC USE

b. AUTO ACCIDENT? YES ☐ NO ☑ PLACE (State)

b. OTHER CLAIM ID (Designated by NUCC)

c. RESERVED FOR NUCC USE

c. OTHER ACCIDENT? YES ☐ NO ☑

c. INSURANCE PLAN NAME OR PROGRAM NAME
MEDICARE

d. INSURANCE PLAN NAME OR PROGRAM NAME
AARP SECONDARY POLICY

10d. CLAIM CODES (Designated by NUCC)

d. IS THERE ANOTHER HEALTH BENEFIT PLAN?
YES ☑ NO ☐ If yes, complete items 9, 9a, and 9d.

READ BACK OF FORM BEFORE COMPLETING & SIGNING THIS FORM.

12. PATIENT'S OR AUTHORIZED PERSON'S SIGNATURE I authorize the release of any medical or other information necessary to process this claim. I also request payment of government benefits either to myself or to the party who accepts assignment below.
SIGNED SIGNATURE ON FILE DATE 01/14/20XX

13. INSURED'S OR AUTHORIZED PERSON'S SIGNATURE I authorize payment of medical benefits to the undersigned physician or supplier for services described below.
SIGNED SIGNATURE ON FILE

14. DATE OF CURRENT ILLNESS, INJURY, or PREGNANCY (LMP) MM DD YY QUAL.

15. OTHER DATE QUAL. MM DD YY

16. DATES PATIENT UNABLE TO WORK IN CURRENT OCCUPATION FROM MM DD YY TO MM DD YY

17. NAME OF REFERRING PROVIDER OR OTHER SOURCE
ROBERT WILSON, MD

17a.
17b. NPI 11122233344

18. HOSPITALIZATION DATES RELATED TO CURRENT SERVICES FROM MM DD YY TO MM DD YY

19. ADDITIONAL CLAIM INFORMATION (Designated by NUCC)

20. OUTSIDE LAB? YES ☐ NO ☐ $ CHARGES

21. DIAGNOSIS OR NATURE OF ILLNESS OR INJURY Relate A-L to service line below (24E) ICD Ind.
A. E11.22 B. C. D.
E. F. G. H.
I. J. K. L.

22. RESUBMISSION CODE ORIGINAL REF. NO.

23. PRIOR AUTHORIZATION NUMBER

24. A. DATE(S) OF SERVICE From MM DD YY	To MM DD YY	B. PLACE OF SERVICE	C. EMG	D. PROCEDURES, SERVICES, OR SUPPLIES (Explain Unusual Circumstances) CPT/HCPCS	MODIFIER	E. DIAGNOSIS POINTER	F. $ CHARGES	G. DAYS OR UNITS	H. EPSDT Family Plan	I. ID. QUAL.	J. RENDERING PROVIDER ID. #
1 01 14 XXXX	01 14 XXXX	11		99213		1	$125 00	1		NPI	11122233344
2										NPI	
3										NPI	
4										NPI	
5										NPI	
6										NPI	

25. FEDERAL TAX I.D. NUMBER 098-76-5432 SSN ☐ EIN ☑

26. PATIENT'S ACCOUNT NO. RW125638

27. ACCEPT ASSIGNMENT? (For govt. claims, see back) YES ☑ NO ☐

28. TOTAL CHARGE $ 125 00

29. AMOUNT PAID $ 0

30. Rsvd for NUCC Use

31. SIGNATURE OF PHYSICIAN OR SUPPLIER INCLUDING DEGREES OR CREDENTIALS (I certify that the statements on the reverse apply to this bill and are made a part thereof.)
Robert Wilson, MD 01/14/XXXX
SIGNED DATE

32. SERVICE FACILITY LOCATION INFORMATION
Feel Better Family Practice
101 Jack Place
New York, NY, 10001
(212) 555-1212
a. 22233344455 b.

33. BILLING PROVIDER INFO & PH # ( )
Robert Wilson, MD
101 Jack Place
New York, NY, 10001
(212) 555-1212
a. 11122233344 b.

NUCC Instruction Manual available at: www.nucc.org PLEASE PRINT OR TYPE APPROVED OMB-0938-1197 FORM 1500 (02-12)

Fig. 14.2 CMS 1500 (02-12) insurance claim form. (From the US Department of Health and Human Services, Centers for Medicare and Medicaid Services.)

B. Medicare

1. Requires the provider to report to the primary carrier on the CMS-1500 form
2. Filing deadline is December 31 of the year following service

C. Medicaid

1. File this claim as soon as possible after service
2. Providers treating Medicaid patients must accept the assignment and accept Medicaid reimbursements as payment in full for the service
3. Patients cannot be billed for qualified services, regardless of the Medicaid amount reimbursed to the provider
4. Services not covered by Medicaid may be billed directly to the patient
5. Keep a copy of the patient's Medicaid identification card within his or her chart

D. Workers' Compensation

1. Form completed in quadruplicate at patient's first visit to report the injury; copies are sent to the state workers' compensation board, compensation carrier, and employer; a copy is also inserted in the patient's chart
2. Filing deadlines may vary by state
3. Progress reports should be a narrative and should indicate any significant changes in the patient's current status
4. If an established patient seeks treatment for a work-related condition, create a separate chart and ledger card for the work-related condition
5. Provider must accept assignment and reimbursement as payment in full

E. Reasons Claims Can Be Delayed or Rejected

1. Coding errors
2. Typographical errors
3. Missing dates
4. Incorrect identification or policy numbers
5. Diagnosis does not support treatment rendered
6. Patient name does not match policyholder's name
7. Dates of treatments do not correspond with dates on the documents
8. Missing attachments
9. Defacement of bar code area of the claim form
10. Submission of claim to the wrong carrier
11. Patient ineligible for benefits
12. Fee total calculated incorrectly

15

Infection Control and Asepsis

I. Medical Asepsis

A. Definition

1. Object or area clean and free from infection

B. Microorganisms/Microbes

1. Definition
   a. Plants or animals that cannot be seen with the naked eye
2. Two types
   a. Nonpathogens: do not cause disease
   b. Pathogens: cause disease; disease-causing agents
3. Growth requirements
   a. Nutrition: living or nonliving substances
   b. Oxygen: most need oxygen (aerobes); some do not (anaerobes)
   c. Temperature: 98.6°F
   d. Darkness: grow best in dark
   e. Moisture: required for metabolism
   f. pH: neutral pH

II. Infection Process Cycle (Chain of Infection) (Fig. 15.1)

A. General

1. Growth of microorganisms in cycle
2. Break the cycle, break the process

B. Reservoir Host

1. Start of the chain
2. May be an insect, animal, or human

3. Supplies nutrition to the microorganism
4. May not cause disease in the reservoir

C. Means/Portal of Exit

1. How the organism escapes the reservoir host
2. Exits include the mouth, nose, eyes, ears, intestines, urinary tract, reproductive tract, and open wounds

D. Means/Modes of Transmission

1. Way organisms are spread
   a. Direct transmission: occurs from contact with an infected person or discharges of an infected person
   b. Indirect transmission: occurs from droplets in the air, vectors (insects) that harbor pathogens, contaminated food or drink, and fomites (contaminated objects)

E. Means/Portals of Entry

1. How the organism gains entry into a new host
2. Entries include the mouth, nose, eyes, intestines, urinary tract, reproductive tract, and open wounds

F. Susceptible Host

1. One that is capable of supporting the growth of a microorganism
2. Factors that affect susceptibility
   a. Location of entry
   b. Dose of organisms
   c. Physical condition/level of immunity of individual
3. If conditions are right, susceptible host becomes reservoir host; the chain or cycle begins again

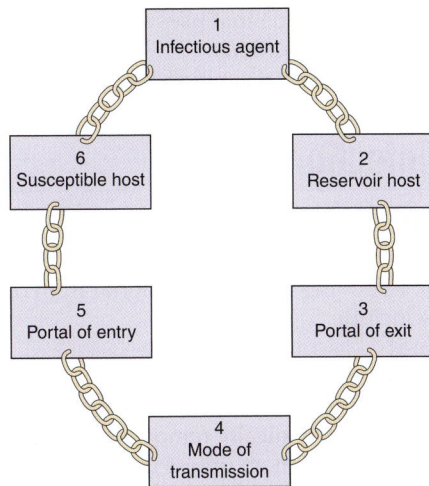

Fig. 15.1 The chain of infection. (From Niedzwiecki B et al: *Kinn's The medical assistant: an applied learning approach*, ed 14, 2020, Elsevier.)

G. Inflammation

1. Trauma to the body alerts the protective mechanisms
2. The body responds
   a. Blood vessels at the site dilate; the number of white blood cells in the area increases, which causes redness
   b. White blood cells overpower and consume microorganisms (phagocytosis), which causes swelling
   c. Fluids in tissues increase and put pressure on nerves, which causes pain
   d. Blood supply to area increases and causes heat
3. The process creates four classic signs of inflammation: redness, swelling, pain, and heat

H. Protective Mechanisms of the Body

1. Body's own way of preventing entrance of pathogens
2. Help break the infection process cycle
3. Include
   a. Skin: most important barrier
   b. Mucous membranes: protect against invasion in the nose, throat, respiratory tract, gastrointestinal tract, and genital tract
   c. Mucus and cilia: trap microorganisms that enter through the nose and respiratory tract
   d. Coughing and sneezing: force out pathogens
   e. Tears and sweat: aid in removal
   f. Urine and vaginal secretions: acidic fluids that are incompatible with pathogen growth
   g. Hydrochloric acid: secreted by stomach; provides acidic environment

III. Occupational Safety and Health Administration Standards

A. General

1. Occupational Safety and Health Administration (OSHA) sets standards and protocols for health and safety

B. Blood-Borne Pathogens

1. Disease-causing microorganisms that may be present in the blood or bodily fluids
2. Concerned mainly with hepatitis B virus (HBV), hepatitis C virus (HCV), and human immunodeficiency virus (HIV)
3. Blood-borne pathogens are transmitted when infected blood comes into contact with nonintact skin or mucous membranes

C. Standard Precautions

1. Concept of treating all blood and body fluids as if they are infected
2. Includes blood, body fluids, excretions, and secretions

D. Prevention of Exposure

1. Immunization: all persons who come in contact with blood or body fluids should receive the hepatitis B series
2. Engineering controls: mechanical devices designed to minimize exposure; include
   a. Eyewash stations
   b. Sharps containers
   c. Biohazard waste containers and labels
   d. Handwashing stations
3. Personal protection equipment: equipment that minimizes exposure beyond engineering controls; includes
   a. Gloves
   b. Laboratory coats
   c. Eye or face shields and masks

E. Exposure Control

1. Contaminated sharps placed in sharps container (puncture-resistant and leak-proof container) immediately after use
2. Do not bend, break, or recap used needles
3. Work surfaces and equipment should be cleaned and decontaminated with disinfectant after each use
4. Contaminated waste (except sharps) should be discarded in a clearly labeled biohazard waste container ("red bag trash")
5. Employee exposure incidents should be reported as directed and properly followed up to ensure that they do not occur again

F. Postexposure Follow-Up

1. If exposed through accidental needlestick, human bite, exposure to broken skin, or splash or splatter onto mucous membranes
   a. Immediately flush or wash exposed area
   b. Report to supervisor
   c. Receive confidential medical evaluation; all documentation kept confidential
   d. Incident report filled out
   e. Source, if known, screened for HIV for HBV and for HCV; consent may or may not be required depending on state law

f. Exposed worker tested for HIV and HBV
g. Exposed worker must receive health counseling
h. Exposed worker may/may not start medication
2. Follow Safety Data Sheet (SDS) guidelines

IV. Hand Hygiene

A. General

1. Most important defense against transmission of microorganisms
2. Proper and effective handwashing depends on friction and running water
3. Hands should be washed
   a. Between patients
   b. After handling specimens
   c. Before and after using the restroom
   d. After handling contaminated materials
   e. Before eating or drinking
   f. Before leaving the clinic at the end of the day
4. Handwashing procedure
   a. Remove all jewelry except plain wedding band
   b. Using warm water, thoroughly wet the hands
   c. Apply soap; lather while keeping the fingers pointed downward
   d. Rub, using friction for 30 seconds; wash between the fingers
   e. Rinse; allow water to flow from the wrist to the fingertips
   f. Thoroughly dry the hands with paper towels, and turn off the faucet or faucets with the paper towels
   g. Apply lotion if desired

B. Alcohol-Based Hand Sanitizers

1. Used when hands are not visibly soiled
2. Remove transient bacteria
3. Sanitizer should be spread over all surfaces of the hands and fingers, around and under nails, up to ½ inch above wrists; rub until hands feel dry

C. Gloves

1. Clean, disposable gloves worn when contact with body substance likely
2. Worn when administering injections, performing venipuncture, and performing lab testing
3. Gloves changed between patients

V. Sanitization

A. General

1. Process of cleaning or removing materials from objects
2. Requires scrubbing objects with detergents and brushes
3. First step in sterilization process
4. Methods
   a. Detergents: agents that remove bacteria, fats, oils, and protein substances (blood)

b. Ultrasound: machine that uses sound waves through a liquid to cause vibrations
c. Antiseptic: agent that sanitizes the skin

VI. Disinfection

A. General

1. Process of removing infectious material from objects
2. Processes include
   a. Chemical
      1) Surface germicide
      2) Used on inanimate objects sensitive to heat
         a) Soap: mechanically removes bacteria but does not destroy them unless the soap is germicidal
         b) Alcohol: commonly used on skin
         c) Acids: solutions containing phenol
         d) Alkalis: bleach; used in the laboratory on flat surfaces
         e) Formalin: solution requires rinsing
   b. Ultraviolet (UV) radiation: UV light can have an effect on surfaces but does not penetrate surfaces
   c. Desiccation: drying; does not kill spores
   d. Boiling: kills most bacteria; does not kill some spores and viruses

VII. Sterilization

A. General

1. Complete destruction of all microorganisms and spores
2. Processes include
   a. Chemical
      1) May be used for heat-sensitive materials
      2) Objects must be completely submerged for long periods
      3) Glutaraldehyde solutions commonly used
   b. Steam under pressure
      1) Autoclave
      2) Most common and effective sterilization method
   c. Gas: special chamber that uses a gas
   d. Oven: dry heat

VIII. Use of the Autoclave

A. Preparing Instruments and Supplies

1. Instruments are sanitized and dried before wrapping
2. Wrapping materials
   a. Muslin
   b. Disposable paper
   c. Peel-back pouches
3. Open any hinged instruments to allow steam to reach all surfaces
4. Items to be wrapped are placed in the center of the wrapping material, with corners of the wrap at the top, bottom, and sides; bring the bottom of the wrapper up over the instrument, folding back a small corner for a handle;

bring in the sides, one at a time, also folding back the small corners; the top of the wrapper is brought around the object and secured with sterilizer tape

5. Label the tape with the identity of the contents, date, and operator's initials
6. Packs should be no larger than $12 \times 12 \times 20$ inches
7. Sterilization indicator should be included in the pack to show that the proper time and temperature were achieved

B. Loading the Autoclave

1. Packs should be placed vertically, 1–3 inches apart, away from the sides of the chamber
2. Place hard goods underneath soft goods
3. Open glassware should be placed on its side

C. Autoclave Procedure

1. Autoclave is a piece of equipment that provides steam under pressure
2. Autoclave is normally run at 250°F, 20–30 lb of pressure, for 15–30 minutes
3. Moist heat in the form of steam circulates in a pattern throughout the autoclave chamber
4. Check the autoclave water level; add distilled water if necessary
5. Properly load the autoclave
6. Close the autoclave door securely; turn the unit on
7. Begin timing when the proper temperature and pressure are achieved
8. After the autoclave cycle is completed, vent the autoclave chamber
9. Open the autoclave door just slightly to allow the contents to dry
10. Remove the dry items and check the indicator on the sterilizer tape; wrapped items may be handled with clean hands
11. Store sterilized items in a clean, dust-proof area; the shelf life of sterilized items is approximately 30 days (resterilize items after 30 days)

Vital Signs and Anthropometric Measurements

I. Vital Signs

A. General

1. Measurements that indicate a patient's general state of health and homeostasis
2. Can indicate a change in health or the presence or disappearance of a disease
3. Accuracy is essential
4. Includes temperature, pulse, respiration (TPR) and blood pressure (BP) (cardinal signs)
5. Can also include pain assessment and pulse oximetry (saturation of peripheral oxygen [SpO_2])

B. Temperature

1. Balance between heat lost by the body and heat that the body produces
2. Heat is produced by metabolism
3. In illness, metabolism increases, increasing internal heat production and increasing the body temperature
4. Variation in a patient's baseline temperature may be the first warning of an illness or change in condition
5. Body temperature is regulated by the hypothalamus
6. Factors affecting body temperature
    a. Age: body heat decreases with age
    b. Environment: exposure, wind chill, and temperature
    c. Activity: physical activity increases body temperature
    d. Diurnal variation: body temperature is lowest in the morning and highest in the evening
    e. Emotions: agitation increases body temperature; depression lowers body temperature
    f. Physiologic processes: body temperature increases with digestion, ovulation, and pregnancy
7. Normal ranges
    a. Oral: 97°F–99°F (36°C–37.8°C)

b. Rectal: 1°F higher than oral (most accurate measurement)
    c. Axillary: 1°F lower than oral (least accurate measurement)
    d. Tympanic (aural): 1°F higher than oral
    e. Temporal artery: 1°F higher than oral
8. Characteristics
    a. Fever: pyrexia; temperature >100°F; temperature ≥105°F can cause brain damage or death if untreated
    b. Febrile: having fever
    c. Afebrile: without fever
    d. Intermittent: fluctuation among normal, abnormal, and fever
    e. Remittent: elevated fluctuations that do not return to normal
    f. Lysis: gradual return to normal
    g. Crisis: sudden return to normal
    h. Fever of unknown origin (FUO): temperature >100.9°F that lasts for 3 weeks in adults and 1 week in children without a known related diagnosis
9. Stages of fever:
    a. Onset: temperature first begins to increase; may be slow or sudden; the patient may experience cold/chills, and pulse and respiration rates may increase
    b. Course of a fever: temperature rises and falls; the patient feels warm to the touch, and pulse and respiration rates increase
    c. Subsiding: the patient's temperature returns to normal
10. Equipment: thermometer; a device used to measure body temperature
    a. Electronic: consists of a battery-powered unit and a probe covered by a disposable plastic cover; temperature is displayed digitally; unit has blue (oral) and red (rectal) probes
    b. Tympanic (aural): handheld processor unit with a tympanic probe covered by a disposable cover; picks up infrared energy from the tympanic membrane; proper technique is important for correct results (Fig. 16.1)

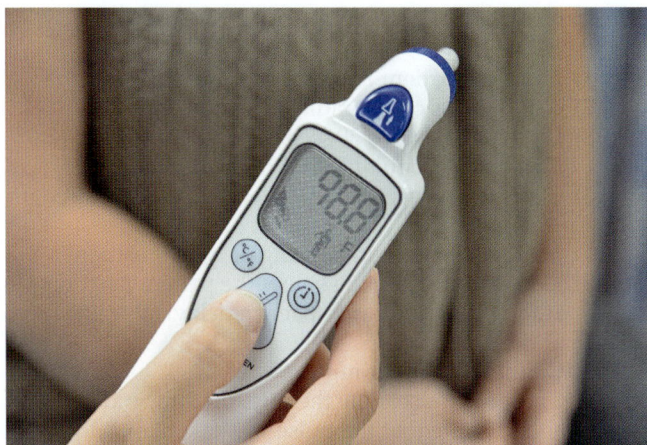

Fig. 16.1 Tympanic membrane thermometer. (From Niedzwiecki B et al: *Kinn's The medical assistant: an applied learning approach*, ed 14, 2020, Elsevier.)

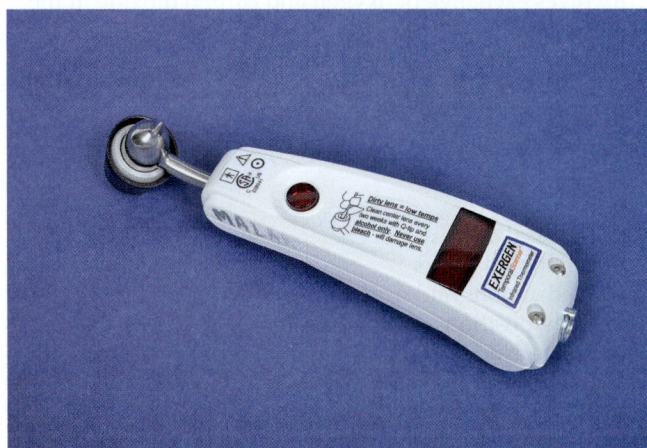

Fig. 16.2 Temporal artery thermometer. (From Niedzwiecki B et al: *Kinn's The medical assistant: an applied learning approach*, ed 14, 2020, Elsevier.)

Fig. 16.3 Charting a temperature reading in SimChart for the medical office.

   c. Temporal artery: electronic device consisting of a probe attached to a portable unit; the probe is slowly moved across the patient's forehead; the sensor picks up infrared heat given off by the temporal artery (Fig. 16.2)
   d. Chemical, single use: contains chemicals that are heat sensitive; dots containing chemicals change color in response to body heat; placed under the tongue
   e. Temperature-sensitive strips: reusable plastic strip that contains heat-sensitive liquid crystals that change color; strip is pressed onto the forehead
11. Charting
   a. Record the patient's temperature within the patient record either in the paper-based record or in the electronic medical record (Fig. 16.3)
   b. Indicate (after the number) what method was used to record patient's temperature: oral—no need to indicate the site, rectal (R), axillary (A), tympanic (T), or temporal artery (TA)
12. Procedure
   a. Oral: place thermometer under the patient's tongue; instruct the patient to keep the lips closed around the thermometer and to breathe through the nose
   b. Axillary: wipe the axilla dry; place the thermometer under the patient's arm

   c. Rectal: apply lubricating jelly to the thermometer; insert into the rectum approximately 1 inch
   d. Tympanic
      1) For adult: gently pull the pinna up and back; insert the probe into the ear canal
      2) For child: gently pull the pinna down and back; insert the probe into the ear canal
   e. Temporal artery
      1) Move probe gently and slowly across patient's forehead

C. Pulse

1. Palpable beat of arteries as they expand with the beat of the heart
2. Pulse in any artery usually is the same as the heartbeat
3. Rate and characteristics can give information about the cardiovascular system
   a. Anxiety, stress, and nervousness
4. Factors affecting pulse
   a. Increased pulse rate: pain, fever, infection, and hyperthyroidism
   b. Decreased pulse rate: chronic pain, central nervous system disorders, and hypothyroidism
5. Characteristics
   a. Rate: number of beats per minute (bpm)
   b. Rhythm: time between beats
   c. Volume: force of beats
   d. Condition of arterial wall: springy, resilient, and elastic
6. Normal ranges
   a. Birth: 120–160 bpm
   b. 1–3 years: 90–140 bpm
   c. 3–6 years: 80–110 bpm
   d. 6–12 years: 75–105 bpm
   e. 12–18 years: 60–100 bpm
   f. Adult (up to age 60): 60–100 bpm
   g. Adult (after age 60): 67–80 bpm
   h. Athlete: 40–60 bpm

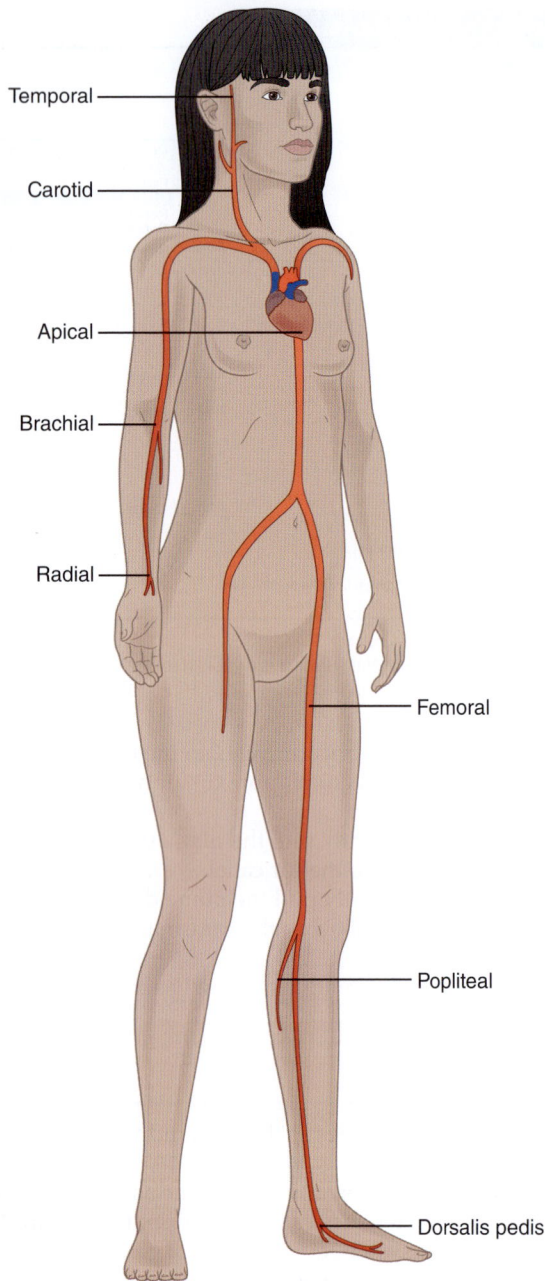

Fig. 16.4 Pulse sites. (From Niedzwiecki B et al: *Kinn's The medical assistant: an applied learning approach*, ed 14, 2020, Elsevier.)

7. Pulse sites (Fig. 16.4)
   a. Radial: most common; located on the thumb side of the wrist
   b. Carotid: located in the groove of the neck between the larynx and the sternocleidomastoid muscle; used in emergencies and during cardiopulmonary resuscitation (CPR)
   c. Brachial: located in the antecubital space; reference for BP
   d. Femoral: located in the groin
   e. Temporal: located over the temporal bone
   f. Popliteal: located at the back of the knee
   g. Dorsalis pedis: located on the top of the foot
   h. Apical: located just below the left nipple on the left side of the chest; taken with a stethoscope for 1 full minute; used for infants, young children, and cardiac patients

8. Procedure
   a. Radial pulse
      1) Have the patient in a sitting or lying position
      2) Gently press on the radial artery until the pulse is felt
      3) Count the beat for 30 seconds and multiply by 2; if the beat is irregular, count for 1 minute
      4) Chart the pulse; note the rate, rhythm, and strength
   b. Apical pulse
      1) Have the patient in a sitting or lying position
      2) Place the stethoscope below the patient's left nipple at the fifth intercostal space midclavicular line (apex of the heart)
      3) Count for 1 full minute
      4) Chart the pulse: note the rate, rhythm, and strength and indicate that the pulse was taken apically (A)

D. Respiration

1. Involves exchange of oxygen and carbon dioxide in the lungs
2. Cycle consists of one inspiration and one expiration
3. Controlled by the medulla oblongata; the breathing rate is determined by the carbon dioxide level in the blood
4. Factors affecting respiration
   a. Disease
   b. Age
   c. Physical activity
   d. Emotional status
   e. Medications and drugs
   f. Body position
5. Characteristics
   a. Rate: number of respirations per minute
   b. Rhythm: breathing pattern
   c. Depth: amount of air being inhaled
6. Normal ranges (breaths per minute)
   a. Birth to 1 year: 30–40 breaths/minute
   b. 1–3 years: 23–35 breaths/minute
   c. 3–6 years: 20–30 breaths/minute
   d. 6–12 years: 18–26 breaths/minute
   e. 12–18 years: 12–20 breaths/minute
   f. Adult: 12–20 breaths/minute
7. Breathing patterns
   a. Eupnea: normal breathing
   b. Dyspnea: difficult, painful, or labored breathing
   c. Apnea: absence of breathing; temporary condition
   d. Orthopnea: difficulty breathing while lying down
   e. Hyperpnea: increased rate of breathing
   f. Tachypnea: excessively rapid breathing
   g. Rales: gurgling sounds caused by secretions
   h. Rhonchi: rattling sounds
   i. Cheyne-Stokes respirations: alternating periods of apnea and tachypnea; can indicate impending death
8. Procedure
   a. Respiration can be consciously controlled; the respiration rate should be counted without the patient's knowledge so that the patient is unaware of your respiration count; continue to act as if you are taking the pulse
   b. Watch the rise and fall of the patient's chest; count one inhalation and one exhalation as one respiration
   c. Count for 30 seconds and multiply by 2; if irregular, count for 1 minute
   d. Chart the respiration: note the rate, depth, and rhythm; note any irregularities

E. Pulse Oximetry

1. Noninvasive procedure used to measure oxygen saturation of hemoglobin, in arterial blood
2. Pulse oximeter: computerized device with a cliplike probe connected by a cable to a monitor (Fig. 16.5)
3. Normal range: 95%–99%
4. Reading recorded as SpO_2 (saturation of peripheral oxygen)
5. Can also measure pulse rate (bpm)
6. Factors affecting pulse oximetry
   a. Incorrect positioning of probe
   b. Dark fingernail polish or artificial nails
   c. Poor peripheral blood flow
   d. Ambient (surrounding) light
   e. Patient movement
7. Procedure
   a. Probe attached at peripheral site that is highly vascular and skin is thin (i.e., fingertip, toe, and earlobe)
   b. Leave probe in place until oximeter displays reading

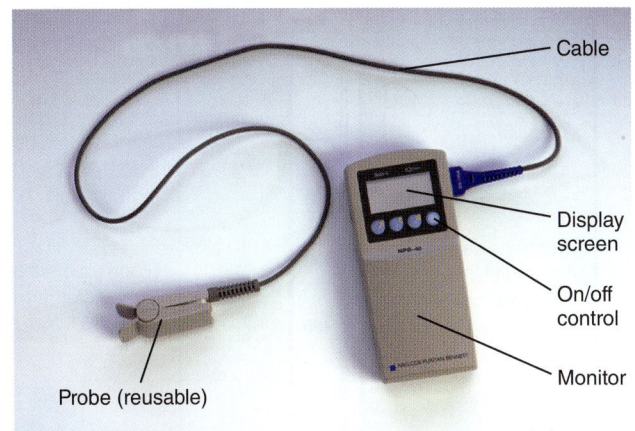

Fig. 16.5 Pulse oximeter. (From Bonewit-West K, Hunt S: *Today's medical assistant*, ed 4, 2021, Saunders.)

F. Blood Pressure

1. Measurement of the pressure of the blood against the walls of the arteries
2. Two readings
   a. Systolic pressure (systole): highest pressure; occurs when the heart contracts
   b. Diastolic pressure (diastole): lowest pressure; occurs when the heart relaxes
3. Systole + diastole = one cardiac cycle
4. Measured in millimeters of mercury (mm Hg)
5. Recorded as a fraction: systolic/diastolic
6. Factors affecting BP
   a. Age: BP increases with age
   b. Activity: BP increases with physical activity
   c. Gender
   d. Diurnal variation: BP is lower in the morning than it is at other times of the day
   e. Stress
   f. Disease state
   g. Medication
7. Normal ranges
   a. Newborn: 50/30 mm Hg
   b. 1–6 years: 95/65 mm Hg
   c. 6–12 years: 100/65 mm Hg
   d. 16 years to adult: 118/75 mm Hg
   e. Adult: 120/80 mm Hg (average); normally ranges from 90/60 to < 140/90 mm Hg
   f. Older adult: 130/80 mm Hg
8. Characteristics
   a. Hypertension (HTN): high BP
      1) BP > 130/80 mm Hg
      2) Essential HTN: unknown cause
      3) Secondary HTN: associated with other disease processes
      4) Malignant: life-threatening severe form of hypertension
   b. Hypotension: low BP, < 90/60 mm Hg
   c. Orthostatic hypotension: temporary decrease in BP that occurs when a patient rapidly changes from a lying or sitting position to a standing position

   d. Pulse pressure
      1) Difference between systolic and diastolic pressure
      2) Average is 40 mm Hg
9. Equipment
   a. Sphygmomanometer: consists of an inflatable cuff (various sizes for different-sized patients) with an inflation bulb (with control valve) and pressure gauge (mercury column or aneroid dial)
   b. Stethoscope: instrument used to listen to pulse
   c. Automatic method requires a monitor that is either portable or wall mounted; no stethoscope is required
10. Procedure (Fig. 16.6)
    a. Objective
       1) Use of the inflatable cuff causes circulation in the artery to disappear
       2) As the cuff is slowly deflated, blood flow resumes, and cardiac cycle sounds are heard through the stethoscope
       3) Gauge readings are taken when the first sound is heard (systolic) and when the last sound is heard (diastolic)
    b. Palpate the brachial artery in the antecubital space
    c. Place the cuff snugly around the patient's arm approximately 1–2 inches above the arm fold, with the arrow on the cuff pointing to the brachial artery
    d. Place the stethoscope over the brachial artery
    e. Close the valve, and inflate the cuff to approximately 200 mm Hg
    f. Slowly release the valve to deflate the cuff; the gauge needle should drop 2 mm Hg/s for proper release rate
    g. Note the gauge reading when the first beat is heard (systolic)
    h. Continue deflating the cuff until the last beat is heard (diastolic)
    i. Fully release the bulb valve, deflate the cuff, and remove it from the patient
    j. Record the result in the patient's chart; indicate which arm was used for reading (right or left); may also indicate the patient's position (sitting, standing, and lying)
    k. Follow manufacturer's instructions for procedure

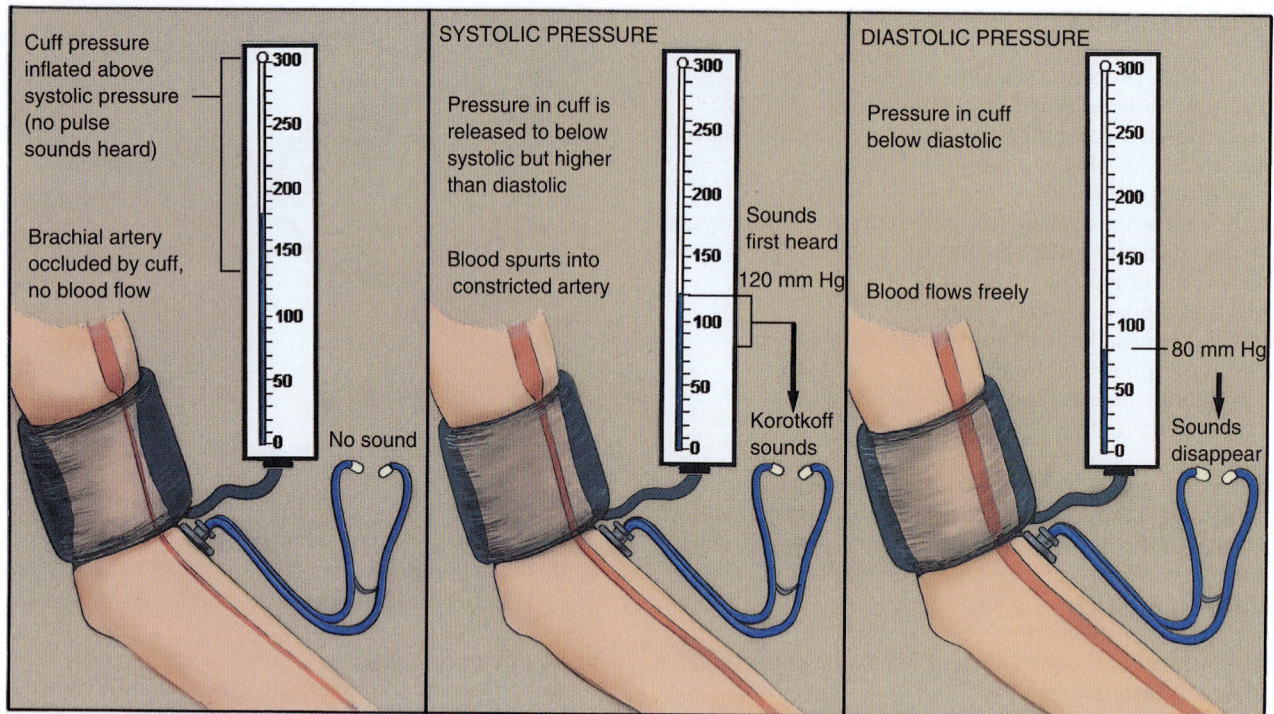

Fig. 16.6 Measurement of blood pressure using a sphygmomanometer and stethoscope. (From Applegate EJ: *The anatomy and physiology learning system*, ed 4, 2011, Saunders.)

11. Korotkoff sounds: sounds heard during the measurement of BP
    a. Phase I: the first sound heard as the cuff deflates; systolic reading
    b. Phase II: swishing sound; blood is flowing through the artery, and sounds may completely disappear and reappear later (auscultatory gap)
    c. Phase III: sharp, tapping sounds return and continue rhythmically
    d. Phase IV: a soft tapping sound that becomes muffled and begins to grow fainter; may be recorded as the fading sound and recorded between the systolic and diastolic (e.g., 130/85/70 mm Hg)
    e. Phase V: sounds disappear; the last sound heard; diastolic reading

II. Pain

A. Definition

1. Unpleasant sensory and emotional experience arising from actual or potential tissue damage
2. Approximately half of patients seek medical attention because of pain
3. Can arise from any organ system
4. Subjective and personal
5. Can reveal tremendous amount of information about the health status of the patient

B. Effects of Pain

1. Disturbs sleep patterns
2. Affects eating patterns and appetite
3. Affects activity patterns
4. Affects mood and emotions
5. Can affect family relationships
6. Can alter physical appearance, sexual function, and energy levels

C. Factors That Influence Pain Experience

1. Nature of illness or injury
2. Physical and emotional health of the patient
3. Whether symptoms are acute or chronic
4. Social status or cultural upbringing of the patient
5. Memory and personality of the patient

D. Symptoms and Diagnosis (Colder)

1. C: character of the pain
2. O: onset of the pain
3. L: location of the pain
4. D: duration of the pain
5. E: what exacerbates the pain
6. R: what relieves the pain

E. Assessment Tools

1. Wong-Baker FACES Pain Rating Scale (Fig. 16.7)
2. Numerical pain scale
    a. Scale of 0–10 (0 represents no pain; 10 represents the worst pain imaginable)

F. Pain Management

1. Analgesic medication
2. Tactile stimulation

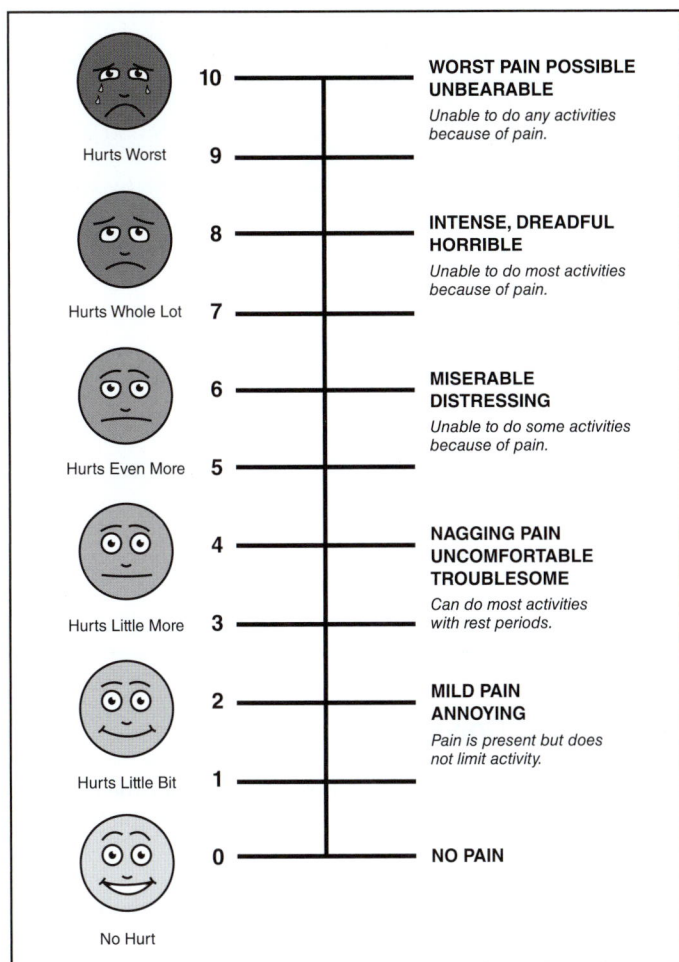

Fig. 16.7 Wong-Baker FACES Pain Rating Scale. (From Niedzwiecki B et al: *Kinn's The medical assistant: an applied learning approach*, ed 14, 2020, Elsevier.)

3. Relaxation techniques
4. Diversion

III. Anthropometric Measurement

A. General

1. Deals with the measurement of size, weight, and proportion of the human body
2. Often included with vital signs

B. Weight

1. May be measured in pounds or kilograms
   a. Place a paper towel on the base of the scale if the patient removes his or her shoes; the patient should be weighed consistently with or without shoes, depending on office procedure
   b. Have the patient stand erect in the center of the base of the scale
   c. Move the large weight to the 50-lb notch nearest to, but under, the patient's weight
   d. Move the smaller weight to the right until the balance needle is in the middle of the frame
   e. Add the large and small weights together; record the result, in pounds, on the patient's chart to the nearest 1/4 lb
   f. Return both weights to zero after the patient leaves the scale
   g. 1 kg = 2.2 lb; 1 lb = 0.45 kg
   h. May also use electronic scale

C. Height

1. May be measured in inches, feet/inches, or centimeters
   a. Place a paper towel on the base of the scale if the patient removes his or her shoes (as previously described)
   b. Have the patient stand erect in the center of the base of the scale
   c. Lower the height bar until it rests on the top of the patient's head
   d. Note the height indicated on the height bar; record the result, in inches, on the patient's chart to the nearest 1/4 inch
   e. Return the height bar to the lowest position
   f. 1 inch = 2.54 cm; 1 cm = 0.39 inch

D. Body Composition

1. Measures percentage of body fat; percentage of body fat may be an indicator of cardiovascular disease, health, vitality, and appearance
2. Methods
   a. Body mass index (BMI)
      1) Height/weight ratio
      2) Correlates with total body fat
      3) Determined by comparing patient's height and weight against a BMI table
   b. Body fat percentage
      1) Caliper method
         a) Measures the thickness of a fold of fat tissue to give total percentage of body fat
         b) Measurements are taken in three to four sites; most common are triceps, biceps, subscapular, and suprailiac
         c) Normal range for males: 15%–19%
         d) Normal range for females: 22%–25%
      2) Bioelectrical impedance method
         a) Electrodes placed on the patient and hooked up to computer
         b) Computer determines body fat percentage on an impedance monitor
      3) Water displacement method
         a) Patient is submerged under water; amount of water displaced is measured
         b) Most accurate and most difficult

17

Assisting With the Physical Examination

I. General

A. Purpose

1. The purpose of the physical examination is to determine the patient's overall state of health and well-being
2. All major organ systems are checked and evaluated

B. Preparation

1. The medical assistant prepares the patient for examination by gowning, positioning, and draping
2. The medical assistant prepares the examination room by setting out the correct equipment and supplies
3. The medical assistant may take the medical history and record the findings in the medical record

II. Gowning

A. General

1. Patient must undress and put on a gown; makes performing the procedure easier for the healthcare provider
2. Principle of gowning: expose only the body part that needs to be exposed for the examination

B. Considerations of Gowning

1. Patient's need for privacy and comfort
2. Type of examination or procedure to be performed
3. Patient's age and gender
4. Accessibility of the body part to be exposed for the examination

C. Types of Gowns

1. Usually all patient clothing is removed under the gown
2. Gown has an opening either in the back or in the front
   a. Full gown
      1) Knee length
      2) Opening extends the full length of the gown
      3) Closures are Velcro or ties
      4) Can be paper or cloth material
   b. Partial gown
      1) Covers only the chest, back, and shoulders
      2) Opening extends the full length of the gown
      3) Can be paper or cloth material

III. Positioning and Draping

A. General

1. Patient is generally positioned on an examination table
2. Table should be long and wide enough to support patients of all sizes
3. Table is covered with a paper covering or a cloth sheet; covering is changed after each patient

B. Positions (Fig. 17.1)

1. Erect
   a. Standing
   b. Patient is upright with arms at sides
   c. Used to examine the musculoskeletal system and the nervous system
2. Sitting (see Fig. 17.1A)
   a. Patient sits upright on the table with legs dangling over the edge of the table
   b. Used to examine the head, chest, EENT, heart, lungs, breasts, axilla, and upper extremities
   c. Draping: drape the sheet across the lap

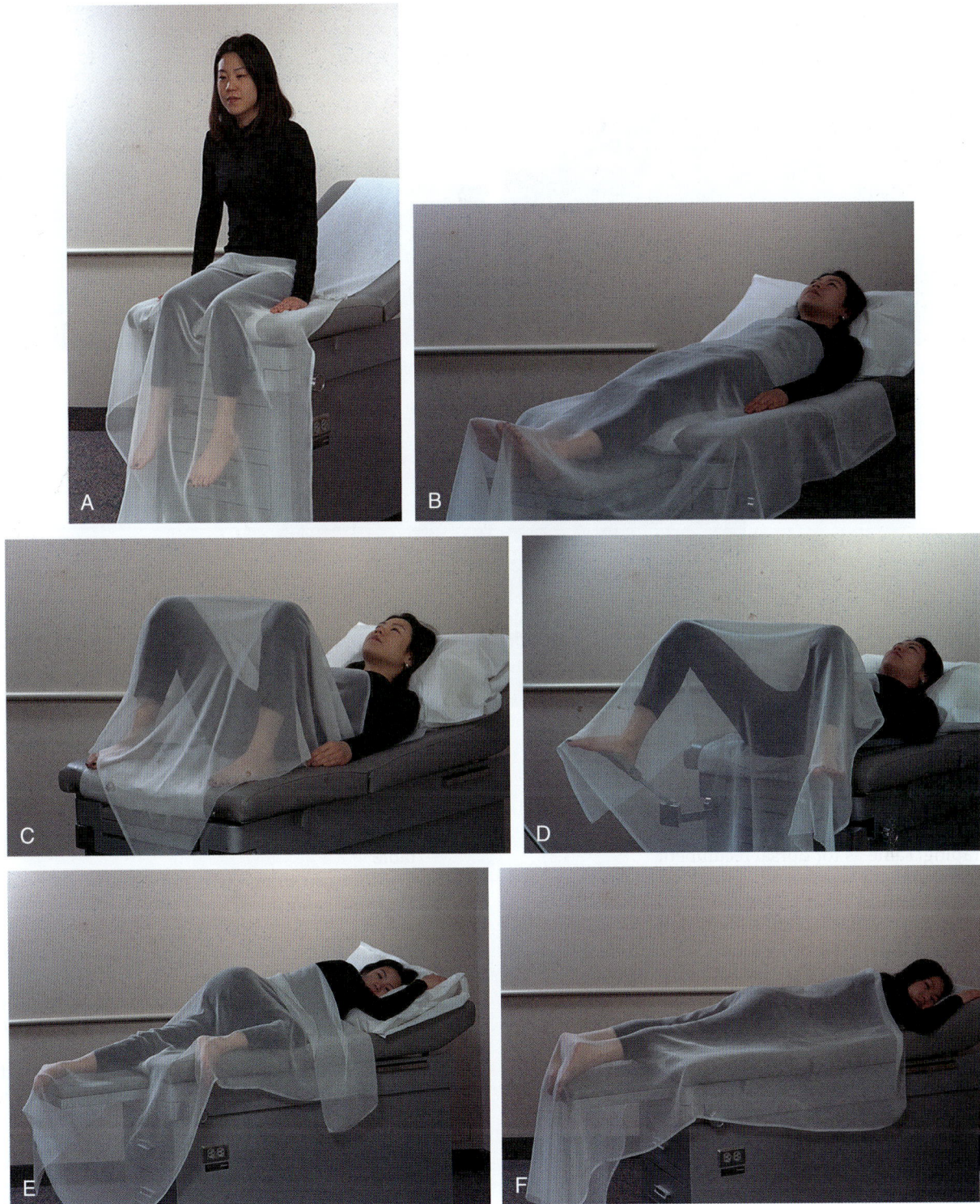

Fig. 17.1 Positions for examination. (From Niedzwiecki B, et al: *Kinn's The medical assistant: an applied learning approach*, ed 14, 2020, Elsevier.)

3. Supine (see Fig. 17.1B)
   a. Patient lies flat on the back with arms at the sides
   b. Used to examine the chest, abdominal area, heart, and extremities
   c. Draping: drape sheet extends from under the arms
4. Dorsal recumbent (see Fig. 17.1C)
   a. Patient is supine with legs bent at the knees and feet flat on the table
   b. Used to examine the genital and rectal areas

   c. Draping: drape sheet is placed over the patient in a diamond-shaped fashion with side corners wrapped around each leg; the upper and lower corners cover the chest, abdominal, and pubic areas
5. Lithotomy (see Fig. 17.1D)
   a. Patient is in dorsal recumbent position except that the feet are placed in stirrups; knees are bent; buttocks are moved to the end of the table

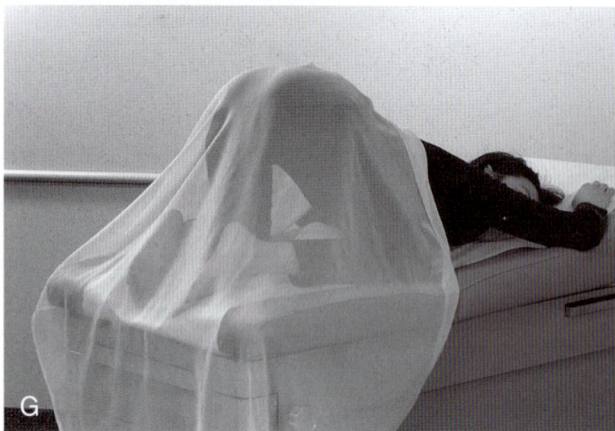

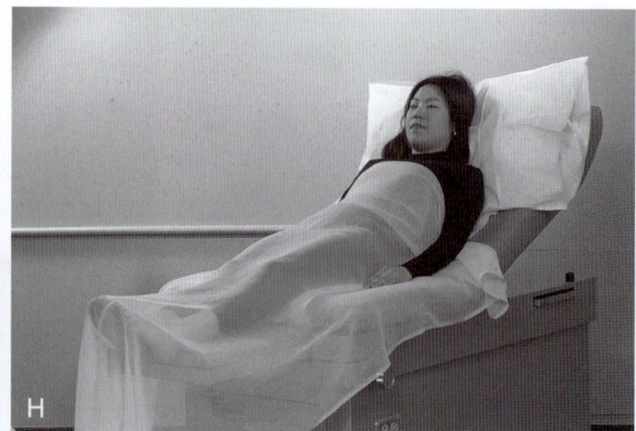

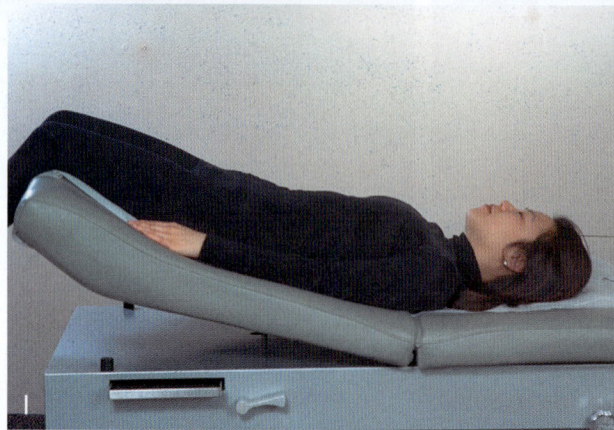

Fig. 17.1, cont'd

b. Used for vaginal examination, pelvic examination, and Papanicolaou (Pap) smear procedure
c. Draping: same as for dorsal recumbent
6. Lateral recumbent (see Fig. 17.1E)
   a. Lateral position
   b. Patient lies on the left side with the left arm behind the body and the right arm forward; both legs are flexed at the knees, but the right leg is sharply bent and positioned next to the left leg
   c. Used to examine the rectal area, perform enemas and douches, and insert suppositories
   d. Draping: drape sheet covers the patient from the shoulders to the toes; adjust to expose the necessary area
7. Prone (see Fig. 17.1F)
   a. Patient lies flat on the abdomen with the head turned to the side; arms are positioned above the head or at the sides of the body
   b. Used to examine the back, spine, and lower extremities
   c. Draping: drape sheet covers the patient from the waist to the knees; adjust to expose the necessary area
8. Knee-chest (see Fig. 17.1G)
   a. Genupectoral
   b. Patient assumes a kneeling position with the buttocks elevated, with head and chest on the table
   c. Used for proctologic examination
   d. Draping: drape sheet covers the buttocks; adjust to expose the necessary area

9. Proctologic
   a. Knee-chest position facilitated by the use of a special table
   b. Used for proctological examination
   c. Draping: same as for knee-chest
10. Fowler
    a. Patient sits on the examination table with the back supported at a 90-degree angle
    b. Used for examination and treatment of the head, neck, and chest, helpful for patients with breathing difficulties or heart conditions
    c. Draping: drape sheet covers the patient from the shoulders down; adjust to expose the necessary area
11. Semi-Fowler (see Fig. 17.1H)
    a. Modification of Fowler; back supported at a 45-degree angle
    b. Used for postsurgical examinations and for patients with head trauma or head pain
    c. Draping: same as for Fowler
12. Trendelenburg (see Fig. 17.1I)
    a. Patient is in supine with the foot of the table elevated 45 degrees (head lower than feet)
    b. Used for shock or abdominal surgery
    c. Draping: drape sheet covers the patient from underarms to below the knees; neck, head, and hands are left uncovered

C. General Considerations

1. Expose only the body part being examined or treated
2. Keep the patient as comfortable as possible
3. Provide a blanket for comfort and warmth
4. Modify the position to accommodate a weak or painful body part
5. Prevent the patient from falling from the table
6. A female medical assistant should be present when a male provider examines a female patient
7. Provide special assistance for patients with special needs (wheelchair-bound, elderly, mentally challenged)

IV. Complete Physical Examinations

A. General

1. Normally performed on new patients to assess their health status and to establish the patient's baseline
2. Also performed on established patients for health maintenance
3. Medical assistant must be familiar with the process, principles, and methods to prepare the patient and to assist the provider

B. Methods of Examination

1. Inspection
   a. Process of visual observation
   b. Includes looking for abnormalities in size, shape, color, continuity, symmetry, or position
2. Palpation
   a. Process of touching and feeling
   b. Can detect abnormalities of size, shape, texture, and tenderness
3. Percussion
   a. Process of tapping or striking the body
   b. Done with fingers or small hammer
   c. Aids in determination of size, position, or density of an organ or body cavity
4. Manipulation
   a. Forceful passive movement of a joint to determine the range of motion
5. Auscultation
   a. Process of listening to the body using a stethoscope
6. Mensuration
   a. Process of measurement

C. Commonly Used Equipment (Fig. 17.2)

1. Ophthalmoscope
   a. Instrument used to illuminate the internal eye for visual inspection
   b. Runs off power source (battery or wall unit)
2. Otoscope
   a. Instrument used to illuminate the external and internal ear for visual examination
   b. Runs off power source (battery or wall unit)
3. Pocket flashlight or headlight
   a. Instrument used to illuminate the mouth, throat, and nose for visual examination
4. Tape measure
   a. Instrument used to measure body structures
5. Tongue depressor
   a. Instrument used to control tongue movement while examining the mouth and throat
   b. Disposable; nonsterile
6. Stethoscope
   a. Instrument used to listen to the sounds of the body
7. Gloves and lubricant
   a. Used for rectal and pelvic examinations

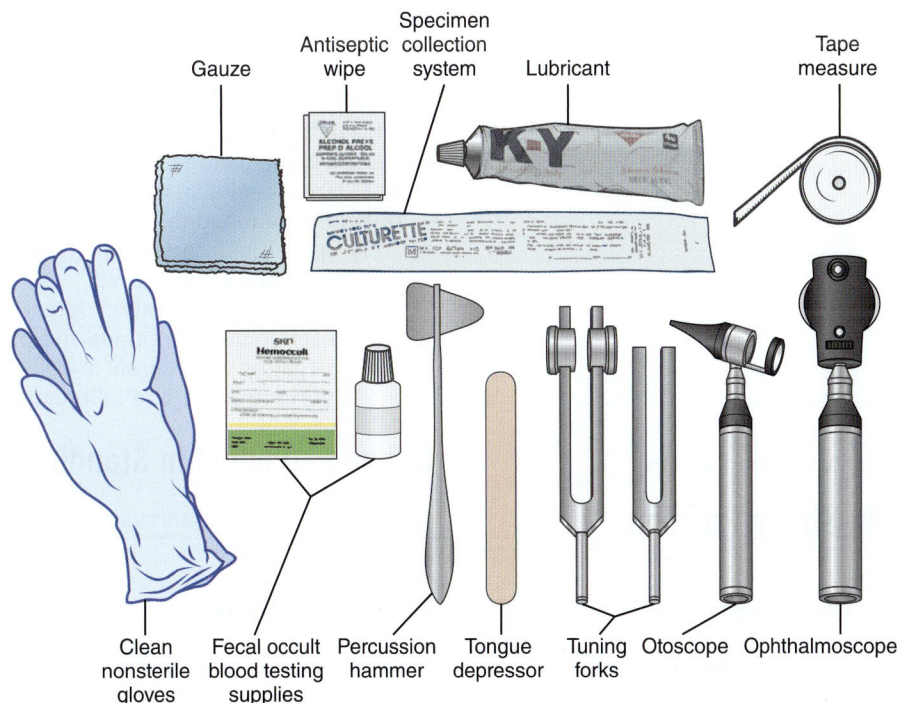

Fig. 17.2 Common instruments and supplies used during the physical examination. (From Niedzwiecki B, et al.: *Kinn's The medical assistant: an applied learning approach*, ed 14, 2020, Elsevier.)

8. Vaginal speculum
   a. Instrument inserted into the patient's vagina to allow visualization of the cervix and vagina
9. Percussion hammer
   a. Rubber-tipped hammer is used to test a patient's reflexes
10. Tuning fork
    a. Instrument used to test the patient's hearing; vibrates when struck to produce sound
11. Miscellaneous
    a. Cotton-tipped applicators
    b. 2-inch × 2-inch gauze squares
    c. Glass slides
    d. Specimen and slide fixative
    e. Tissues

D. Sequence of Events

1. Patient health history
2. Vital signs and anthropometric measurements
3. Physical examination
4. Specimen collection
   a. Includes urine, blood, or other body fluids
   b. Examination may be more comfortable if the patient's bladder is empty
5. Diagnostic tests
   a. Includes electrocardiogram, x-ray, spirometry, and immunizations
6. Patient consultation or discussion with a provider

V. Provider Assessment During the Physical Examination

A. Presenting Appearance (Patient's General Appearance)

1. General assessment of the patient's state of health
2. Includes
   a. Signs of distress
   b. Appearance of the skin
   c. Posture, gait, and motor activity
   d. General grooming
   e. Presence of odors
   f. Speech patterns
   g. Body language and facial expressions
   h. Weight and height

B. Skin

1. Color, vascularity, and lesions
2. Temperature, moisture, turgor, and texture

C. Head—Patient in Sitting Position

1. Hair, scalp, and face
2. Eyes: ophthalmoscope is used to examine the retina and vessels visually
3. Ears: otoscope is used to examine the external ear and tympanic membrane

4. Nose and sinuses: otoscope or nasal speculum is used to examine the nares and sinus cavities
5. Mouth and throat
   a. Lips, gums, teeth, and tongue
   b. Light source, tongue depressor (blade), and laryngeal mirror used to examine the throat visually
6. Neck: inspect and palpate the thyroid, trachea, and lymph nodes

D. Thorax—Patient in Sitting Position

1. Back
   a. Spine and muscles of the back are visually inspected
   b. Lungs are auscultated with a stethoscope
2. Chest
   a. Visually inspected for symmetry and expansion
   b. Inspirations auscultated
   c. Axillary nodes palpated
3. Heart
   a. Stethoscope is used to listen to heart sounds
   b. Complete silence in the examination room is necessary to interpret the sounds
4. Breasts
   a. Examined for masses, tenderness, symmetry, and discharge
   b. May also be examined with the patient in the supine position

E. Abdomen—Patient in Supine Position

1. Auscultated for the presence or absence of bowel sounds
2. Visually inspected for symmetry and contour
3. Manipulated and palpated for contours of the organs
4. Area needs to be relaxed for proper examination

F. Genital and Rectal—Patient in Supine Position

1. Inguinal area: palpated for lymph nodes and hernias
2. Male genital and rectal: penis, scrotum, prostate, and anus palpated and inspected
3. Female genital and rectal: patient in lithotomy position
   a. External genitalia, vagina, cervix, and anus inspected
   b. Pelvic examination
      1) Speculum inserted into the vagina to visualize the vaginal wall and cervix
      2) Bimanual examination done with a gloved hand inserted into the vagina and the other hand palpating the external abdomen to examine the uterus, ovaries, and fallopian tubes

G. Legs—Patient in Standing Position

1. Inspected for pulse and varicosities
2. Inspect toenails

H. Neurological

1. Determination of mental status and level of consciousness
2. Test reflexes

VI. Steps in Diagnosis (Fig. 17.3)

A. Symptoms

1. Conditions and feelings experienced by the patient

B. Signs

1. Observable characteristics by healthcare providers
2. May also be noticed by the patient

C. Differential Diagnosis

1. Comparing certain diseases with others that have similar signs and symptoms
2. Process of ruling out (R/O)

D. Impression

1. Working diagnosis
2. Subject to change as the provider adds data from other diagnostic tools

E. Diagnostic Tools

1. Patient history
2. Physical examination
3. Vital signs
4. Laboratory and diagnostic tests
5. Patient's communications
6. Physician's perceptions

F. Final Diagnosis

1. The provider's final conclusion

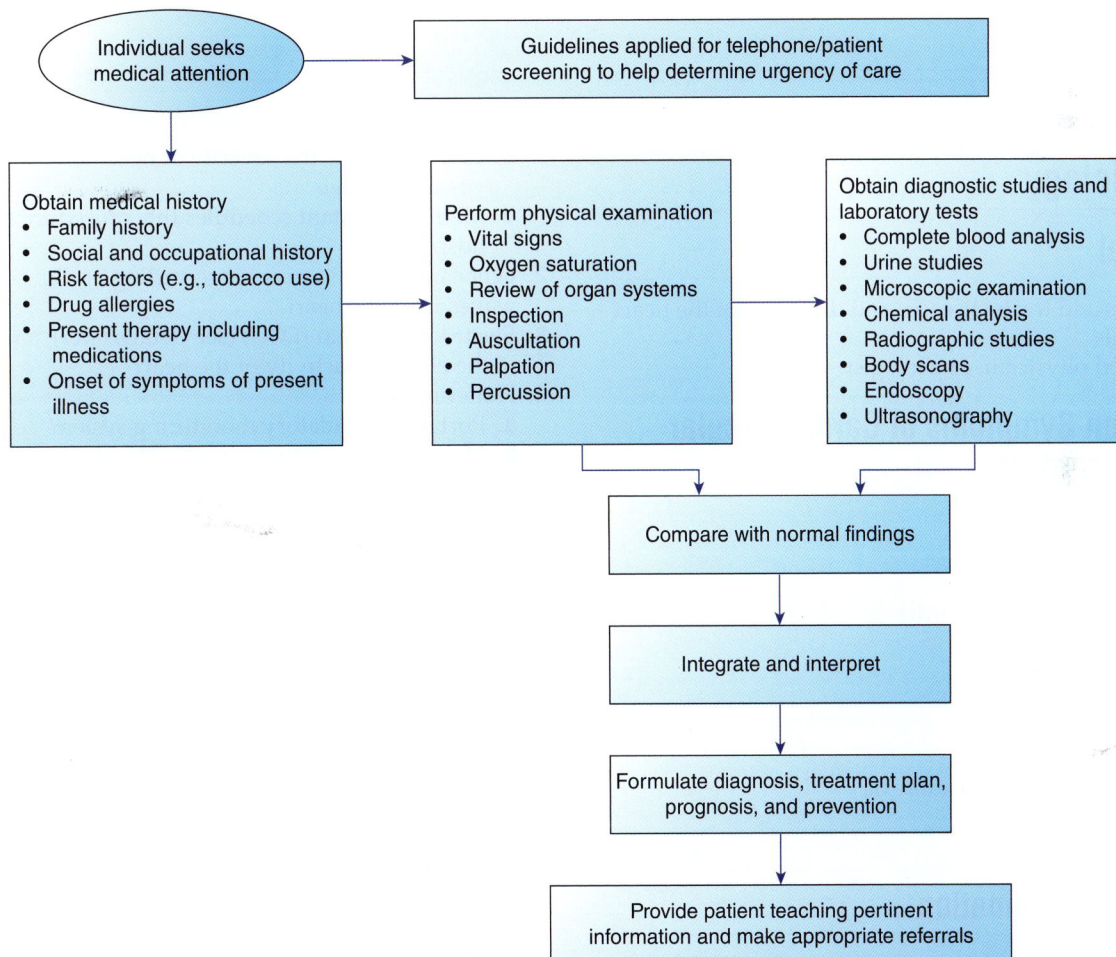

Fig. 17.3 Essential steps in diagnosis. (From Frazier MS, Drzymkowski J: *Essentials of human diseases and conditions*, ed 6, 2016, Elsevier.)

18

Assisting With Medical Specialties

I. Cardiology

A. General

1. Diagnoses and treats diseases and disorders of the heart and vessels
2. Specialized physician: cardiologist

B. Common Symptoms of Cardiovascular System Disorders

1. Chest pain
2. Dyspnea
3. Fatigue and weakness
4. Palpitations and tachycardia
5. Bradycardia
6. Pallor and cyanosis
7. Edema
8. Syncope
9. Unusual sweating
10. Nausea, vomiting, and anorexia
11. Headache
12. Anxiety

C. General Examination

1. Listening to the heart with a stethoscope; noting heart sounds, rate, and rhythm

D. Diagnostic Procedures

1. Cardiac catheterization
   a. Intensive study of the heart
   b. Catheters are used to perform angiocardiography or pressure-and-flow measurements
   c. Can determine the severity of heart disease and/or vessel blockage
   d. Medical assistant schedules this procedure at the hospital
2. Echocardiogram: a graphic recording of ultrasound waves from the heart
3. Electrocardiogram (ECG) (see details later): a recording of the electrical activity of the heart
4. Holter monitor
   a. Portable ambulatory monitoring system
   b. Monitors ECG activity over a 24-hour period
   c. Designed so that the patient is able to maintain usual daily activities with minimal inconvenience while being monitored
   d. Device is connected to the patient by electrodes placed on the patient's chest and a special portable magnetic tape recorder that continually monitors the heart's activity
   e. Recorder is in a protective case that is either worn on a belt around the patient's waist or hung over the shoulder by a strap
   f. Patient may complete an activity diary; all activities and emotional states are recorded along with any symptoms experienced (e.g., chest pain, vertigo, and palpitations)
   g. Monitor is removed from patient after a 24-hour period, and the tape is evaluated and analyzed
   h. Electrodes (floating electrodes) are placed as follows:
      1) Right border of the sternum (manubrium)
      2) Left border of the sternum (manubrium)
      3) Right sternal border at the level of the fifth rib
      4) Fifth rib space at the left anterior axillary line
      5) Fifth rib space at the right anterior axillary line
5. Treadmill: motorized machine that allows patient to walk in place; allows evaluation of the patient's heart function while exercising

6. Angiography: x-ray of blood vessels after an injection of radiopaque material
7. Arterial blood gases (ABGs): oxygen, carbon dioxide, and metabolic balance are measured in an arterial blood sample
8. Cardiac enzymes
    a. Creatine phosphokinase (CPK): enzyme released into the blood when the heart or skeletal muscles are injured
    b. Aspartate aminotransferase (AST) (formerly serum glutamic-oxaloacetic transaminase [SGOT]): found in high concentrations in heart muscle and the liver
    c. Lactic dehydrogenase (LDH): enzyme found in heart muscle, skeletal muscles, kidneys, liver, and red blood cells
9. Prothrombin time (PT): tests coagulation of blood

E. Treatment Procedures

1. Angioplasty: surgical repair of a blood vessel
2. Defibrillation (cardioversion): brief charges of electricity applied to the chest to stop cardiac arrhythmia
3. Coronary artery bypass: open-heart surgery for the purpose of bypassing an obstructed coronary artery
4. Endarterectomy: removal of the interior portion of an artery and occluding fatty deposits
5. Vein stripping: removal of a diseased portion of a vein

F. Medications

1. Diuretics
    a. Promote urination; decrease blood pressure
    b. Examples: Bumex, Dyazide, Lasix, and Hydro-Diuril
2. Antihypertensives
    a. Decrease blood pressure
    b. Examples: Inderal, Lanoxin, Procardia, Tenormin, and Minipress
3. Antilipemics
    a. Decrease cholesterol levels in blood
    b. Examples: Lopid, Mevacor, Crestor, and Lipitor
4. Antianginals
    a. Decrease chest pain
    b. Examples: Nitrostat and Transderm-Nitro

G. Electrocardiogram (Fig. 18.1)

1. Cardiac electrical activity is generated, spreads through the heart, and creates an electrical wave
2. Electrical wave is measured as an ECG
    a. Electrical system of the heart
        1) Sinoatrial (SA) node (pacemaker)
        2) Atrioventricular (AV) node
        3) Bundle of His
        4) Right and left bundle branches
        5) Purkinje fibers

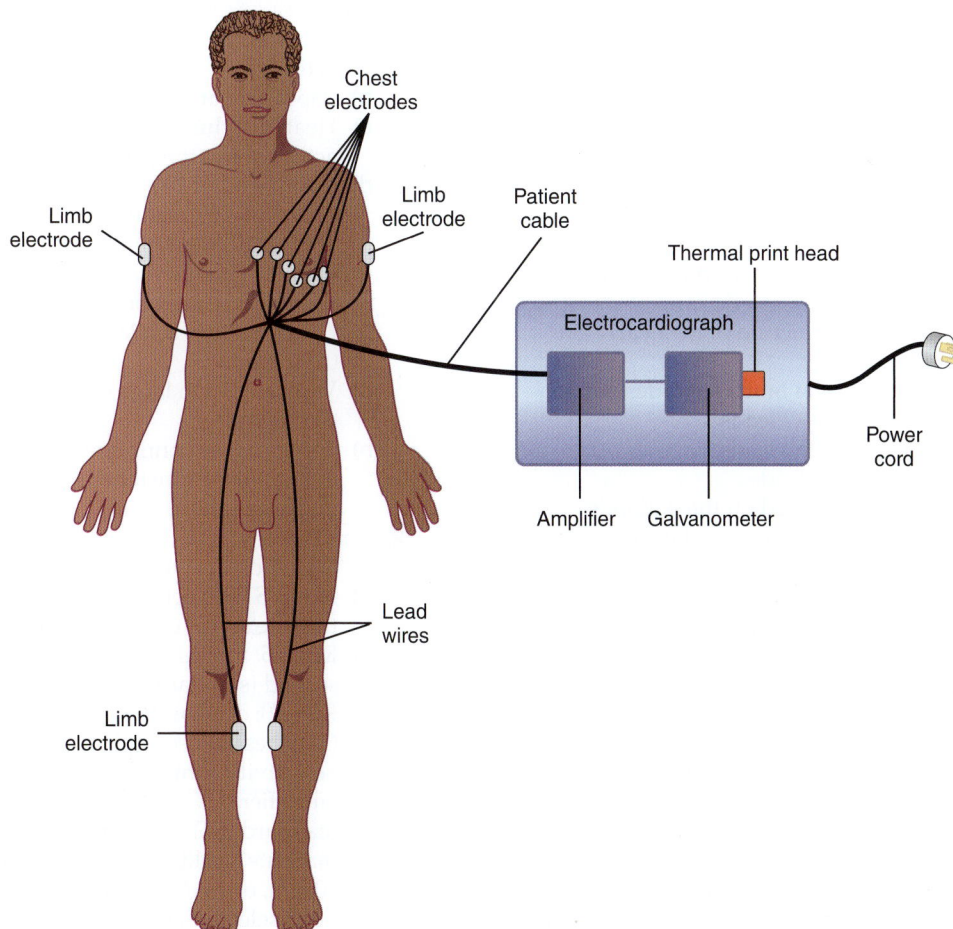

Fig. 18.1 Basic components of the electrocardiograph. (From Bonewit-West K, Hunt S: *Today's medical assistant*, ed 4, 2021, Saunders.)

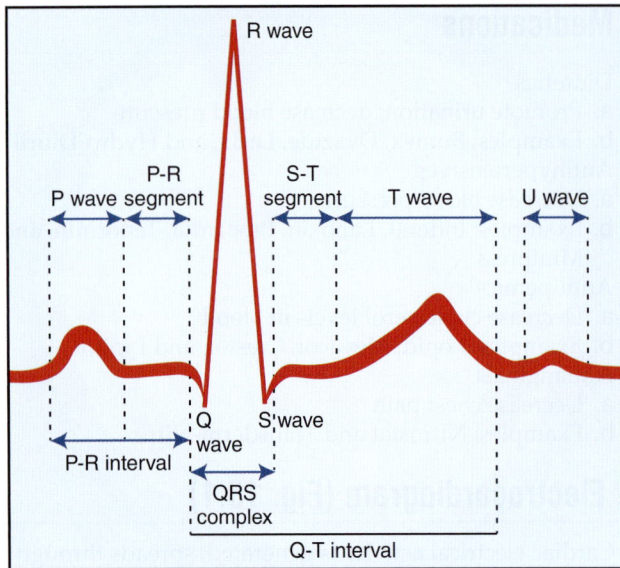

Fig. 18.2 Cardiac cycle.

b. Electrical states of the heart
   1) Polarization: cardiac muscle cells are resting
   2) Depolarization: cardiac muscle cells contract
   3) Repolarization: cardiac muscle cells transform from active to resting state for recharging
c. Normal ECG (Fig. 18.2): all heartbeats appear as a pattern, consisting of
   1) P wave: impulse starting in the atria
   2) QRS complex: impulse going through ventricles
   3) T wave: repolarization of ventricles
d. ECG leads (Fig. 18.3)
   1) Externally applied electrodes
   2) Relative to an axis (a direct line) between two poles
   3) Each lead makes up one positive pole, one negative pole, and one ground
   4) Leads give an electrical picture of the heart from different angles
   5) ECG uses 10 electrodes (4 limb electrodes and 6 chest electrodes) to give 12 leads
      a) Bipolar (standard) limb leads
         (1) Six of the twelve leads
         (2) Electrodes are placed on the patient's extremities (upper arms and inside of calves)
         (3) Measures cardiac electrical activity between two extremities (negative and positive poles)
         (4) Right electrode is used for the ground
            (a) Lead I: measures activity from the right arm to the left arm (RA to LA)
            (b) Lead II: measures activity from the right arm to the left leg (RA to LL)
            (c) Lead III: measures activity from the left arm to the left leg (LA to LL)
      b) Unipolar (augmented) limb leads: measure cardiac electrical activity between the heart and one extremity
         (1) aVR: right side

      (2) aVL: left side
      (3) aVF: left foot
   c) Precordial (chest) leads (Fig. 18.4)
      (1) Provide points of reference across the chest wall
      (2) Differentiate left-sided and right-sided heart events
         (a) Lead V1: electrode placed at the fourth intercostal space to the right of the sternum
         (b) Lead V2: electrode placed at the fourth intercostal space to the left of the sternum
         (c) Lead V3: electrode placed midway between leads V2 and V4
         (d) Lead V4: electrode placed at left midclavicular line in the fifth intercostal space
         (e) Lead V5: electrode placed at the level of V4 at axillary line
         (f) Lead V6: electrode placed at the level of V5 at the midaxillary line
   d) Leads in relation to the anatomy of the heart
      (1) Right side of the heart: V1 and aVR
      (2) Left side of the heart: V5, V6, I, and aVL
      (3) Transition from right to left side of the heart: V2, V3, and V4
      (4) Inferior heart: II, III, and aVF
e. ECG equipment
   1) Paper
      a) Records visible record of the heart's electrical activity
      b) Paper is heat sensitive
      c) Heated stylus on the machine traces the heart activity onto the paper
      d) Composed of 1-mm squares: every fifth line is darkened, creating large blocks five squares wide and five squares high
      e) Cardiac voltage is measured on the vertical scale; time is measured on the horizontal scale
      f) Horizontally, each large block represents 0.2 seconds
      g) Vertically, each large block represents 0.5 mV of electricity
      h) Paper moves continuously through the machine at the rate of 1 inch per second on the standard machine setting
   2) Controls
      a) Main power switch: turns the machine on and off
      b) RUN/STOP: activates (or stops) the amplifier so that the stylus can react to the heartbeat
      c) Run-25: moves the paper 25 mm (1 inch) per second (standard speed)
      d) Run-50: doubles the paper's speed to 50 mm (2 inches) per second
      e) Sensitivity control: regulates the output of the amplifier
      f) Standard (STD) button: manually checks the machine's calibration (stylus should deflect 10 mm, or two large squares)
      g) Lead selector: changes leads
      h) Marker button: allows manual identification of leads; uses codes of dots or dashes

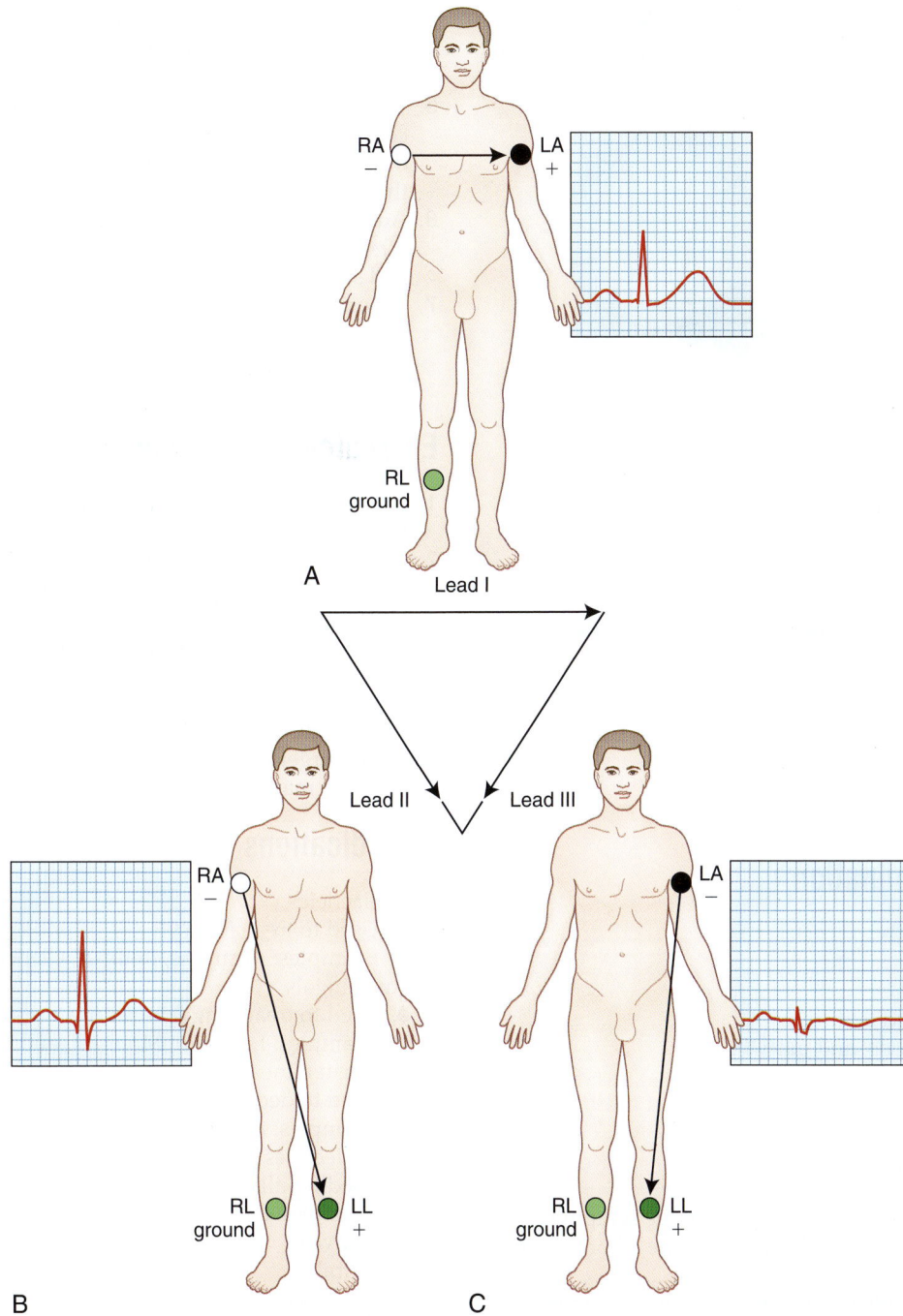

Fig. 18.3 Electrocardiogram leads, wires, and tracings. (A) Lead I. (B) Lead II. (C) Lead III. *LA*, Left arm; *LL*, left leg; *RA*, right arm; *RL*, right leg.

3) Artifacts: abnormal ECG tracings not caused by heart activity

    a) Somatic tremor: caused by the patient's muscle movement

    b) Alternating current (AC) interference: caused by nearby operation of electrical equipment

    c) Wandering baseline: caused by electrodes applied too loosely or too tightly

II. Dermatology

A. General

1. Diagnoses and treats disorders of the skin, hair, glands, nails, and subcutaneous tissue
2. Specialized physician: dermatologist

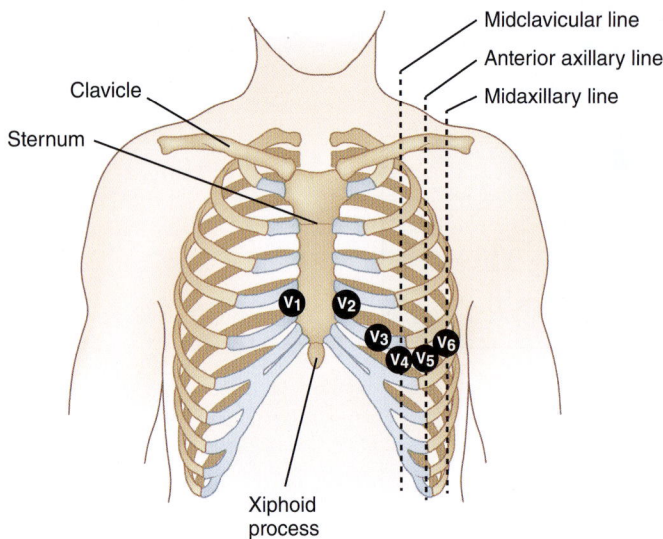

Fig. 18.4 Precordial (chest) electrocardiogram leads: V1–V6.

B. Common Symptoms of Skin Disorders

1. Lesions and/or eruptions
2. Pruritus and/or hives
3. Inflammation
4. Edema
5. Discomfort
6. Erythema

C. General Examination

1. Skin, hair, and nails
2. Examine for
   a. Color
   b. Consistency and texture
   c. Eruptions, lesions, and growths
   d. Tenderness
   e. Irregularities

D. Diagnostic Procedures

1. Fungal, bacterial, and viral cultures: tissue scrapings, purulent material, and exudate sent to the laboratory to identify pathogenic organisms
2. Potassium hydroxide (KOH) smears: skin scrapings immersed in 20% KOH; sample examined for fungus
3. Biopsy
   a. Excisional: removal of the entire section of tissue for microscopic examination
   b. Incisional: removal of a portion of the tissue for microscopic examination
   c. Punch: use of an instrument (dermal punch) to remove only a small amount of tissue for microscopic examination
4. Allergy testing
   a. Patch test: a small piece of gauze with a small amount of allergen is placed on the skin; a positive reaction occurs if the skin becomes red or blistered after 48 hours
   b. Scratch test: a minute amount of allergen is placed, by scratch, in the skin; a positive reaction occurs if the scratch becomes red and swollen

   c. Intradermal: a small amount of allergen is injected intradermally; a positive reaction is determined by measuring the size of the wheals produced
5. Wood light examination: detects fluorescent characteristics of certain fungi; the skin is viewed in a darkened room under ultraviolet light that is filtered through Wood glass
6. Antinuclear antibody (ANA) titer: blood test used to screen for cutaneous and systemic lupus erythematosus and similar connective tissue diseases
7. Tuberculin (TB) skin testing: tests patient for tuberculosis antibodies
   a. Mantoux: intradermal injection using purified protein derivative (TST)

E. Treatment Procedures

1. Cryosurgery: the use of extreme cold (liquid nitrogen) to freeze and destroy unwanted tissue
2. Curettage: removal of the surface of the skin or a lesion by scraping with a sharp, spoon-shaped instrument (curette)
3. Dermabrasion: removal of scars or lesions by the use of mechanical or chemical abrasives
4. Electrodesiccation: destruction of growths, warts, or unwanted areas of tissue with electrical current (diathermy)
5. Mohs surgery: removal and microscopic examination of layers of malignant growth

F. Medications

1. Antiacneics
   a. Used to treat acne
   b. Examples: Accutane, Retin-A, Cleocin, and Persa-Gel
2. Antifungals
   a. Used to treat fungal infections
   b. Examples: Lotrimin, Monistat, and Nizoral
3. Antihistamines
   a. Used to decrease allergic reactions
   b. Examples: Atarax and Benadryl
4. Antiinfectives
   a. Used to kill microorganisms
   b. Examples: Erythromycin, Keflex, Mycolog II, and Sumycin
5. Antivirals
   a. Used to inhibit viruses
   b. Example: Zovirax
6. Scabicides and pediculicides
   a. Used to kill scabies and lice
   b. Examples: Lindane and Kwell
7. Topical steroids
   a. Used externally to decrease inflammation
   b. Examples: Aristocort, Medrol, Topicort, and Kenalog

III. Endocrinology

A. General

1. Diagnoses and treats diseases and disorders of the endocrine system
2. Specialized physician: endocrinologist

B. Common Symptoms of Endocrine System Disorders

1. Mental deviations
2. Changes in energy levels
3. Growth abnormalities
4. Skin, hair, and nail changes
5. Muscle weakness and atrophy
6. Emotional disturbances
7. Edema
8. Changes in blood pressure and heart irregularities
9. Sexual irregularities
10. Changes in urinary output

C. General Examination

1. Complete physical examination

D. Diagnostic Procedures

1. Radioactive iodine uptake: measures the uptake of a dose of radioactive iodine by the thyroid gland
2. Thyroid scan
   a. Administration of a radioactive compound to visualize the thyroid gland
   b. Used to detect tumors and nodules
3. Computer tomography (CT) scans
   a. Can visualize the endocrine glands
   b. Can detect disease processes and masses
4. Ultrasonography: the use of sound waves to obtain images
5. Blood tests
   a. Used to diagnose and manage endocrine disorders
   b. Blood tests for
      1) Adrenocorticotropic hormone (ACTH): from the pituitary
      2) Aldosterone: from the adrenal cortex
      3) Thyroxine: from the thyroid
      4) Calcium: from the parathyroid
      5) Cortisol: from the adrenal cortex
      6) Electrolytes (sodium, potassium, and chloride): from the adrenal cortex
      7) Estradiol: from the ovaries
      8) Follicle-stimulating hormone (FSH): from the pituitary
      9) Growth hormone (GH): from the pituitary
      10) Glucose: from the pancreas
      11) Insulin: from the pancreas
      12) Luteinizing hormone (LH): from the pituitary
      13) Parathyroid hormone: from the parathyroid
      14) Triiodothyronine (T_3) and thyroxine (tetraiodothyronine [T_4]): from the thyroid
      15) Testosterone: from the testes
6. Basal metabolic rate (BMR)
   a. Test infrequently ordered
   b. Measures energy exchange rate of the body in a state of rest
7. Glucose tolerance test (GTT)
   a. Blood is tested at specific intervals after the patient ingests a measured amount of glucose

E. Treatment Procedures

1. Oophorectomy: surgical removal of the ovaries
2. Orchiectomy: surgical removal of the testes
3. Thyroidectomy: total or partial removal of thyroid gland

F. Medications

1. Thyroid medications
   a. Replace thyroid hormones
   b. Examples: Synthroid and Euthroid
2. Corticosteroids
   a. Decrease inflammation
   b. Examples: cortisone, Aristocort, Kenalog, Medrol, and Decadron
3. GH
   a. Stimulates growth
   b. Example: Humatrope
4. Antidiuretic hormones
   a. Reduce urine volume; treat diabetes insipidus
   b. Example: vasopressin (Pitressin)
5. Oral antidiabetics
   a. Lower blood glucose levels in type 2 diabetes
   b. Examples: Orinase, Glucotrol, Diabinese, and Glucophage
6. Insulin
   a. Lowers blood glucose levels by increasing glucose uptake
   b. Examples: Humulin, Novolin, and Lantus

IV. Ear, Nose, and Throat (Otorhinolaryngology)

A. General

1. Diagnosis and treatment of diseases and disorders of the ear, nose, and throat (ENT)
2. Specialized physician: otorhinolaryngologist

B. Common Symptoms of ENT Disorders

1. Loss of hearing
2. Vertigo and dizziness
3. Tinnitus
4. Earache, increased ear pressure
5. Sore throat
6. Fever, malaise, and headache
7. Epistaxis
8. Nasal congestion and rhinorrhea

C. General Examination

1. Examination of the ear with an otoscope
2. Examination of the nasal structures, throat, and sinuses

D. Diagnostic Procedures

1. Audiometry
   a. Use of an audiometer to deliver sound frequencies
   b. Determines the patient's hearing threshold

2. Laryngoscopy: visual examination of the larynx with a laryngoscope
3. Otoscopy: visual examination of the ear with an otoscope
4. Throat culture: inflamed areas of the throat are swabbed and analyzed for various pathogens
5. Nasal smear: removal of a specimen and analysis for pathogens
6. Skull, mastoid, sinus, and chest x-rays: standard views of specific body parts
7. Rapid strep test: test for beta-hemolytic *Streptococcus*

E. Treatment Procedures

1. Adenoidectomy: surgical excision of adenoids
2. Myringotomy: an incision into the eardrum
3. Myringotomy with tubes: incision into the eardrum with placement of ventilation tubes
4. Rhinoplasty: reconstruction or plastic surgery of the nose
5. Tonsillectomy: surgical excision of tonsils
6. Tonsilloadenoidectomy (T&A): surgical removal of the tonsils and adenoids
7. Ear irrigation: washing of external ear canal

F. Medications

1. Antibiotics
   a. Kills or inhibits the growth of microorganisms
   b. Examples: Amoxil, Ceclor, erythromycin, and Keflex
2. Otics
   a. Treat otitis externa
   b. Examples: Cipro HC, Ciprodex, and Floxin Otic

V. Gastroenterology

A. General

1. Diagnoses and treats diseases and disorders of the digestive tract
2. Specialized physician: gastroenterologist

B. Common Symptoms of Gastrointestinal Disorders

1. Anorexia and weight loss
2. Abdominal pain
3. Nausea and vomiting
4. Change in bowel habits
5. Flatulence
6. Blood and mucus in feces
7. Fever
8. Heartburn, indigestion, and difficulty swallowing
9. Diaphoresis

C. General Examination

1. Examination of the mouth
2. Palpation of the abdomen and intestines
3. Inspection of the rectum (can be accomplished with a scope)

D. Diagnostic Procedures

1. Colonoscopy: visual examination of the colon using a lighted scope
2. Liver biopsy: removal of a tissue sample from the liver for microscopic examination
3. Proctoscopy (sigmoidoscopy): visual examination of the anus, the rectum, and part of the sigmoid colon
4. Barium enema (BE): infusion of barium into the rectum for visualization by x-ray
5. Cholecystogram: x-ray examination of the gallbladder
6. Upper gastrointestinal (GI) series: x-ray study of the esophagus, stomach, and duodenum; contrast medium is orally administered
7. Gastric analysis: aspiration of the stomach contents by a tube placed into the stomach, through the nose; contents analyzed
8. Occult blood (guaiac) test: a test for hidden blood in the stool; Hemoccult
9. Ova and parasites (O&P): analysis of a stool sample for the presence of eggs and parasites
10. Liver function tests: tests performed to diagnose liver-related diseases or disorders

E. Treatment Procedures

1. Appendectomy: removal of the appendix
2. Cholecystectomy: removal of the gallbladder
3. Colostomy: creation of an opening between the colon and the body surface
4. Hemorrhoid ligation: removal of hemorrhoids by using tying off (ligating)
5. Hemorrhoidectomy: excision of hemorrhoids
6. Vagotomy: surgical transection of the vagus nerve to decrease stomach acid secretion in patients with ulcers

F. Medications

1. Anthelmintics
   a. Kill helminths (worms)
   b. Example: Vermox
2. Antibiotics
   a. Kill microorganisms
   b. Examples: Sumycin and Flagyl
3. Antispasmodics
   a. Decrease spasms of the GI tract
   b. Examples: Bentyl, Librax, and Donnatal
4. Antidiarrheals
   a. Decrease or slow diarrhea
   b. Examples: Imodium, Lomotil, and Pepto-Bismol
5. H_2 antagonists
   a. Decrease stomach acids
   b. Examples: Tagamet, Zantac, Axid, and Pepcid
6. Laxatives
   a. Encourage bowel movements
   b. Examples: Colace, Dulcolax, Ex-Lax, and Milk of Magnesia

VI. Geriatrics

A. General

1. Treats and provides health maintenance for older adults
2. Specialized physician: gerontologist and internist

B. Aging

1. Complex physiologic, psychological, and social process
2. Aging is not an illness; it is a normal life process
3. Changes occur in
   a. Appearance
   b. Abilities
   c. Vision
   d. Hearing
   e. Taste
   f. Smell

C. Caring for Older Patients

1. Speak slowly and distinctly if the patient is hearing impaired
2. Use indirect lighting in examination rooms to decrease glare
3. Do not carry on conversations with the patient where a large amount of background noise is present
4. Do not patronize the older patient
5. Touch the older patient politely and affectionately, not in a controlling manner
6. Use eye contact when conversing with the older patient
7. Offer assistance to the older patient as needed
8. Treat the older patient as an individual
9. Reinforce treatment instructions by writing them down
10. Never approach a visually impaired patient without making your presence known; identify yourself and others in the room

D. Problems Associated With Aging

1. Inability to perform personal care, including bathing, dressing, eating, getting out of bed, and using the toilet
2. Inability to live independently, including preparing meals, shopping, managing money, using the telephone, and doing housework
3. Functioning such as walking, climbing the stairs, lifting, and standing for periods of time

VII. Hematology

A. General

1. Diagnoses and treats blood disorders, bone marrow, and coagulation
2. Specialized physician: hematologist

B. Common Symptoms of Blood Disorders

1. Cold and numb extremities
2. Fatigue
3. Dyspnea
4. Headache
5. Anorexia
6. Edema
7. Pallor
8. Syncope
9. Bone pain
10. Easy bleeding and bruising

C. General Examination

1. Obtain blood or bone marrow samples for testing
2. Palpation of the spleen and liver

D. Diagnostic Procedures

1. Bone marrow aspiration: insertion of a large needle into the sternum or iliac crest to remove bone marrow for testing
2. Blood cell counts (red blood cell [RBC] and white blood cell [WBC]): a blood test to determine the number of RBCs and WBCs per cubic millimeter of blood
3. Differential: blood smear on glass slide; stain is applied to the smear; the smear is studied under a microscope to differentiate the types of WBCs
4. Hematocrit (Hct): measures the percentage of RBCs in volume of blood
5. Hemoglobin (Hgb): measures the grams of hemoglobin in volume of blood
6. Platelet count: estimates the number of platelets in volume of blood
7. PT: measures coagulation time of blood

E. Medications

1. Anticoagulants
   a. Prevent blood from clotting
   b. Examples: warfarin (Coumadin), heparin, and Eliquis
2. Stimulating factors
   a. Stimulate production of blood cells
   b. Examples: Neupogen and Leukine
3. Thrombolytic agents
   a. Dissolve clots
   b. Examples: Abbokinase and Streptase
4. Antianemics
   a. Treat anemias
   b. Examples: Epogen, Slow-Fe, and vitamin B_{12}
5. Antiplatelet agents
   a. Inhibit platelet aggregation; prolonged bleeding time
   b. Example: Plavix

VIII. Neurology

A. General

1. Diagnoses and treats diseases and disorders of the nervous system
2. Specialized physician: neurologist

B. Common Symptoms of Nervous System Disorders

1. Headaches
2. Nausea and vomiting
3. Weakness and motor disturbances
4. Mood swings and memory impairment
5. Drowsiness, stupor, and coma
6. Seizures, paralysis, convulsions, and numbness
7. Muscle rigidity and flaccidity
8. Disturbances in speech, vision, hearing, and taste
9. Tremors
10. Radiating pain

C. General Examination

1. Mental status: includes assessment of intelligence; assessment of memory; orientation to person, place, and time; and general appearance
2. Evaluation of all cranial nerves
3. Motor nerves: includes coordination, strength, Romberg test, walking, and finger-to-nose exercise
4. Sensory nervous system
5. Reflexes

D. Diagnostic Procedures

1. Electroencephalogram (EEG)
   a. Study of the electrical activity of the brain
   b. Uses electrodes attached to the scalp
2. Electromyography (EMG): the study of the contraction of a muscle as a result of electrical stimulation
3. Lumbar puncture: a procedure to remove cerebrospinal fluid for analysis
4. Brain scan: a procedure that uses radioactive chemicals and specialized machines to record the passage through, and absorption into, brain lesions
5. Myelography: an x-ray of the spinal cord
6. Skull series: standard x-ray views of the skull
7. Cervical, thoracic, and lumbosacral spine series: standard x-ray views of specific portions of the spine

E. Treatment Procedures

1. Craniotomy: surgical opening into the cranium
2. Laminectomy: removal of laminae to decompress pinched spinal nerve roots
3. Halo traction: traction device for neck stability

F. Medications

1. Anticonvulsants
   a. Decrease seizure activity
   b. Examples: Depakote, Dilantin, and Tegretol
2. Antiemetics (antivertigo agents)
   a. Decrease vomiting and dizziness
   b. Examples: Antivert, Compazine, and Dramamine
3. Anti-Parkinson agents
   a. Decrease symptoms of Parkinson disease
   b. Examples: Artane, Cogentin, and Sinemet

4. Antidepressants
   a. Counteract depression
   b. Examples: Paxil, Prozac, and Celexa

IX. Obstetrics and Gynecology

A. General

1. Diagnoses and treats diseases and disorders of the female reproductive system and pregnancy
2. Specialized physician: obstetrician (pregnancy and childbirth) or gynecologist (female reproductive system)

B. Common Symptoms of Female Reproduction System Disorders

1. Sexually transmitted diseases/sexually transmitted infections (STIs)
   a. Pelvic or genital pain
   b. Dysuria, hematuria, and purulent discharge
   c. Burning or itching on urination
   d. Urinary frequency and incontinence
   e. Dyspareunia
   f. Fever and malaise
   g. Lesions in genital area
2. Infertility
   a. Abnormal pregnancies
   b. Endometriosis
   c. Congenital malformations
   d. Decreased sperm count
3. Specific to female reproductive system
   a. Fever
   b. Abnormal vaginal discharge, itching, or both
   c. Pain in lower abdomen or pelvic region

C. General Examination

1. Inspection and palpation of the breasts
2. Inspection of the external genitalia, vagina, and cervix
3. Palpation of the uterus, ovaries, and fallopian tubes
4. Prenatal: includes initial general examination and periodic examinations to monitor fetal growth and development

D. Diagnostic Procedures

1. Amniocentesis
   a. Puncture of the amniotic sac with a needle to withdraw amniotic fluid for analysis
   b. Can detect genetic disorders
2. Cervical biopsy: removal of tissue to evaluate the presence of abnormalities
3. Colposcopy: examination of the cervix with a scope
4. Dilation and curettage (D&C): expansion of the cervix so that the uterine wall can be scraped
5. Fetal monitoring: recording of the fetal heart rate
6. Laparoscopy: examination of the abdomen by insertion of a laparoscope through the abdominal wall
7. Human chorionic gonadotropin (HCG)

a. Hormone produced by the placenta during pregnancy
b. Basis for pregnancy testing
c. Testing performed on blood or urine
8. Chorionic villi sampling (CVS)
   a. Use of ultrasound to guide a needle into the uterine wall to obtain a sample of chorion
   b. Can detect chromosomal abnormalities
9. Endovaginal ultrasound: sound probe placed in the vagina for a closer, sharper view of the pelvis
10. Hysterosalpingography: x-ray of the uterus and fallopian tubes, using radiopaque material
11. Pelvimetry: measurement of the dimensions of the pelvis
12. Papanicolaou (Pap) smear (ThinPrep)
    a. Scrapings from the cervix used to detect tissue changes
    b. Screening test for cervical cancer

E. Treatment Procedures

1. Abortion
   a. Premature termination of pregnancy
   b. May be spontaneous or therapeutic
2. Cauterization: the use of heat to destroy abnormal tissue
3. Cesarean section (C-section): birth of an infant through a surgical incision into the uterus
4. Conization: removal of a cone-shaped wedge of tissue from the cervix for examination
5. Cryosurgery: use of cold to destroy abnormal tissue
6. Hysterectomy: surgical removal of the uterus through the abdominal wall or vagina
7. Hysteroscopy: insertion of a scope into the uterus to view the endometrial cavity
8. Kegel exercises: simple exercises to strengthen the pubococcygeal muscles
9. Tubal ligation
   a. Tying off the fallopian tubes
   b. Female sterilization procedure

F. Medications

1. Hormone replacement
   a. Examples: Premarin, Depo-Provera, and Ogen
2. Ovulation stimulants
   a. Example: Clomid
3. Oral contraceptives
   a. Prevent pregnancy
   b. Examples: Triphasil, Ovral, Ortho-Novum, and Ortho Tri-Cyclen
4. Supplements
   a. Vitamins and iron
   b. Examples: Ferro-Sequels and Natalins
5. Antifungals
   a. Treat fungal or yeast infections
   b. Examples: Monistat and Gyne-Lotrimin

G. Contraception

1. Prevents fertilization of ovum
2. Commonly referred to as birth control
3. No method is 100% effective
4. Various methods

a. Hormonal
   1) Prevents ovulation
   2) Can be in the form of oral contraceptives (pills); injection (Depo-Provera); intrauterine device/intrauterine contraceptive (Mirena); vaginal ring (NuvaRing); long-acting implants (Implanon)
b. Nonhormonal/barrier
   1) Blocks entrance of sperm into the uterus
   2) Can be in the form of condoms (male and female); cervical cap with spermicide; diaphragm with spermicide; spermicidal creams, foams, and suppositories
c. Surgical
   1) Permanent
   2) Vasectomy: performed on the male vas deferens; results in no sperm in seminal fluid
   3) Tubal ligation: performed on the female fallopian tubes; results in no eggs reaching the tubes
d. Behavioral
   1) Abstinence: no intercourse
   2) Rhythm: avoidance of intercourse for several days near the time of ovulation
   3) Withdrawal (coitus interruptus): penis withdrawn before ejaculation

X. Oncology

A. General

1. Treats patients with tumors or cancer
2. Specialized physician: oncologist

B. Common Signs and Symptoms of Cancer (*CAUTION*)

1. *C*hange in bowel and bladder habits
2. *A* sore that does not heal
3. *U*nusual bleeding or discharge
4. *T*hickening or lump in a breast or elsewhere
5. *I*ndigestion or difficulty swallowing
6. *O*bvious change in a wart or mole
7. *N*agging cough or hoarseness

C. Tumors

1. Malignant: cancerous tumor
   a. Cells multiply rapidly
   b. Invasive
   c. Undifferentiated
   d. Metastatic
2. Benign: noncancerous tumor
   a. Slow growing
   b. Encapsulated and noninvasive
   c. Well differentiated
   d. Nonmetastatic
3. Carcinoma: a malignant tumor derived from epithelial tissue (skin, glands)
4. Sarcoma: a malignant tumor derived from connective tissue (bone, muscle, fat)
5. Lymphoma: a malignant tumor that develops in lymphatic tissue

6. Leukemia: a malignancy of the bone marrow
7. Myeloma: a malignant tumor of the plasma cells in bone marrow
8. Mixed tumors: a combination of cells
9. Carcinoma in situ (CIS): cancer cells have not invaded the organ of origin

D. Staging and Grading Tumors

1. To treat cancer, the provider must determine severity (grade) and size and spread (stage)
2. Grading
   a. Grade I: well-differentiated tumor
   b. Grade II: moderately differentiated tumor
   c. Grade III: poorly differentiated tumor
   d. Grade IV: undifferentiated tumor
3. Staging
   a. TNM system
      1) T: size of tumor
      2) N: number of lymph nodes involved
      3) M: presence of distant metastasis
      4) Numbers after the letters denote size and degree of involvement (0 through 4)

E. Diagnosis

1. Patient history
2. Tumor markers
3. Biopsy
4. Imaging
5. Self-detection

F. Treatment

1. Surgery
   a. Cautery: the burning of tissue to destroy it
   b. Cryosurgery: the use of cold to destroy tissue
   c. En bloc resection: removal of the tumor and large amount of surrounding tissue
   d. Excisional biopsy: removal of the tumor and margin of normal tissue
   e. Incisional biopsy: removal of a piece of the tumor for examination to determine the diagnosis
2. Radiation therapy (radiation oncology)
   a. Goal: deliver the maximum dose of radiation to the tumor and minimal dose to surrounding tissue
   b. Can produce undesirable side effects
      1) Alopecia
      2) Nausea and vomiting
      3) Xerostomia (dry mouth)
      4) Myelosuppression
      5) Mucositis
3. Chemotherapy
   a. Treatment of cancer using chemicals or drugs
      1) Alkylating agents
      2) Antibiotics
      3) Antimetabolites
      4) Antimitotics
      5) Hormonal agents

G. Clinical Procedures

1. Used to detect and treat malignancies
   a. Bone marrow biopsy
   b. Bone marrow/stem cell transplant
   c. Fiberoptic colonoscopy
   d. Cytology
   e. Laparoscopy
   f. Mammography
   g. Needle biopsy

XI. Ophthalmology

A. General

1. Diagnoses and treats diseases and disorders of the eye
2. Specialized physician: ophthalmologist

B. Common Symptoms of Eye Disorders

1. Visual disturbances
2. Redness
3. Pain or burning around the eye

C. General Examination

1. Inspection and measurement of the external eye, eyelids, and accessory structures
2. Measurement of eye movements and pupillary distance

D. Diagnostic Procedures

1. Keratometry (K-readings): measurement of the steepness of the cornea
2. Ophthalmoscopy: visual examination of the interior eye using an ophthalmoscope
3. Visual acuity: sharpness of vision
   a. Determines amount of myopia, hyperopia, or astigmatism
   b. Uses Snellen eye chart
4. Near visual acuity: assesses the patient's ability to read close objects
5. Slit lamp examination: examines the cornea, conjunctiva, iris, lens, and vitreous humor using a slit light and biomicroscope
6. Tonometry
   a. Measures intraocular tension
   b. May indicate the presence of glaucoma
7. Ishihara color vision test: tests color vision

E. Treatment Procedures

1. Blepharoplasty: surgical repair of the eyelids
2. Cataract extraction: removal of the lens of the eye
3. Enucleation: removal of the eye from the socket
4. Glaucoma operation: a procedure that relieves increased intraocular pressure

F. Medications

1. Antibiotics
   a. Treatment of bacterial infections
   b. Examples: Tobrex and bacitracin ophthalmic
2. Corticosteroids
   a. Reduces inflammation
   b. Examples: Decadron and Opticrom
3. Glaucoma treatment
   a. Reduces intraocular pressure
   b. Examples: Timoptic, Propine, and Betagan

XII. Orthopedics

A. General

1. Diagnoses and treats disorders of the musculoskeletal system
2. Specialized physician: orthopedist and orthopod

B. Common Symptoms of Musculoskeletal Disorders

1. Joint stiffness, pain, inflammation, and swelling
2. Weight loss
3. Bone mass loss; deformation of bones
4. Fatigue, malaise, weakness, and fever
5. Tenderness and swelling of joints and bones
6. Loss of motion and immobility

C. General Examination

1. Observes for
   a. Decreased range of motion (ROM)
   b. Tenderness and swelling
   c. Unequal or decreased strength
   d. Deformities or growths

D. Diagnostic Procedures

1. Arthrocentesis: removal of joint fluid with a needle for analysis of fluid
2. Arthroscopy: examination of a joint with a viewing scope (arthroscope)
3. Electromyography (EMG): recording the strength of muscle contraction as a result of electrical stimulation
4. Muscle biopsy: removal of muscle tissue for examination
5. Bone scan: use of a machine to measure the uptake of a radioactive substance injected intravenously
6. Computed tomography (CT) scan: computer-assisted x-ray technique used to distinguish pathologic conditions such as tumors or fractures; a noninvasive method of viewing inside the body
7. Magnetic resonance imaging (MRI): production of detailed pictures of internal structures, using magnetism and computers; a noninvasive method of viewing inside the body
8. Skeletal x-ray: plain x-ray of a body part

9. Erythrocyte sedimentation rate (ESR; sed rate): blood test that determines whether inflammation is present within the patient's body
10. Latex fixation: test for the presence of rheumatoid factor present in rheumatoid arthritis

E. Treatment Procedures

1. Wrap: cloth or elastic material used to immobilize limbs or joints
2. Splint: rigid material used to immobilize limbs or joints; may be movable or immovable
3. Cast: application of material (e.g., plaster, resin, and fiberglass) molded to the affected limb and allowed to harden; holds the affected limb or joint in a fixed position until healing is complete
4. Arthroscopic surgery: surgical procedures performed on joints using an arthroscope
5. Reduction: restoration of a fracture to its normal position
   a. Closed reduction: manipulation without an incision
   b. Open reduction: an incision is made at the fracture site
6. Physical therapy: use of exercise, heat, cold, and other physical means to reduce pain and swelling, increase movement and circulation, and promote healing

F. Medications

1. Analgesics
   a. Used to reduce pain
   b. Examples: aspirin and acetaminophen (Tylenol)
2. Narcotic analgesics
   a. Used to reduce pain with narcotics
   b. Examples: Lortab and Percodan
3. Antibiotics
   a. Used to kill microorganisms
   b. Examples: Cipro and Keflex
4. Nonsteroidal antiinflammatory drugs
   a. Used to reduce inflammation without the use of steroids
   b. Examples: Advil, Motrin, Naprosyn, Indocin, and Clinoril
5. Muscle relaxants
   a. Used to relax skeletal muscles
   b. Examples: Flexeril and Valium

XIII. Pediatrics

A. General

1. Diagnosis and treatment of diseases and disorders associated with childhood and provides health maintenance for infants, children, and adolescents
2. Specialized physician: pediatrician

B. General Examination

1. Similar to a complete physical examination for an adult
2. Examinations fall into two general categories
   a. Well-child (well-baby) visit

1) Evaluates a child's growth and development
2) Physical examination is performed at this time
3) Necessary immunizations are administered
b. Sick-child (sick-baby) visit
1) Child shows signs and symptoms of a disease process or injury
2) Provider diagnoses and prescribes treatment

C. Growth Chart

1. Chart used to plot the physical growth pattern of a child
2. Includes height, weight, and head circumference
3. Identifies the percentile into which the child's growth falls compared with measurements listed on the standardized chart
4. Should be plotted at each well-baby visit
5. Separate charts
   a. Girls, birth to 36 months (Fig. 18.5)
   b. Girls, 2–20 years
   c. Boys, birth to 36 months (Fig. 18.6)
   d. Boys, 2–18 years
6. Body mass index (BMI) charts for infants and young adults
   a. $BMI = \dfrac{wt\,\|\,lbs\,\|\,\times 703}{Ht\,\|\,in\,\|^{2}}$

D. Common Pediatric Diseases and Disorders

1. Colic: abdominal distress
2. Diarrhea: loose stools; two or more watery or abnormal stools within 24 hours
3. Failure to thrive: an infant or young child whose weight is consistently below the 3rd percentile on growth charts; medical and social factors must be evaluated
4. Obesity: BMI for age is between 85th and 95th percentiles
5. Common cold: a highly contagious viral disease spread through droplets
6. Otitis media: infection or inflammation of the middle ear; can be serous or suppurative
7. Croup: viral inflammation of the larynx and trachea causing edema and spasms of the vocal cords
8. Bronchiolitis: viral infection of the small bronchi and bronchioles
9. Asthma: result of bronchospasm and inflammation
10. Influenza: highly contagious viral infection of the respiratory tract
11. Conjunctivitis: pink eye; a highly contagious bacterial infection that affects the conjunctiva
12. Tonsillitis: inflammation of the tonsils most frequently caused by streptococcus A
13. Fifth disease: erythema infectiosum; "slapped cheek disease"; caused by parvovirus B19
14. Varicella: chickenpox; a viral disease caused by a herpesvirus; transmitted by droplets; vaccine available for protection
15. Meningitis: inflammation of the membranes that cover the brain and spinal cord; can be caused by bacteria, fungi, or viruses; Hib vaccine available (Hib) for protection

16. Hepatitis B: viral infection that can be transmitted across the placenta or during the birth process if the mother is infected; vaccine available for protection
17. Reye syndrome: cause unknown; linked to use of aspirin during a viral illness

E. Immunizations (Fig. 18.7)

1. Always refer to the Centers for Disease Control and Prevention (CDC) guidelines for current schedule
   a. Childhood diphtheria-tetanus-acellular pertussis vaccine (DTaP)
      1) Five doses required by law between 2 months and 6 years of age
      2) Administer: 0.5 mL intramuscularly (IM)
      3) Trade names: Daptacel and Infarix
   b. Adolescent tetanus-diphtheria toxoids vaccine (Td): 11 and 12 years of age, Td booster
   c. Adult tetanus vaccine (Td)
      1) Given as a booster from age 7 through adulthood
      2) Adults are given one dose every 10 years for life
      3) For severe or dirty wounds, a booster is given if the last normal dose was more than 5 years ago
      4) For minor or clean wounds, a booster is given if the last normal dose was given 10 or more years ago
   d. *Haemophilus influenzae* type b (Hib)
      1) Four doses administered between 2 months and 18 months of age
      2) Administer: 0.5 mL IM
      3) Vaccine consists of killed virus grown in chicken embryo tissue
      4) Trade names: COMVAX, PedVaxHIB, ActHIB, and Hiberix
   e. Inactivated poliovirus (poliomyelitis) vaccine (IPV)
      1) Four doses administered between 2 months and 4–6 years of age
      2) Administer: 0.5 mL IM or subcutaneously (SC)
      3) Trade name: Ipol
   f. Hepatitis B vaccine (HepB)
      1) Three doses administered between birth and 18 months of age
      2) Administer: 0.5 mL IM
      3) Two doses of Recombivax HB 1 mL may be given to 11- to 15-year-olds
      4) Trade names: Engerix-B and Recombivax HB
   g. Mumps, measles, and rubella (MMR) vaccine
      1) Two doses administered between 12 months and 11–12 years of age
      2) Administer: 0.5 mL SC
      3) Vaccine consists of attenuated measles, mumps, and rubella virus
      4) Trade name: M-M-R II
   h. Varicella vaccine (Var; chickenpox)
      1) Two doses: first administered after 12 months of age; second at 4–6 years
      2) Administer: 0.5 mL SC
      3) Trade name: Varivax
   i. Pneumococcal vaccine (PCV)
      1) Three doses administered before age 12 months; last dose given after 12 months and before age 5

2 to 20 years: Girls
Stature-for-age and Weight-for-age percentiles

NAME _____

RECORD # _____

Mother's Stature _____ Father's Stature _____

Date	Age	Weight	Stature	BMI*

*To Calculate BMI: Weight (kg) ÷ Stature (cm) ÷ Stature (cm) x 10,000
or Weight (lb) ÷ Stature (in) ÷ Stature (in) x 703

AGE (YEARS)

STATURE

WEIGHT

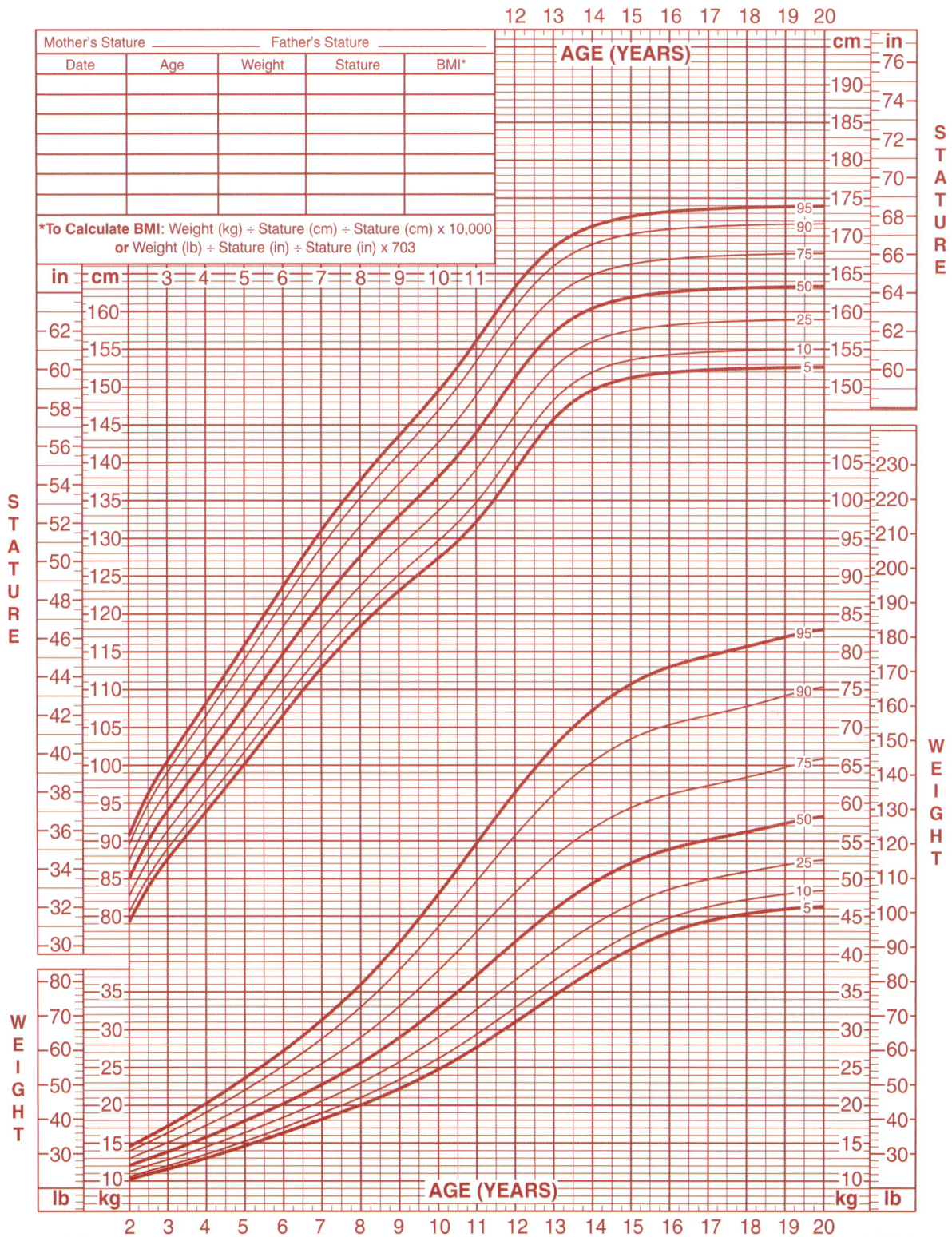

Published May 30, 2000 (modified 11/21/00).
SOURCE: Developed by the National Center for Health Statistics in collaboration with
the National Center for Chronic Disease Prevention and Health Promotion (2000).
http://www.cdc.gov/growthcharts

CDC
SAFER · HEALTHIER · PEOPLE™

Fig. 18.5 Growth chart for girls from 2 to 20 years.

Birth to 36 months: Boys
Length-for-age and Weight-for-age percentiles

NAME _____

RECORD # _____

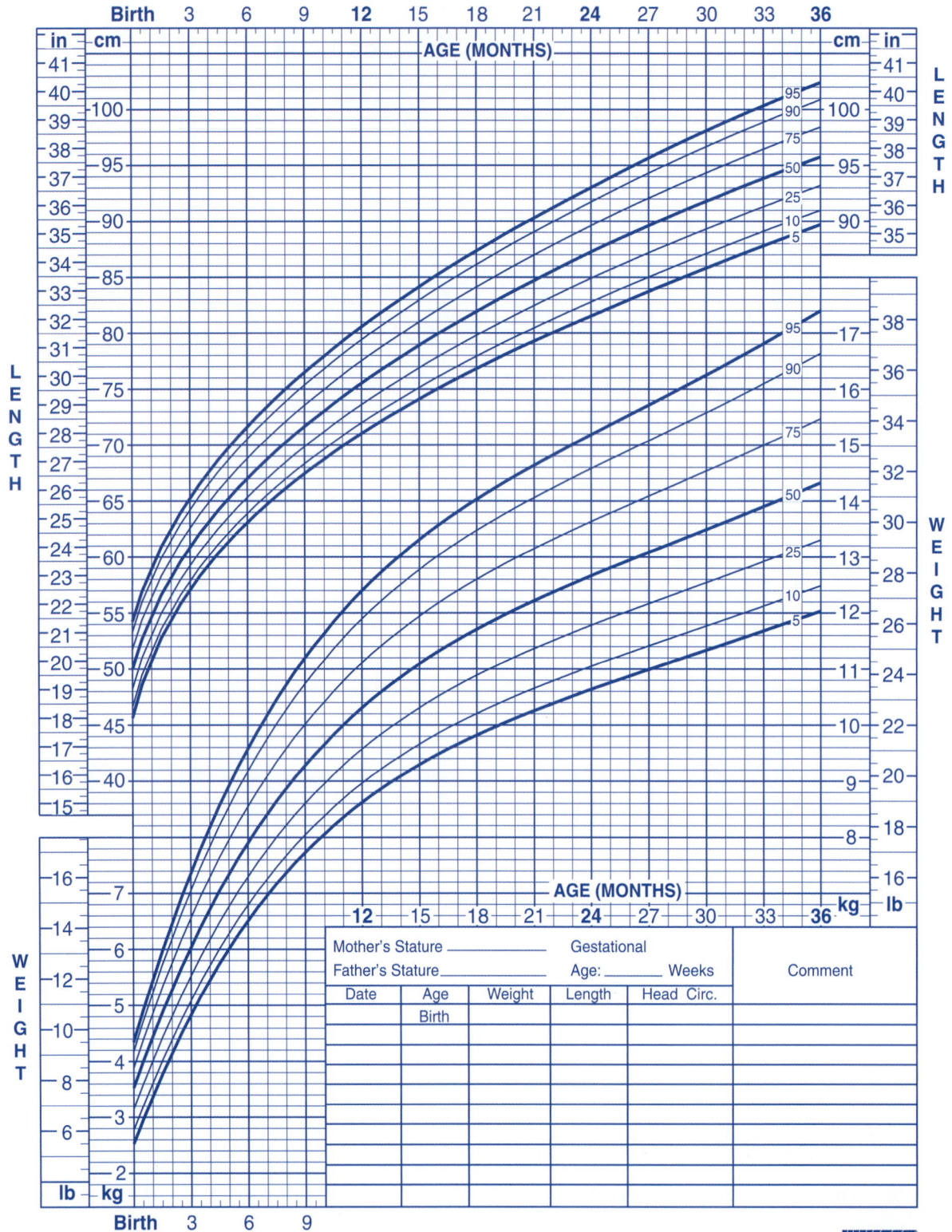

Published May 30, 2000 (modified 4/20/01).
SOURCE: Developed by the National Center for Health Statistics in collaboration with
the National Center for Chronic Disease Prevention and Health Promotion (2000).
http://www.cdc.gov/growthcharts

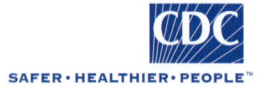

Fig. 18.6 Growth chart for boys from birth to 36 months.

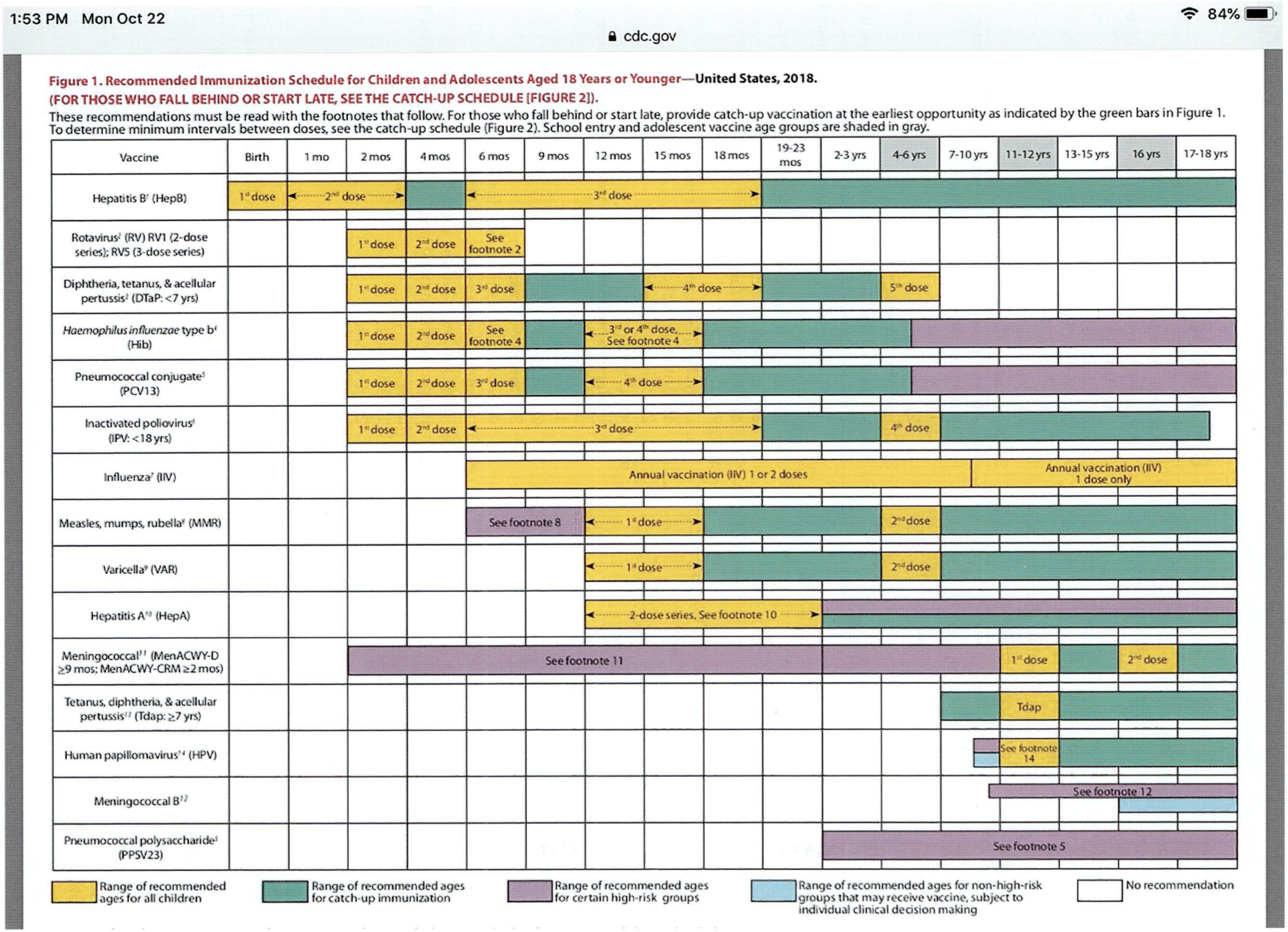

Figure 1. Recommended Immunization Schedule for Children and Adolescents Aged 18 Years or Younger—United States, 2018.

(FOR THOSE WHO FALL BEHIND OR START LATE, SEE THE CATCH-UP SCHEDULE [FIGURE 2]).

These recommendations must be read with the footnotes that follow. For those who fall behind or start late, provide catch-up vaccination at the earliest opportunity as indicated by the green bars in Figure 1. To determine minimum intervals between doses, see the catch-up schedule (Figure 2). School entry and adolescent vaccine age groups are shaded in gray.

Vaccine	Birth	1 mo	2 mos	4 mos	6 mos	9 mos	12 mos	15 mos	18 mos	19-23 mos	2-3 yrs	4-6 yrs	7-10 yrs	11-12 yrs	13-15 yrs	16 yrs	17-18 yrs
Hepatitis B[1] (HepB)	1st dose	2nd dose			3rd dose												
Rotavirus[2] (RV) RV1 (2-dose series); RV5 (3-dose series)			1st dose	2nd dose	See footnote 2												
Diphtheria, tetanus, & acellular pertussis[3] (DTaP: <7 yrs)			1st dose	2nd dose	3rd dose			4th dose				5th dose					
Haemophilus influenzae type b[4] (Hib)			1st dose	2nd dose	See footnote 4		3rd or 4th dose, See footnote 4										
Pneumococcal conjugate[5] (PCV13)			1st dose	2nd dose	3rd dose		4th dose										
Inactivated poliovirus[6] (IPV: <18 yrs)			1st dose	2nd dose	3rd dose							4th dose					
Influenza[7] (IIV)						Annual vaccination (IIV) 1 or 2 doses							Annual vaccination (IIV) 1 dose only				
Measles, mumps, rubella[8] (MMR)					See footnote 8		1st dose					2nd dose					
Varicella[9] (VAR)							1st dose					2nd dose					
Hepatitis A[10] (HepA)							2-dose series, See footnote 10										
Meningococcal[11] (MenACWY-D ≥9 mos; MenACWY-CRM ≥2 mos)					See footnote 11									1st dose		2nd dose	
Tetanus, diphtheria, & acellular pertussis[12] (Tdap: ≥7 yrs)														Tdap			
Human papillomavirus[14] (HPV)													See footnote 14				
Meningococcal B[12]														See footnote 12			
Pneumococcal polysaccharide[5] (PPSV23)														See footnote 5			

Legend:
- Range of recommended ages for all children
- Range of recommended ages for catch-up immunization
- Range of recommended ages for certain high-risk groups
- Range of recommended ages for non-high-risk groups that may receive vaccine, subject to individual clinical decision making
- No recommendation

Fig. 18.7 Recommended immunization schedule for children ages birth to 18 years. (From http://www.cdc.gov/vaccines/schedules/downloads/child/0-18yrs-child-combined-schedule.pdf.)

    2) Administer 0.5 mL IM or SC

    3) Trade names: Pneumovax 23 and Prevnar 13

  j. Human papillomavirus (HPV2 and HPV4)

    1) Three doses of HPV2 over a 6-month period to female patients 9–26 years

    2) Three doses HPV4 to male and female patients 9–26 years

    3) Administer: 0.5 mL IM

    4) Trade names: Gardasil 9 (males and females) and Cervarix (females only)

  k. Influenza, live attenuated

    1) One dose yearly up to age 50 years

    2) Administer: 0.5 mL IM

    3) Trade names: Afluria, Fluad, Flublok, Flucelvax, FluLavel, Fluarix, Fluvirin, and Fluzone

  l. Hepatitis A (HepA)

    1) Two doses 6 months apart

    2) Administer: 0.5 mL IM for patients younger than 18 years; 1.0 mL IM for patients older than 19 years

    3) Trade names: Havrix and Vaqta

  m. Rotavirus (RV1)

    1) Two doses between 2 and 6 months of age

    2) Administer: 0.5 mL IM

    3) trade name: Rotarix

  n. COVID-19

    1) Three doses: dose 2, 3 weeks after dose 1; dose 3, >8 weeks after dose 2

    2) Administer 0.25 mL

    3) Trade Names: Moderna COVID-19; Pfizer-BioNTech; Novavax; Oxford-AstraZeneca

2. Combination vaccines

  a. DTaP + HepB + IPV (Pediarix): 0.5 mL IM

  b. DTaP + Hib + IPV (Pentacel): 0.5 mL IM

  c. DTaP + Hib (TriHIBit): 0.5 mL IM

  d. DTaP + IPV (Kinrix): 0.5 mL IM

  e. Hib + HepB (Comvax): 0.5 mL IM

  f. MMR + Var (ProQuad): 0.5 mL SC for patients younger than 12 years

  g. HepA + HepB (Twinrix): 1 mL IM for patients older than 18 years

XIV. Psychiatry

A. General

1. Diagnoses, prevents, and treats mental illness

2. Specialized physician: psychiatrist

3. Psychologist: nonmedical person trained in methods of therapy

B. Common Signs and Symptoms of Mental Disorders

1. Stress, anxiety, and depression

2. Withdrawal from society

3. Disorganized thinking and hallucinations

4. Inappropriate or violent behavior

5. Crying, mood swings

6. Sleep disturbances, fatigue, and agitation

7. Loss of concentration

8. Inability to experience pleasure

9. Forgetfulness

10. Inability to place self in environment, person, and place

11. Paranoia

C. Psychiatric Disorders

1. Anxiety disorders

  a. Characterized by anxiety (unpleasant tension, distress, troubled feelings, avoidance behavior)

    1) Panic disorder

    2) Phobic disorders

    3) Obsessive-compulsive disorder (OCD)

    4) Posttraumatic stress disorder (PTSD)

2. Delirium and dementia

  a. Abnormal cognition (mental processes of thinking, perception, reasoning, and judgment)

    1) Delirium

    2) Dementia

3. Dissociative disorders

  a. Chronic or sudden disturbances of memory, identity, consciousness, and perception of environment

    1) Not caused by direct effects of brain damage and drug abuse

    2) Dissociative identity disorder

    3) Dissociative amnesia

    4) Dissociative fugue

4. Eating disorders

  a. Disturbances in eating behavior

    1) Anorexia nervosa

    2) Bulimia nervosa

5. Mood disorders

  a. Prolonged emotion that dominates person's entire mental life

    1) Bipolar I

    2) Bipolar II

    3) Depressive disorder

    4) Seasonal affective disorder (SAD)

6. Personality disorders

  a. Inflexible and rigid personality traits causing impairment of functioning, distress, and conflict with others

    1) Antisocial

    2) Histrionic

    3) Narcissistic

    4) Paranoid

    5) Schizoid

7. Schizophrenia

  a. Characterized by withdrawal from reality into an inner world of conflict and disorganized thinking

  b. Symptoms

    1) Delusions

    2) Hallucinations

    3) Disorganized thinking

    4) Flat affect

    5) Impaired interpersonal functioning and relationships

8. Sexual and gender identity disorders

  a. Sexual disorders

    1) Paraphilias: recurrent intense sexual urges, fantasies, and behaviors

2) Sexual dysfunctions: disturbances in sexual desire and response
b. Gender identity disorders
1) Strong, persistent cross-gender identification with opposite sex
9. Somatoform disorders
a. Patient's mental conflicts expressed as physical symptoms
1) Conversion disorder
2) Hypochondriasis
10. Substance-related disorders
a. Symptoms, behavioral changes associated with regular use of substances that affect the central nervous system
b. Prolonged use produces dependence
1) Alcohol
2) Amphetamines
3) Cannabis
4) Cocaine
5) Hallucinogens
6) Opioids
7) Sedatives
c. Common signs and symptoms of substance abuse
1) Changes in weight and sleep habits
2) Impaired memory
3) Illogical thinking
4) Mood swings, irritability, depression, and anger
5) Anxiety and overreaction to difficult situations
6) Changes in vital signs
7) Runny nose, nasal stuffiness, bloodshot eyes, and sweating
8) Changes in friends and appearance

D. Therapeutic Techniques

1. Psychotherapy
a. Treatment of emotional problems using psychological techniques
2. Cognitive behavior therapy
3. Family therapy
4. Group therapy
5. Hypnosis
6. Play therapy
7. Psychoanalysis
8. Sex therapy
9. Supportive psychotherapy
10. Electroconvulsive therapy (ECT)
a. Electrical current applied to brain while patient is anesthetized and ventilated
b. Used mainly for serious depression and bipolar disorder
11. Drug therapy
a. Use of medications to treat psychiatric disorders
1) Antianxiety agents: lessen anxiety, tension, and agitation
a) Examples: Xanax, Valium, Buspar, Paxil, and Ativan
2) Antidepressants: reverse depressive symptoms; produce feelings of well-being
a) Examples: Prozac, Paxil, Elavil, Wellbutrin, and Celexa
3) Anti–obsessive-compulsive agents: relieve symptoms of OCD
a) Examples: Anafranil and Zoloft

4) Antipsychotics: modify psychotic symptoms and behavior
a) Examples: Haldol, Zyprexa, and Risperdol
5) Hypnotics: produce sleep
a) Examples: Ambien, Restoril, and Halcion
6) Mood stabilizers: treat manic episodes of bipolar illness
a) Examples: Eskalith, Tegretol, Lithium, and Lamictal
7) Stimulants: prescribed for attention deficit hyperactivity disorder (ADHD) in children
a) Examples: Ritalin and Cyclert

XV. Pulmonology

A. General

1. Diagnoses and treats diseases and disorders of the lungs and respiratory system
2. Specialized physician: pulmonologist

B. Common Symptoms of Respiratory System Disorders

1. Pain in respiratory tract including chest pain and sore throat
2. Dyspnea, wheezing, rales, and cyanosis
3. Cough, productive or nonproductive
4. Dysphonia
5. Fatigue and malaise
6. Chills, fever, and headache
7. Hemoptysis and epistaxis

C. General Examination

1. Inspection of the nose, face, and throat
2. Examination of the mucous membranes
3. Inspection and palpation of the sinuses, neck, and lymph nodes
4. Auscultation of the lungs

D. Diagnostic Procedures

1. Bronchoscopy: visualization of the bronchi through a bronchoscope
2. Spirometry: measurement of breathing capacity of the lungs
3. Lung biopsy: biopsy of tissue taken from the lungs
4. Pulmonary function test (PFT): evaluates how the patient breathes; determines lung volumes, pulmonary gas exchange, and flow rates
5. Thoracentesis: puncture of the chest wall with a needle to obtain fluid for testing
6. Tracheostomy: emergency or elective procedure that creates an opening through the neck into the trachea
7. Chest x-ray: full view of the lungs from the back (posteroanterior [PA]) and sides (lateral)
8. Sputum culture: collection of a sputum sample and testing it for microorganisms
9. ABGs: measurement of hydrogen, carbon dioxide, pH, and oxygen pressure from an arterial blood sample

E. Treatment Procedures

1. Endotracheal intubation: a procedure that establishes an airway by inserting a tube through the nose, pharynx, and larynx into the trachea
2. Thoracotomy: surgical insertion of a tube into the chest to drain fluid or air
3. Nebulizer: a machine that produces a fine mist of water and medication; the patient receives the medication by inhaling the mist

F. Medications

1. Antibiotics
   a. Kill microorganisms
   b. Examples: Amoxil, ampicillin, Biaxin, Ceclor, and Keflex
2. Antihistamines
   a. Counteract the effects of histamine
   b. Examples: Benadryl, Phenergan, and Seldane
3. Bronchodilators
   a. Dilate bronchial tubes
   b. Examples: albuterol (Proventil and Ventolin) and aminophylline
4. Expectorants
   a. Produce productive cough
   b. Example: Humibid
5. Decongestants
   a. Decrease congestion in the nose and nasal passages
   b. Examples: Entex, Afrin, and Sudafed

XVI. Urology

A. General

1. Diagnoses and treats diseases and disorders of the male and female urinary systems and the male reproductive system
2. Specialized physician: urologist

B. Common Symptoms of Urinary System Disorders

1. Anorexia, nausea, and vomiting
2. Malaise, fatigue, and lethargy
3. Nocturia, hematuria, pyuria, and proteinuria
4. Dysuria, urgency, frequency, and incontinence
5. Pain in lumbar region or flank
6. Edema and ascites
7. Hypertension and shortness of breath

C. General Examination

1. Palpation of the kidneys and bladder
2. Inspection of the external genitalia
3. Palpation of the prostate gland through the rectum

D. Diagnostic Procedures

1. Cystoscopy: visual examination of the bladder with a cystoscope
2. Retrograde pyelogram: x-ray of the kidney after introducing a contrast medium through the ureter
3. Intravenous pyelogram (IVP): study of the kidney using an intravenous contrast medium
4. Renal ultrasound: an ultrasound of the kidneys
5. X-ray of the kidney, ureter, and bladder (KUB): x-ray done without injection of air or contrast medium; shows size and location of the organs
6. Urinalysis (UA): analysis of urine to determine physical, chemical, and microscopic properties
7. Blood urea nitrogen (BUN): measures the amount of urea in the blood; kidney function test
8. Semen analysis: measures the quantity and motility of sperm
9. Prostate-specific antigen (PSA): blood test to check for the presence of prostate cancer
10. Helicobacter pylori: stool test to detect *H. pylori* that can cause stomach ulcers
11. Clostridium difficile: stool test for *C. diff* infection

E. Treatment Procedures

1. Dialysis: artificial means of removing waste products from the blood when the kidneys have failed
2. Lithotripsy: procedure to crush or break up stones in the urinary tract
3. Catheterization: introduction of a flexible tube through the urethra into the urinary bladder
4. Circumcision: removal of the foreskin of the penis
5. Prostatectomy: removal of the prostate
6. Transurethral resection of the prostate (TURP): prostatic tissue removed through an endoscope introduced through the urethra
7. Vasectomy: removal of a segment of the vas deferens; male sterilization technique

F. Medications

1. Antibiotics
   a. Destroy microorganisms
   b. Examples: Bactrim, Furadantin, Gantrisin, and Rocephin
2. Analgesics
   a. Reduce pain
   b. Example: Pyridium
3. Gonadotropins
   a. Stimulate gonads
   b. Example: Pergonal
4. For impotence
   a. Example: Viagra

19

Nutrition and Health Promotion

I. Nutrition

A. Definition

1. All processes involved in the intake and use of nutrients
2. Can indicate the condition of the body resulting from the use of nutrients
3. Good health is a state of emotional and physical well-being that can be mostly determined by diet and lifestyle factors
4. "We are what we eat"

B. Nutrients

1. Organic and inorganic chemicals in foods
2. Supply the energy and raw materials for cellular activities
3. Include:
   a. Carbohydrates
   b. Fats
   c. Proteins
   d. Vitamins
   e. Minerals
   f. Water
4. Perform one or more of the three basic functions in the body
   a. Provide a source of fuel or energy
   b. Supply material for the growth and repair of tissues
   c. Regulate metabolic processes

C. Health Problems Related to Poor Nutrition and Lifestyle Choices

1. Anemia: low iron or folate intake
2. Cancers: high-fat, low-fiber diet; high alcohol and sodium intake; sedentary lifestyle; tobacco use
3. Constipation: low fiber; inadequate fluids; high-fat diet; sedentary lifestyle
4. Type 2 diabetes: high-calorie, high-fat diet; obesity; sedentary lifestyle
5. Hypercholesterolemia and atherosclerosis: high-fat, low-fiber diet; high sugar and alcohol intake; tobacco use; sedentary lifestyle
6. Hypertension: high-calorie, high-fat diet; high sodium intake; sedentary lifestyle; obesity; stress
7. Osteoporosis: low calcium intake; inadequate vitamin D; high alcohol intake; sedentary lifestyle; tobacco use
8. Stroke: high-fat, low-fiber diet; high alcohol intake; tobacco use; stress

D. Reasons for Food Choices

1. Convenience
2. Cost
3. Emotional comfort
4. Routine
5. Positive experiences
6. Ethnic and regional influences
7. Health and weight

E. Nutrition Terms

1. Added Sugars: sugar added to food during preparation
2. Antioxidant: molecule that inhibits the oxidation of other molecules
3. Bariatrics: branch of medicine that deals with obesity and diseases associated with obesity
4. Complete protein: protein that contains all of the essential amino acids that the body needs
5. Empty calorie food: food that provides calories but no nutrition
6. Essential amino acid: amino acid required by the body that the body cannot make
7. Glocogen: storage form of glucose in the body
8. Incomplete protein: protein that lacks one or more amino acids that the body needs

9. Macronutrients: nutrients that the body needs in small amounts
10. Micronutrients: nutrients that the body needs in small amounts
11. Mineral: naturally occurring inorganic substance essential for body function
12. Nutrient: chemical substance found in food that is needed by the body
13. Saturated fat: fat that is solid at room temperature; comes from animal sources
14. Unsaturated fat: fat that is liquid at room temperature; comes from plant sources
15. Vitamin: organic compound that the body requires for growth and development

II. Components of Nutrients

A. Carbohydrates (CHO)

1. Organic compounds primarily from plants
2. Supply fuel for energy and all basic cellular functions
3. Three groups
   a. Simple sugars (table sugar, molasses, candy, milk): easily digested and absorbed
   b. Complex carbohydrates (whole grains, cereal, pasta, rice, vegetables): easily digested and absorbed
   c. Dietary fiber (bran, oatmeal, beans, vegetables, seeds): indigestible, passes through the digestive tract unchanged
4. Recommended consumption (per US Food and Drug Administration [FDA])
   a. 55%–57% of total calories per day

B. Fats

1. Storage form of fuel; backup for carbohydrates as energy source
2. Provide essential fatty acids for the absorption of fat-soluble vitamins
3. Support and protect vital organs
4. Help regulate body temperature
5. Protect nerve fibers and help relay nerve impulses
6. Crucial to cell membrane development
7. Stored in adipose (fat) tissue
8. Cholesterol: nonessential nutrient that plays a vital role in metabolic activities
   a. Manufactured in the liver
   b. Found only in animal tissues, not plants
   c. High-density lipoprotein (HDL): "good" fat; carries cholesterol from body tissues to the liver for metabolism and excretion
   d. Low-density lipoprotein (LDL): "bad" fat; carries cholesterol to the cells; can collect as plaques on blood vessel walls
9. Recommended consumption (per the FDA)
   a. 20%–35% of total calories per day

C. Protein

1. Large molecules made up of amino acids
2. Builds and repairs body tissue, including new tissue, blood, and hormones

3. Aids in the body's defense mechanisms against disease
4. Regulates fluid and electrolyte balance
5. Provides energy when carbohydrates and fat stores are depleted
6. Found in meat, fish, poultry, and eggs
7. Recommended protein consumption
   a. No more than 18% of total calories per day

D. Vitamins (Table 19.1)

1. Organic substances that occur in minute quantities in plant and animal tissue
2. Function as catalysts to help or allow metabolic reactions
3. Regulate synthesis of the bone, skin, glands, nerves, and blood
4. Aid in the metabolism of protein, carbohydrates, and fats
5. Prevent nutritional deficiency diseases
6. Provide for good health at all ages
7. Do not cure diseases
8. Two groups:
   a. Fat soluble: A, D, E, K
   b. Water soluble: B complex, C

E. Minerals (Table 19.2)

1. Naturally occurring inorganic substances
2. Body requires two types:
   a. Major minerals (needed in larger amounts)
   b. Trace minerals (needed in smaller amounts)
3. Supplied through food and supplements
4. Contribute to the body's water balance and acid/base balance
5. Electrolytes
   a. Minerals with electrical charge

F. Water

1. Body can survive longer without food than without water
2. Part of almost every vital body function
3. Plays a key role in the maintenance of body temperature
4. Solvent and medium for biochemical reactions
5. Vehicle to transport substances, such as nutrients, hormones, antibodies, and wastes
6. Acts as a lubricant for joints and mucous membranes
7. Lost from the body in urine, feces, sweat, and expiration

III. MyPlate

A. Purpose

1. Developed by the US Department of Agriculture (USDA) to explain dietary guidelines
2. Good nutrition is a balance among
   a. Carbohydrates
   b. Protein
   c. Vitamins
   d. Minerals
   e. Fiber
   f. Water
   g. Exercise

TABLE 19.1   Vitamins

Vitamin	US RDA[a]	Best Sources	Functions	Deficiency Symptoms[b]	Toxic?	Processing Tips	Did You Know?
A (carotene)	5000 IU/day	Yellow or orange fruits and vegetables, green leafy vegetables, fortified oatmeal, liver, dairy products	Formation and maintenance of skin, hair, and mucous membranes; helps vision in dim light; bone and tooth growth	Night blindness, dry and scaly skin, frequent fatigue	Yes, in high doses, but beta-carotene is nontoxic	Serve fruits and vegetables raw and keep covered and refrigerated; steam vegetables; broil, bake, or braise meats	Low-fat and skim milks are often fortified with vitamin A, which was removed with the fat
B$_1$ (thiamine)	1.5 mg/day	Fortified cereals and oatmeal, meats, rice and pasta, whole grains, liver	Helps body release energy from carbohydrates during metabolism; growth and muscle tone	Heart irregularity, fatigue, nerve disorders, mental confusion	No, high doses are excreted by the kidneys	Do not rinse rice or pasta before and after cooking; cook in minimal water	Pasta and breads made of refined flours have B$_1$ added because it is lost in the milling process
B$_2$ (riboflavin)	1.7 mg/day	Whole grains, green leafy vegetables, organ meats, milk, eggs	Helps body release energy from protein, fat, and carbohydrates during metabolism	Cracks in corners of mouth, rash, anemia	No toxic effects reported	Store food in containers that light cannot enter; cook vegetables in minimal water; roast or broil meats	Most ready-to-eat cereals are fortified with 25% of US RDA for B$_2$
B$_6$ (pyridoxine)	2 mg/day	Fish, poultry, lean meats, bananas, prunes, dried beans, whole grains, avocados	Helps build body tissue and aids in metabolism of protein	Convulsions, dermatitis, muscular weakness, skin cracks, anemia	Long-term megadoses may cause nerve damage in hands and feet	Serve fruits raw or cook for shortest time in little water; roast or broil meats	Because B$_6$ aids in use of protein in the body, the need for B$_6$ increases with protein intake
B$_{12}$ (cobalamin)	6 μg/day	Meats, milk products, seafood	Aids cell development, functioning of the nervous system, metabolism of protein and fat	Anemia, nervousness, fatigue, and, in some cases, neuritis and brain degeneration	No toxic effects reported	Roast or broil meat and fish	Vegetarians who do not eat any animal products may need a supplement
Biotin	0.3 mg/day	Cereal/grain products, yeast, legumes, liver	Involved in metabolism of protein, fats, and carbohydrates	Nausea, vomiting, depression, hair loss, dry scaly skin	No toxic effects reported	Storage, processing, and cooking do not appear to affect this vitamin	Biotin deficiency is extremely rare in the United States
Folate (folacin, folic acid)	0.4 mg/day	Green leafy vegetables, organ meats, dried peas, beans, and lentils	Aids in genetic material development and is involved in red blood cell production	Gastrointestinal disorders, anemia, cracks on lips	Some evidence of toxicity in high doses	Store vegetables in refrigerator and steam, boil, or simmer in minimal water	Deficiencies can occur in premature infants and pregnant women
Niacin	20 mg/day	Meat, poultry, fish, enriched cereals, peanuts, potatoes, dairy products, eggs	Involved in carbohydrate, protein, and fat metabolism	Skin disorders, diarrhea, indigestion, general fatigue	Nicotinic acid form should be taken only under a physician's care	Roast or broil beef, veal, lamb, and poultry; cook potatoes in minimal water	Niacin is formed in the body by converting an amino acid found in proteins

(Continued)

TABLE 19.1   Vitamins—cont'd

Vitamin	US RDAª	Best Sources	Functions	Deficiency Symptomsᵇ	Toxic?	Processing Tips	Did You Know?
Pantothenic acid	10 mg/day	Lean meats, whole grains, legumes, vegetables, fruits	Helps in release of energy from fats and carbohydrates	Fatigue, vomiting, stomach stress, infections, muscle cramps	No toxic effects reported	Eat fruits and vegetables raw	It is believed that some pantothenic acid is produced in the gastrointestinal tract
C (ascorbic acid)	60 mg/day	Citrus fruits, berries, vegetables—especially peppers	Essential for structure of bones, cartilage, muscle, and blood vessels; helps maintain capillaries and gums; aids in absorption of iron	Swollen or bleeding gums, slow wound healing, fatigue/depression, poor digestion	Intakes of ≥1 g can cause nausea, cramps, and diarrhea	Do not store or soak fruits and vegetables in water; refrigerate juices and store only 2–3 days	Smokers may benefit from increased intake of vitamin C
D	400 IU/day	Fortified milk, sunlight, fish, eggs, butter, fortified margarine	Aids in bone and tooth formation; helps maintain heart action and nervous system	In children, rickets and other bone deformities; in adults, calcium loss from bones	High intakes may cause diarrhea and weight loss	Storage, processing, and cooking do not appear to affect this vitamin	Sunlight starts vitamin D production in the skin
E	30 IU/day	Fortified and multigrain cereals, nuts, wheat germ, vegetable oils, green leafy vegetables	Protects blood cells, body tissue, and essential fatty acids from harmful destruction in the body	Muscular wasting, nerve damage, anemia, reproductive failure	Relatively nontoxic	Store in airtight containers away from light	Most fortified cereals have 40% of FDA requirements
K	—ᶜ	Green leafy vegetables, fruit, dairy products, grain products	Essential for blood-clotting functions	Bleeding disorders in newborns and patients on blood-thinning medications	Not toxic as found in food	Store in containers away from light	Vitamin K is also formed by bacteria in the colon

Vitamins A, D, E, and K are fat soluble; the other vitamins in this table are water soluble.
ªFor adults and children older than 4.
ᵇMany of the symptoms outlined under this heading can also be attributed to problems other than vitamin deficiency. If you have these symptoms and they persist, consult your physician.
ᶜThere is no US RDA for vitamin K; however, the recommended dietary allowance is 1 µg/kg of body weight.
FDA, US Food and Drug Administration; *RDA,* recommended daily allowance.
From the US Food and Drug Administration, American Institute for Cancer Research, and US Department of Agriculture/Human Nutrition Information Service.

B. MyPlate Symbol (Fig. 19.1)

1. In June 2011, MyPlate replaced MyPyramid as the government's primary food group symbol
2. Shows ideal plate proportions of main food groups
3. Explaining MyPlate (choosemyplate.gov) to patients encourages healthy eating habits

IV. Nutrition Therapy (Diets)

A. General

1. Some illnesses and diseases can be cured, and recovery can be facilitated with special diets/nutrition plans

2. Consider the patient's lifestyle, cultural influences, and background
3. Normal diet is modified to create a therapeutic diet by either restricting or increasing the needed nutrients
4. Diet: food consumed by a person; specific intake of nutrition for health or weight management
5. Nutrition therapy: application of nutrition to promote health and to treat illness

B. Therapeutic Diets

1. Liquid
   a. Two types
      1) Clear liquid: broth, tea, gelatin
      2) Full liquid: all foods on a clear diet plus milk, custard, strained cream soup, milkshakes, all juices

TABLE 19.2 Minerals

Functions	Sources	Deficiency Symptoms	Toxicity Symptoms
Mineral and Elemental Symbol: Calcium (Ca^{2+})			
Helps the muscles contract and relax, helping regulate the heartbeat; plays a role in the normal functioning of the nervous system; aids in blood coagulation and functioning of some enzymes; helps build strong bones and teeth	Primarily found in milk and milk products; also found in dark green, leafy vegetables, tofu and other soy products, sardines, salmon with bones, and hard water	Poor bone growth and tooth development, leading to stunted growth and increased risk of dental caries, rickets (bowing of legs) in children, osteomalacia (soft bones) and osteoporosis (brittle bones) in adults, poor blood clotting, and possible hypertension	Kidney stones
Mineral and Elemental Symbol: Chloride (Cl$^-$)			
Involved in the maintenance of fluid and acid-base balance; provides an acid medium, in the form of hydrochloric acid, for activation of gastric enzymes	Major source is table salt (sodium chloride); also found in fish and vegetables	Disturbances in acid-base balance, with possible growth retardation, psychomotor defects, memory loss	Disturbances in acid-base balance
Mineral and Elemental Symbol: Magnesium (Mg^{2+})			
Helps build strong bones and teeth; activates many enzymes; participates in protein synthesis and lipid metabolism; helps regulate heartbeat	Raw, dark green vegetables, nuts and soybeans, whole grains and wheat bran, bananas and apricots, seafood, coffee, tea, cocoa, and hard water	Rare but in disease states may lead to central nervous system problems (confusion, apathy, hallucinations, poor memory) and neuromuscular problems (muscle weakness, cramps, tremor, cardiac arrhythmia)	Drowsiness, weakness, and lethargy; in severe toxicity, skeletal paralysis, central nervous system depression, respiratory depression, and ultimately coma and death
Mineral and Elemental Symbol: Phosphorus (PO$_4^-$)			
Helps build strong bones and teeth; present in the nuclei of all cells; helps in the oxidation of fats and carbohydrates (energy metabolism); aids in maintaining the body's acid-base balance	Milk and milk products, eggs, meats, legumes, whole grains, and soft drinks (used to make the "fizz")	Rare but with malabsorption can cause anorexia, weakness, stiff joints, and fragile bones	Hypocalcemic tetany (muscle spasms)
Mineral and Elemental Symbol: Potassium (K$^+$)			
Plays a key role in fluid and acid-base balance; transmits nerve impulses, helps control muscle contractions, and promotes regular heartbeat; needed for enzyme reactions	Apricots, bananas, oranges, grapefruit, raisins, green beans, broccoli, carrots, greens, potatoes, meats, milk and milk products, peanut butter and legumes, molasses, coffee, tea, and cocoa	May cause impaired growth, hypertension, bone fragility, central nervous system changes, renal hypertrophy, diminished heart rate, and death	Hyperkalemia (excess potassium in the blood) with cardiac function disturbances
Mineral and Elemental Symbol: Sodium (Na$^+$)			
Plays a key role in the maintenance of acid-base balance; transmits nerve impulses and helps control muscle contractions; regulates cell membrane permeability	Salt (sodium chloride) is the major dietary source; minor sources occur naturally in milk and milk products and several vegetables	Hyponatremia (too little sodium in the blood)	May cause hypertension, which can lead to cardiovascular diseases and renal (kidney) disease; in the form of salt tablets, can cause gastric irritation
Mineral and Elemental Symbol: Chromium (Cr^{3+})			
Activates several enzymes; enhances removal of glucose from the blood	Liver and other meats, whole grains, cheese, legumes, and brewer's yeast	Weight loss, abnormalities of the central nervous system, and possible aggravation of diabetes mellitus	Inhibited insulin activity
Mineral and Elemental Symbol: Copper (Cu^{2+})			
Aids in production and survival of red blood cells; parts of many enzymes involved in respiration; plays a role in normal lipid metabolism	Shellfish, especially oysters, liver, nuts and seeds, raisins, whole grains, and chocolate	Anemia, central nervous system problems, abnormal electrocardiograms, bone fragility, impaired immune response; may be a factor in failure to thrive in premature infants	In Wilson disease and Huntington chorea (both hereditary diseases), copper accumulation causes neuron and liver cell damage

(Continued)

TABLE 19.2   Minerals—cont'd

Functions	Sources	Deficiency Symptoms	Toxicity Symptoms
Mineral and Elemental Symbol: Fluorine (F⁻)			
Helps the formation of solid bones and teeth, reducing the incidence of dental caries, and may help prevent osteoporosis	Fluoridated water (and foods cooked in fluoridated water), fish, tea, and gelatin	Increased susceptibility to dental caries	Fluorosis and mottling of teeth
Mineral and Elemental Symbol: Iodine (I⁻)			
Helps regulate energy metabolism through being part of thyroid hormones; essential for normal cell functioning, helps keep the skin, hair, and nails healthy	Primarily from iodized salt, also found in saltwater fish, seaweed products, and vegetables grown in iodine-rich soils	Goiter, cretinism in infants born to iodine-deficient mothers, with accompanying mental retardation; diffuse central nervous system abnormalities	Little toxic effect in individuals with normal thyroid gland functioning
Mineral and Elemental Symbol: Iron (Fe^{3+})			
Essential to the formation of hemoglobin, which is important for tissue respiration and ultimately growth and development; part of several enzymes and proteins in the body	Heme sources, organ meats especially liver, red meats, and other meats; nonheme sources, iron-fortified cereals, dark-green leafy vegetables, legumes, whole grains, blackstrap molasses, dried fruit, and foods cooked in iron pans	Iron-deficiency anemia and possible alterations that impair behavior	Idiopathic hemochromatosis, which can lead to cirrhosis, diabetes mellitus, skin pigmentation, arthralgias (joint pain), and cardiomyopathy
Mineral and Elemental Symbol: Manganese (Mn^{2+})			
Needed for normal bone structure, reproduction, normal functioning of cells, and central nervous system; component of some enzymes	Protein-rich foods (meat, eggs, milk), whole grains, seafood, liver and other meats, and garlic	Keshan disease (a human cardiomyopathy) and Kashin-Bek disease (an endemic human osteoarthropathy)	Physical defects of fingernails and toenails and hair loss
Mineral and Elemental Symbol: Zinc (Zn^{2+})			
Plays a role in protein synthesis; essential for normal growth and sexual development, wound healing, immune function, cell division and differentiation, and smell acuity	Whole grains, wheat germ, crabmeat, oyster, liver and other meats, brewer's yeast	Depressed immune function, poor growth, dwarfism, impaired skeletal growth and delayed sexual maturation, acrodermatitis	Severe anemia, nausea, vomiting, abdominal cramps, diarrhea, fever, hypocupremia (low blood serum copper), malaise, fatigue

From Poleman CM, Peckenpaugh NJ: *Nutrition essentials and diet therapy*, ed 6, 1991, Saunders, pp 128–129; Garrison RH, Somer E: *The nutrition desk reference*, 1985, Keats Publishing; and Griffeth HW: *Complete guide to vitamins, minerals and supplements*, 1988, Fisher Books.

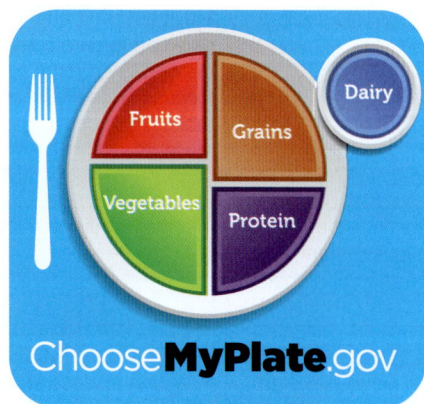

Fig. 19.1 MyPlate. (From US Department of Agriculture: ChooseMyPlate, 2020, www.choosemyplate.gov.)

    b. Indicated for preparation for certain diagnostic tests and postoperatively

2. Soft diet
    a. Foods with roughage (fiber) are eliminated
    b. Eliminate raw fruits and vegetables; strongly flavored/gas-forming vegetables (onions, beans, broccoli, cauliflower)
    c. Indicated postoperatively; certain gastrointestinal (GI) disorders

3. Mechanical soft diet
    a. Regular diet in which foods are ground, chopped, or pureed
    b. Indicated after oral surgery and for patients who have difficulty chewing or swallowing

4. Bland diet
    a. Restricts components that are GI irritants

b. Chemically irritating agents
   1) Caffeine
   2) Pepper
   3) Chili
   4) Alcohol
c. Mechanically irritating agents
   1) High-fiber foods
d. Eliminate fried foods and highly concentrated sweets
e. Indicated for GI problems
5. Elimination diet
   a. Eliminates certain foods to treat allergies
   b. Types
      1) Simple elimination diet: removes only one or two foods
      2) Rowe elimination diet: more extensive diet; begins with a few hypoallergenic foods (rice cereal, apples, pears, carrots, sweet potatoes, lamb, milk substitutes); if no allergic reaction, single food groups are introduced about every 10 days
6. High-fiber or low-fiber diet
   a. Fiber in the diet is either increased or decreased depending on the specific disorder
   b. Low-fiber diets are indicated for GI disorders such as diverticulitis
   c. High-fiber diets are indicated for hypercholesterolemia, diabetes mellitus, and prevention of certain cancers

C. Nutrition Therapy

1. Obesity:
   a. Used to achieve a healthy weight
   b. Reduce the number of calories taken in and increase the number of calories used
   c. Requires lifestyle changes, healthy meals, and control of portion sizes
2. Cardiovascular disease
   a. Goals of diet are to eat foods that reduce cholesterol, decrease LDLs, increase HDLs, and keep blood pressure within normal limits
   b. Includes exercise
3. Hypertension
   a. Goals of diet are to reduce the amount of sodium (salt) taken in
   b. Used for patients with high blood pressure, edema, and cardiovascular disease
4. Diabetes
   a. Basic goal is to control blood glucose levels
   b. Based on an exchange list; objective is to achieve the balance of carbohydrates, proteins, and fats
   c. Diet plan is individual; must take into consideration weight control, patient preferences, exercise patterns, and lifestyle
   d. Glycemic index places carbohydrate foods on a scale from slowest-to-fastest effects on blood glucose levels
5. Lactose intolerance:
   a. Treated by limiting/avoiding food containing lactose
6. Gluten intolerance:
   a. Treated by following gluten-free diet

7. Food Allergies:
   a. Special diets that eliminate allergens
   b. Diets can include elimination diet, rotation diet, and denaturation

V. Food Labels

A. General

1. The FDA requires all food products to carry a nutritional fact label
   a. Found on the back or side of package
   b. Source of nutrition information and nutrients within the package
   c. Mandatory components and order in which they must appear
      1) Serving size
      2) Calories per serving
      3) Calories from fat per serving
      4) Grams of total fat
      5) Milligrams of cholesterol
      6) Milligrams of sodium
      7) Milligrams of potassium
      8) Grams of total carbohydrates
      9) Grams of dietary fiber
      10) Grams of sugars
      11) Grams of protein
      12) Percent of daily values of vitamins A and C
      13) Percent of daily values of calcium and iron

B. Use of Label Information

1. Tells the amount of nutrients in each serving size
2. Tells about the foods eaten
3. Ingredients listed in a descending order of weight (proportion of ingredients)

VI. Eating Disorders

A. Definition

1. Any eating behavior pattern that can lead to a health problem
2. Can damage all body systems and lead to death

B. Anorexia Nervosa

1. Characterized by self-induced starvation
2. Patient is typically an adolescent who is sensitive to failure and criticism and a perfectionist
3. Patient uses avoidance of food as a way of controlling feelings
4. Patient loses 15%–60% of normal body weight, resulting in malnutrition
5. Patient has a distorted body image
6. Patient requires psychotherapy to alleviate depression, deal with emotional issues, and form a positive self-image

C. Bulimia

1. Characterized by cycles of bingeing and purging
2. Patient believes self-worth is related to being thin
3. Intake during binge period can be 20,000 calories
4. Purge period can include vomiting, use of laxatives and enemas, excessive exercise, and food abstinence
5. Treatment: combination of medication, psychotherapy, nutritional counseling to establish healthy eating patterns and improve self-image

D. Obesity

1. Affects more than 60% of the population
2. Obese patients are at risk for hypertension, type 2 diabetes, coronary artery disease, stroke, gallbladder diseases, osteoarthritis, sleep apnea, and certain types of cancer
3. Assessment includes body mass index
4. Treatment can be surgical (bariatric surgery) or by medication (e.g., appetite suppressants, lipase inhibitors)

VII. Health Promotion

A. Definition

1. Includes adequate nutrition, healthy environment, and ongoing health education in an attempt to prevent disease and maintain optimal wellness
2. Uses immunizations, appropriate personal hygiene, environmental sanitation standards, protection against occupational hazards, diet, and periodic health screening and examinations to promote wellness

B. Exercise

1. Defined: physical exertion for the improvement/maintenance of health or for the correction of a physical handicap
2. Improves cardiorespiratory function
3. Maintains musculoskeletal health
4. Relieves stress
5. Used along with diet and rest for good health

C. Stress Management

1. Stress response can lead to health issues if not managed
2. Best managed with exercise

D. Health Screening

1. Routine component of health promotion
2. Every visit should include
   a. Update health history
   b. Weight
   c. Temperature, pulse, and respiration (TPR) and blood pressure (BP) taken/recorded
3. May also include
   a. Tuberculin skin test
   b. Pap smear
   c. Prostate-specific antigen (PSA) level
   d. Hemoccult after age 50
   e. Colonoscopy or sigmoidoscopy every 3–5 years after age 50
   f. Mammogram after age 40
   g. Urinalysis (UA)
   h. Serum cholesterol
   i. Chest x-ray
   j. Electrocardiogram (ECG, EKG)

20

Therapeutic Modalities and Physical Agents to Promote Tissue Healing

I. Therapeutic Modalities

A. General

1. Use of heat, cold, massage, water, exercise, or electricity to restore normal function to injured tissues (Fig. 20.1)
2. Physical therapy program may be prescribed by a provider and implemented by a physical therapist

B. Objectives

1. Relieve pain
2. Increase or improve circulation
3. Increase or restore muscle function
4. Improve strength, range of motion, and joint mobility

II. Heat Application (Thermotherapy)

A. General

1. Relieves pain, inflammation, and congestion
2. Promotes muscle relaxation
3. Local effects
   a. Dilation of blood vessels, resulting in increased blood supply and tissue metabolism
   b. Increases nutrients and oxygen to area and eliminates waste products

B. Heat Therapy

1. Infrared therapy
   a. Administered by a heat lamp
   b. Lamp is placed 2–4 feet from the affected area for 15–20 minutes

2. Diathermy
   a. Electrical field that produces deep heat penetration
   b. Commonly used for muscular injuries and inflammation in joints
   c. Types
      1) Microwave: electromagnetic radiation
      2) Shortwave: high-frequency current
      3) Ultrasound: high-frequency sound waves
3. Ultrasound
   a. High-frequency sound waves used as deep-heating agent
   b. Used for strains, sprains, arthritis, edema, and dislocation
   c. Coupling agent (oil or gel) used to increase conductivity
   d. Ordered by intensity of sound waves per unit of time
4. Paraffin wax
   a. Wax is melted and heated to approximately 125°F
   b. Affected part is immersed in melted wax and lifted out
   c. Wax hardens and holds in the heat
   d. Relieves arthritis, increases circulation, and reduces stiffness
5. Hot water bag
   a. Rubber bag filled approximately one-half full with hot water (115°F–125°F)
   b. Bag is applied to the affected body part for the prescribed period
   c. Place some sort of covering (towel, blanket) over the body part before positioning the hot water bag
6. Hot soaks
   a. Basin is filled with a warmed solution (105°F–110°F)
   b. Body part is immersed in basin for the prescribed period
   c. As solution cools, replace it with more warmed solution
7. Hot compress
   a. Immerse cloth or gauze squares in warm solution (105°F–110°F)

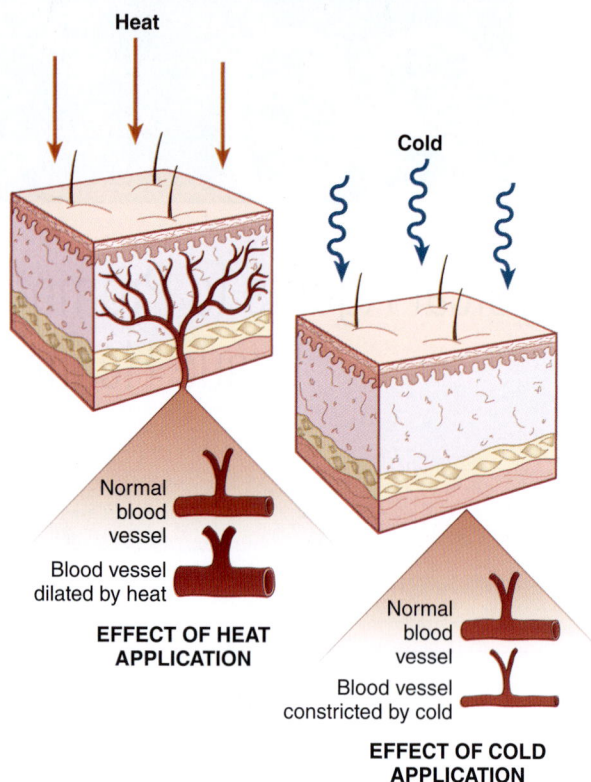

Fig. 20.1 Effects of local application of heat and cold.

b. Wring out excess fluid, and place material over the affected body part
c. Replace the hot compress every 2–3 minutes for the prescribed time
8. Heating pad
   a. Consists of a network of wires that convert electrical energy into heat
   b. Provides even and constant heat application
   c. Must be plugged into an electrical outlet
   d. Pad placed on the affected body part; do not lie on the pad
   e. Used to relieve pain and muscle spasms

III. Cold Application (Cryotherapy)

A. General

1. Prevents edema by constricting vessels
2. Applied immediately after the trauma
3. Relieves pain by numbing
4. Local effects: vascular constriction, which leads to decreased blood supply to the area; decreased tissue metabolism; and decreased accumulation of wastes

B. Types of Cold Therapies

1. Ice bag
   a. Ice bag is filled one-half to two-thirds full of ice
   b. Applied to affected area for the prescribed time
   c. Place some sort of covering (towel, blanket) over the body part before positioning the ice bag
   d. Check for pallor, numbness, or cyanosis, and report any of these signs immediately

2. Cold compress
   a. Immerse cloth or gauze squares in a basin filled with cold water and ice
   b. Wring out excess fluid, and place material over the affected body part
   c. Replace the cold compress every 2–3 minutes for the prescribed time

IV. Hydrotherapy

A. General

1. Use of external water applications for therapeutic purposes
2. Used for
   a. Relaxation
   b. Increased circulation
   c. Improved mobility

B. Types of Hydrotherapies

1. Whirlpool: moist heat with massage action
2. Contrast baths: patient moves affected part from hot, to cold, to hot baths
3. Underwater exercise: buoyant effect of water facilitates exercise

V. Ultraviolet (UV) Therapy

A. General

1. Produced by the sun and sunlamps
2. Capable of killing bacteria
3. Activates the formation of vitamin D in skin
4. Used to treat acne, psoriasis, wound applications, and pressure sores
5. Cover eyes when using UV therapy

B. Types of UV Therapy

1. Exposure to natural sunlight
2. Exposure to UVB rays for prescribed amounts of time in a light box

VI. Exercise Therapy

A. General

1. Use of body motion to help the patient regain function
2. Dose must be constantly adjusted for the patient to benefit

B. Types

1. Active: patient performs the exercise
2. Passive: exercises are performed on the patient by someone else
3. Aided: active exercise helped by a physical aid (e.g., a pool)
4. Active resistance: counterpressure is applied
5. Range of motion: active or passive joint mobility

VII. Massage

A. General

1. Manipulation of external body tissues to promote healing
2. Patient must be relaxed to receive benefit
3. Lubricating oil or cream should be used

B. Approaches

1. Stroking: systematic movement of the hand across the patient's skin
2. Compression: squeezing, kneading, or pressing the patient's soft tissues
3. Percussion: thumping or striking the patient's skin with the hand
4. Effleurage: stroking movement
5. Friction: deep stroking or rubbing that involves the deeper tissues
6. Pétrissage: kneading or rolling type of motion
7. Tapotement: rapidly repeated light percussion or tapping

VIII. Devices to Assist Patient Mobility

A. Crutches

1. Wood or aluminum devices that serve as aids for walking
2. Patient's weight is transferred from the legs to the arms
3. Types
   a. Axillary crutches
      1) Crutch that extends from the patient's axillary region to the ground
      2) Used for temporary assistance
      3) Measured to fit for each individual patient
   b. Lofstrand crutches
      1) Cuff and handgrip that extend from the patient's forearm to the ground
      2) Used by patients who require permanent walking assistance
4. Crutch gaits (Fig. 20.2)
   a. Four-point gait
      1) Patient must be able to bear his or her own weight on both legs
      2) Used for muscle weakness
      3) Right crutch moves forward, left foot moves to the level of the left crutch; left crutch moves forward, and right foot moves to the level of the right crutch
   b. Three-point gait
      1) Used when the patient cannot bear his or her own weight on one leg
      2) Move both crutches and weak leg forward, then move the strong leg forward while balancing on both crutches
   c. Two-point gait
      1) Similar to four-point gait
      2) Move right crutch and left foot forward simultaneously, then move left crutch and right foot forward simultaneously

   d. Swing gait
      1) Used by patients with lower extremity paralysis
      2) Patient moves both crutches forward simultaneously, then swings both legs through

B. Canes

1. Wood or aluminum pole with a handle or handgrip
2. Provides a balance point or support or both to a patient with leg weakness on one side
3. Used on the side of the strong leg
4. Measured so that the handle is level with the greater trochanter; the elbow should be flexed at 25–30 degrees
5. Types
   a. Standard cane: least amount of support; used by patients who require slight assistance
   b. Tripod cane: three legs and a bent shaft; provides greater stability because of wider support base
   c. Quad cane: four legs and a bent shaft; provides the same support as a tripod
6. Gait
   a. Cane is held on the strong side; move the cane forward 12 inches, move the weak leg to the level of the cane, and move the strong leg ahead of the weak leg and the cane
   b. Patient needs to stand erect and not lean on the cane to ensure good balance and support

C. Walkers

1. Aluminum frame consisting of handgrips for both of the patient's hands and four squarely placed legs
2. Provides optimal balance for patients with balance problems
3. Gait: pick up the walker and move it forward 6 inches, move the right foot and then the left foot forward into the walker, and then move the walker again

D. Wheelchairs

1. Lock the wheels so the chair cannot move
2. Fold back the foot rests
3. Patient should back into the chair using the arm rests
4. To leave the chair, lock the chair
5. Patient should place unaffected foot or feet flat on floor and lift his or her body, supporting himself or herself on the arm rests

E. Casts

1. Stiff cylindrical synthetic or plaster casing
2. Used to immobilize a body part
   a. Broken bones
   b. Support and stabilize weak or dislocated joints
   c. Promote healing after surgical correction
   d. Aid nonsurgical correction of deformities
3. Plaster casts
   a. Bandage roll must be soaked in water; becomes pliable to mold to the body
4. Synthetic casts
   a. Made of fiberglass, polyester, and cotton or plastic

Stand with both feet together.

Move one leg together with one crutch on opposite side.

Move other leg with opposing crutch.

A

Move right crutch.

Move left foot.

Move left crutch.

Move right foot.

B

Affected leg

Stand with both feet together.

Move both crutches together with affected leg.

Move unaffected leg.

C

Stand with both feet together.

Move both crutches.

Move both legs by swinging them forward.

D

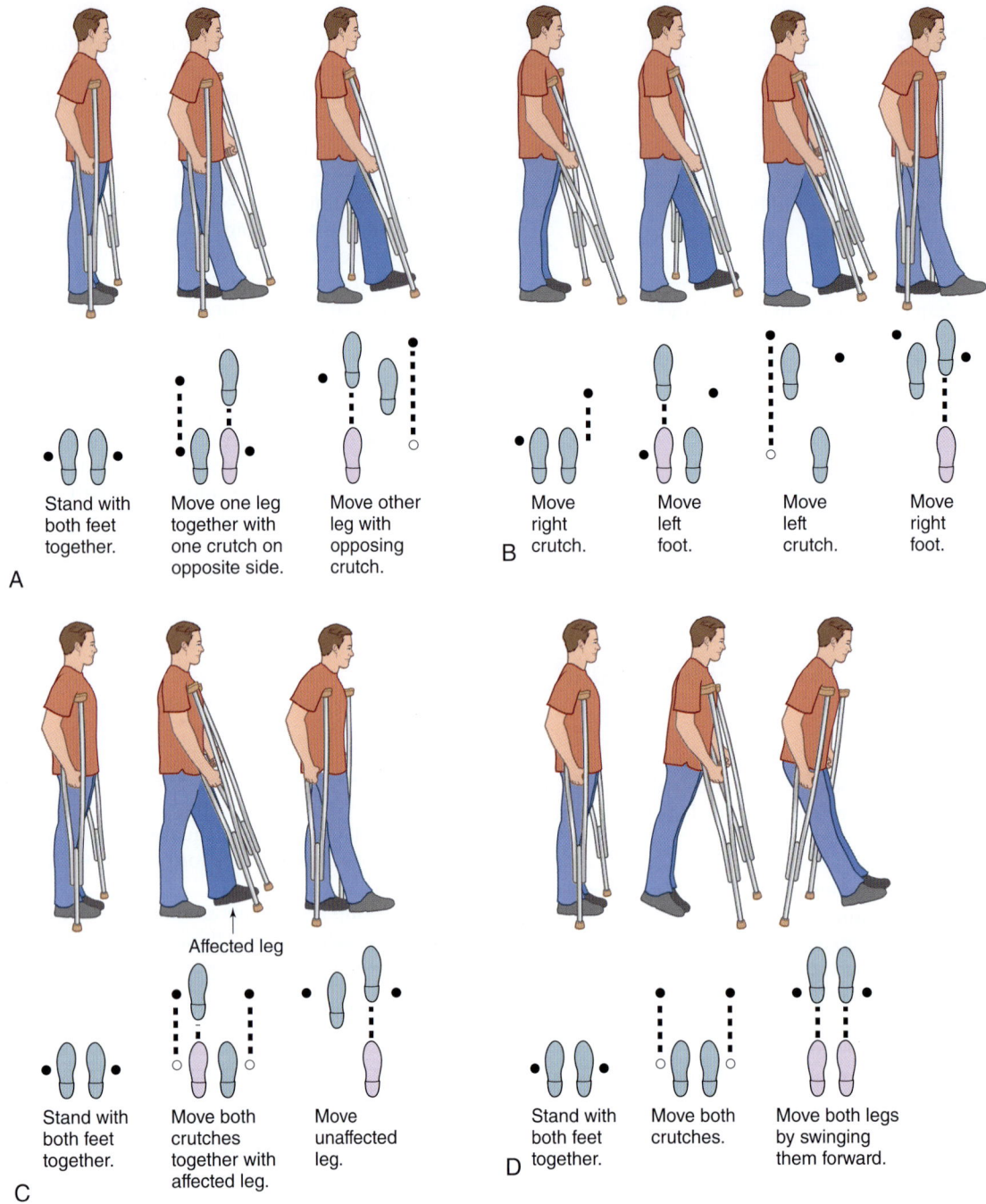

Fig. 20.2 Crutch gaits. (A) Two-point gait. (B) Four-point gait. (C) Three-point gait. (D) Swing-through gait. (From Niedzwiecki B, et al: *Kinn's The medical assistant*, ed 14, 2020, Elsevier.)

F. Splints and Braces

1. Used to assist in the treatment of fractures
2. Splint: rigid removable device used to support and immobilize; can be used for sprains and strains; molded to fit the body part

3. Brace: designed to support the body part in its correct position for functioning while healing takes place

21

Radiography and Diagnostic Imaging

Depending on the location, a medical assistant may or may not be legally permitted to perform x-ray procedures.

I. Introduction to Radiography

A. General

1. High-energy, invisible, electromagnetic waves
2. Able to penetrate body structures
3. Discovered by Wilhelm Konrad Roentgen in 1895
4. X-ray images called radiographs
5. Some states may require a limited radiography license to take films
6. Radiology: branch of medicine that deals with radiant energy in the diagnosis and treatment of disease
7. Radiologist: physician who specializes in the diagnosis and treatment of disease with various forms of radiant energy
8. Radiograph: permanent record of the picture produced on the radiographic film
9. Radiography: taking of permanent records (radiographs) of internal body structures and organs by passing x-rays through them to act on a specially sensitized film

B. Functions

1. Reveals presence of fractures or abnormalities of bones
2. Reveals size and shape of organs
3. Reveals presence and position of foreign bodies
4. Destroys pathologic cells

II. Equipment

A. Table

1. Supports the patient's body
2. Contains grids and Bucky mechanism for film placement

B. X-ray Tube

1. Glass vacuum tube that produces, focuses, and transmits x-rays

C. Collimator

1. Apparatus below tube that permits the radiographer to vary the size of radiation field

D. Control Panel

1. Allows control of x-ray emissions
2. Regulates the machine
3. Should be located behind lead-lined wall so that the operator is protected from x-rays
   a. Main switch: turns machine on and off
   b. Milliamperes (mA) setting: sets the amount of radiation that comes from the tube
   c. Time switch: number of seconds the patient is exposed to x-rays
   d. Kilovolt peak (kVp) setting: penetrating power of x-ray beam
   e. Bucky switch: turns on the Bucky mechanism
   f. Exposure switch: exposes the patient to x-rays

E. Grid

1. Absorbs scattered radiation
2. Prevents blurring of the film
3. Placed between the patient and the film to reduce secondary wave interference

F. Potter-Bucky Diaphragm (Bucky)

1. Framelike structure under the table
2. Holds the grid above the film
3. Used when thicker body parts are exposed to x-rays

G. Cassette

1. Device that holds the film

H. Intensifying Screen

1. Special plates located within the cassette
2. Reduces the amount of exposure required, which reduces the time the patient is exposed to radiation

I. X-ray Film

1. Coated with special material that is sensitive to x-rays
2. Creates a visible record for viewing and archives
3. Film that receives x-ray appears black and gray; film that does not receive x-ray appears white; the more dense the object, the lighter the image is on the film
4. Use only under safety light in a darkroom to avoid exposure
5. Common sizes are 5×7 inches, 8×10 inches, 10×12 inches, 11×14 inches, and 14×17 inches

J. View Box

1. Lighted box for viewing developed x-ray film

K. Caliper

1. Measures the thickness of body parts
2. Used to calculate the amount of x-ray exposure

III. Digital and Computed Radiography

A. Digital Radiography

1. Filmless imaging system; no cassettes or processing involved
2. Images stored in computer system; can be accessed on screen anywhere
3. Conventional radiographs can be scanned and added to the system
4. Images can be printed

B. Computed Radiography

1. Filmless imaging system; special image receptor exposed to conventional x-ray equipment
2. Image displayed on monitor
3. Hard copies can be printed
4. Images stored in computer system

IV. Safety

A. Hazards

1. Radiation has a cumulative effect on the body
2. Exposure damages body cells, especially gametes and the developing fetus

3. Eye exposure can cause cataracts
4. Exposure over a long period may cause cancer, sterility, or genetic defects
5. High exposure over a short period may cause radiation sickness (nausea, vomiting, diarrhea, hair loss)

B. Precautions

1. Keep appropriate equipment in good condition
2. Prevent exposure to gonads by using lead shields or lead aprons on patients and operators
3. Always ask women of childbearing age whether any chance exists that they are pregnant; if so, the physician must approve the x-ray procedure
4. Wear a dosimeter (x-ray badge containing reactive material that is sensitive to radiation); must be checked periodically to measure the technician's exposure level
5. Wear lead shield or lead apron

V. Patient Positioning (Figs. 21.1–21.4)

A. Body Positioning

1. Body part nearest the film gives the greatest detail
2. Anteroposterior (AP): x-ray beam enters the anterior of the body surface and exits the posterior of the body surface before it hits the film
3. Posteroanterior (PA): x-ray beam enters the posterior of the body surface and exits the anterior of the body surface before it hits the film
4. Lateral: x-ray beam passes from one side to the other side before hitting the film; this x-ray order may be right lateral (from the right to the left side) or left lateral (from the left to the right side)
5. Oblique: x-ray beam passes through the body part at an angle

VI. Darkroom

A. General

1. Location where film is handled and developed
2. Lit by a safety light

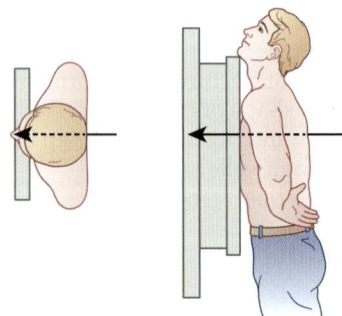

Fig. 21.1 Posteroanterior (PA) projections.

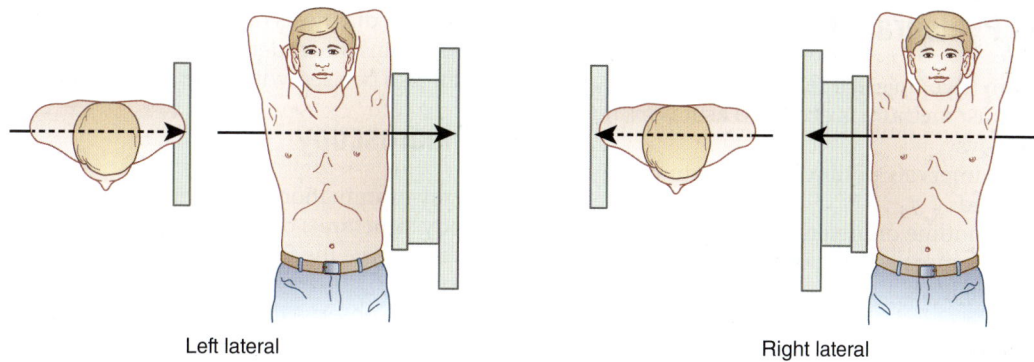

Left lateral   Right lateral

Fig. 21.2 Lateral projections.

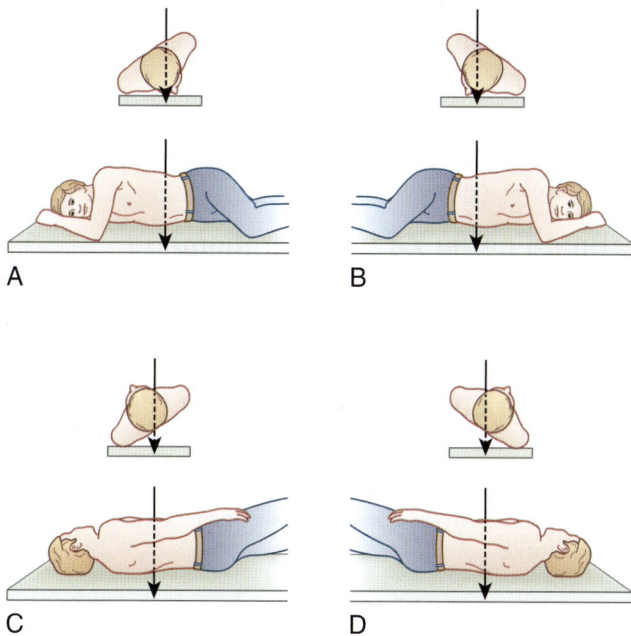

Fig. 21.3 Oblique projections. (A) Right anterior oblique (RAO); (B) left anterior oblique (LAO); (C) left posterior oblique (LPO); (D) right posterior oblique (RPO).

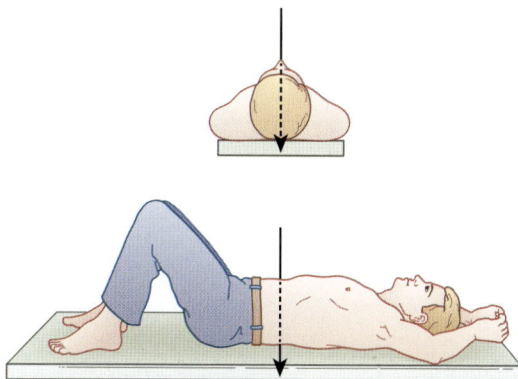

Fig. 21.4 Anteroposterior (AP) projections.

3. Developer may be manual or automatic
4. Film is handled by the edges only
5. After film is dried, put in storage envelope or file
6. Undeveloped film is kept in a lead-lined vault

VII. Special Radiographic Studies

A. Angiogram

1. Contrast medium injected intravenously
2. Can determine cardiovascular disease

B. Arteriogram

1. Similar to angiogram but specifically studies the arteries

C. Barium Enema (Lower Gastrointestinal [GI] Series)

1. Contrast medium is instilled by enema into the colon
2. Used to visualize lower intestines

D. Barium Meal (Upper GI Series)

1. Orally administered contrast medium
2. Used to visualize esophagus, stomach, and duodenum

E. Bronchogram

1. Contrast medium administered through trachea and into bronchial tree
2. Detects cancer and other lung disorders

F. Cholecystogram

1. Tablet form of contrast medium ingested the night before the procedure
2. Gallbladder is observed on film

G. Hysterosalpingogram

1. Contrast medium injected into the fallopian tubes
2. Detects patency of the tubes

H. Kidney, Ureter, Bladder (KUB)

1. Basic flat x-ray of abdominal area
2. Shows size, shape, location, and malformation of kidneys and bladder
3. Used to visualize calculi (stones)

I. Intravenous Pyelogram (IVP)

1. Contrast medium (dye) injected intravenously
2. Pathway of contrast medium is observed as it is excreted through the kidneys
3. Films obtained at intervals until contrast medium is completely excreted
4. Used to visualize outline of ureters and bladder
5. Used to diagnose tumors, calculi, obstructions, and congenital abnormalities

J. Mammogram

1. X-ray of the breast
2. Detects abnormalities, masses, and breast cancer

VIII. Diagnostic Imaging Modalities

A. Computed Tomography (CT)

1. Radiographic technique that produces a picture that represents a detailed cross section of tissue structures
2. More sensitive than other x-rays
3. Wide range of applications, including scans of the brain, spine, abdomen, chest, neck, pelvis, and sinuses
4. Can also be used with contrast media

B. Magnetic Resonance Imaging (MRI)

1. Combines radio waves and magnetic field to produce images of soft tissues
2. Noninvasive
3. Images can be managed in a computer database

4. Used for diagnosis of intracranial or spinal lesions, aneurysms, heart defects, and soft tissue abnormalities
5. Can also be used with contrast medium

C. Fluoroscopy

1. X-ray examination that permits visualization of internal body structures; contrast medium is used
2. Can observe the flow of contrast medium through a body structure
3. Can also observe the motion of a body part

D. Sonography

1. Diagnostic ultrasound
2. Not a radiologic procedure
3. Permits visualization of internal structures by the use of high-frequency sound waves
4. Sound waves echo off the body part and are displayed on a screen
5. Useful for observation of obstetric and soft tissue (brain, eye, breast, reproductive organs)

E. Dual-Energy X-ray Absorptiometry (DEXA) Scan

1. Measures bone density

F. Positron Emission Tomography (PET) Scan

1. Use of radionuclides to reconstruct brain sections and look for diseases in various body systems
2. Can be used to assist in diagnosis of Alzheimer disease and stroke

22

Pharmacology, Medication Administration, and Intravenous Therapy

I. Definition

A. Pharmacology

1. Science that deals with the study of drugs and their actions, uses, properties, and origins

II. Drugs

A. General

1. Any substances that cause a change in body functions or structure

B. Uses

1. Therapeutic: relieves symptoms
2. Prophylactic: helps to lessen or prevent the effects of disease
3. Diagnostic: helps diagnose diseases and disorders
4. Replacement: replaces missing chemicals in the body
5. Preventive: prevents/lessens severity of the disease
6. Palliative: reduces symptoms but does not cure the condition
7. Curative: removes the cause of the disease
8. Maintenance: maintains a condition of health that has been put at risk by a disease process
9. Supportive: maintains the body in homeostasis until the disease can be resolved

C. Sources

1. Plant
   a. Naturally occurring substance from plants
   b. Parts used include roots, stems, leaves, and fruits

2. Animal
   a. Substances obtained from animals
   b. Includes glands, organs, and tissues
3. Mineral: naturally occurring substances obtained from the earth or soil
4. Synthetic
   a. Artificially prepared substances
   b. Prepared using chemicals and techniques in a laboratory

D. Names

1. Chemical name: drug's chemical formula that identifies its molecular structure
2. Generic name
   a. Official name of the drug
   b. Not capitalized
3. Trade name
   a. Brand name
   b. Name owned by the manufacturer and copyrighted (uses registered trademark [])
   c. Always capitalized
4. Official name
   a. Name listed in official publications
   b. Generic name frequently used in place of official name

E. Drug References

1. *Physicians' Desk Reference* (PDR)
   a. Common reference book
   b. Provides information on uses, precautions, indications, and doses for various drugs
   c. Organized in color-coded sections
      1) Section 1 (white)
         a) Manufacturer's Index
         b) Lists manufacturers who have given product information for use in the book

2) Section 2 (pink)
  a) Product Name Index
  b) Lists trade and generic names alphabetically
3) Section 3 (blue)
  a) Product Category Index
  b) Drugs are listed according to their classification
4) Section 4 (yellow)
  a) Generic and Chemical Name Index
  b) Lists drugs alphabetically according to the main ingredient
5) Section 5 (noncolored pages)
  a) Product Identification
  b) Color photographs of the drugs
6) Section 6 (white)
  a) Product Information
  b) Detailed descriptions of drugs
2. Product insert
  a. Folded sheet of paper within the drug container or box
  b. Contains information similar to information on the drug contained in the PDR
3. *United States Pharmacopoeia/National Formulary (USP/NF)*
  a. Published every 5 years
  b. All drugs listed have met federal governmental standards
4. *Physicians' Desk Reference for Nonprescription Drugs and Dietary Supplements*: similar to PDR but for over-the-counter (OTC) medications

F. Forms of Drugs

1. Liquid preparations
  a. Aerosol: drug is suspended in a liquid and administered in a spray or aerosol form
  b. Elixir: drug is dissolved in a mixture of water, alcohol, and sugar
  c. Emulsion: mixture of water and oil; must be shaken to mix before administration
  d. Liniment
    1) Drug is mixed with soap, alcohol, oil, or water
    2) Applied topically to produce a feeling of heat and warmth
  e. Lotion
    1) Topical preparation that is nongreasy
    2) Contains suspended particles of the drug mixed in an aqueous solution
  f. Solution: liquid preparation containing one or more solutes dissolved in a solvent
  g. Suspension: drug that does not dissolve evenly in a liquid; must be shaken to mix before administration
  h. Spirit: drug combined with alcohol solution
  i. Spray: fine stream of medication usually used to treat nasal and throat conditions
  j. Syrup: drug is dissolved in water, mixed with sugar and flavoring
  k. Tincture: drug is dissolved in alcohol
2. Solid preparations
  a. Caplet: capsule-shaped tablet
  b. Capsule: powdered or liquid drug within a gelatin capsule
  c. Chewable Tab: powdered drug pressed into dish and flavored
  d. Cream: semisolid preparation that is absorbed into the tissue in a slow, sustained release.

e. Lozenge (troche): medicine is mixed within a candylike base made to be dissolved within the mouth
f. Ointment
  1) Semisolid preparation
  2) Drug is combined with oil or fat; topically applied
g. Patch: transdermal administration of a medication
h. Sublingual Tab: powdered drug pressed into disk and designed to dissolve under the tongue
i. Suppository
  1) Drug is mixed with a base of fat or wax
  2) Shaped into a cone or cylinder
  3) Made to be inserted into the rectum, vagina, or urethra
  4) Suppository dissolves at body temperature
j. Tablet
  1) Powdered medication is compressed into a disk shape
  2) May be scored for breaking into halves or quarters
  3) May be enteric-coated for dissolution in intestines instead of stomach
k. Time-release tablets, capsules, and patches: medication dissolves or is administered over a time period

G. Transactions

1. Prescribe: an order for a medication by a licensed practitioner
2. Administer: to give a medication that has been prescribed
3. Dispense: to prepare and give out to a patient
4. All practitioners who prescribe, administer, or dispense controlled substances must register and renew with the Drug Enforcement Administration (DEA)
  a. Practitioner receives a DEA registration number that is valid for 3 years
  b. All controlled substances must be stored separately from other medications within the office; must be kept locked
  c. Separate records must be kept of all controlled substances
  d. Controlled substance inventory must be counted and recorded daily, as well as verified by two individuals for count accuracy
  e. Discarded liquid controlled substances must be poured down the sink drain
  f. Discarded solid controlled substances must be crushed and flushed down the toilet

H. Drug Regulations and Controls

1. Controlled Substances Act of 1970
  a. Federal legislation designed to control dispensing of drugs that have a high potential for abuse
  b. Five schedules, based on medical usefulness and potential for abuse
    1) Schedule I
      a) Drugs with a high potential for abuse and no acceptable medical use
      b) Examples: heroin and lysergic acid diethylamide (LSD)
    2) Schedule II
      a) Drugs with some accepted medical use but high potential for abuse
      b) Examples: morphine and cocaine

3) Schedule III
   a) Drugs with moderate abuse potential; require prescription, which is limited to five refills within 6 months
   b) Example: Tylenol with codeine
4) Schedule IV
   a) Drugs with low abuse potential; prescription is limited to five refills within 6 months
   b) Example: Valium, Darvon, and Librium
5) Schedule V
   a) Low abuse potential; may include drug mixtures with a limited amount of narcotics
   b) Examples: cough medicines with codeine, Lomotil
2. Federal Food, Drug, and Cosmetic Act: allows the US Food and Drug Administration (FDA) to protect the public by requiring rigid standards for drug development
3. DEA: responsible for controlling narcotics abuse and illegal sales of drugs

I. Pharmacokinetics

1. Study of how drugs are used within the body
2. Process includes
   a. Absorption
      1) How a drug enters the body
      2) Depends on how drug is administered
   b. Distribution: how a drug is transported from the site of administration to the site or sites of action
   c. Action: changes that the drug causes when it reaches the site or sites of action
   d. Biotransformation
      1) How the drug is inactivated
      2) Usually occurs within the liver
   e. Elimination: route by which the drug is eliminated from the body

III. Prescriptions

A. General

1. An order written by the practitioner for the compounding, dispensing, and administration of a particular drug for a particular patient
2. A prescription is a legal document
3. Using common or accepted abbreviations is acceptable when writing a prescription; check with the agency for approved abbreviations
4. Electronic health records can be used to create, print paper copies, and/or send the prescription to the pharmacy

B. Parts of a Prescription (Fig. 22.1)

1. Preprinted physician's name, address, telephone number, and DEA number
2. Date the prescription was written
   a. Prescriptions must be filled within 12 months of writing or may be refilled for 12 months after initial filling
3. Patient's name, address, telephone number, and age (if a child)
4. Superscription: symbol Rx means "take thou" or "recipe"
5. Inscription: name, form, quantity, and strength of drug prescribed
   a. Active ingredient shown in milligrams in each dosage form
6. Subscription
   a. Practitioner's instructions to the pharmacist
   b. Includes the number of doses prescribed and special preparations

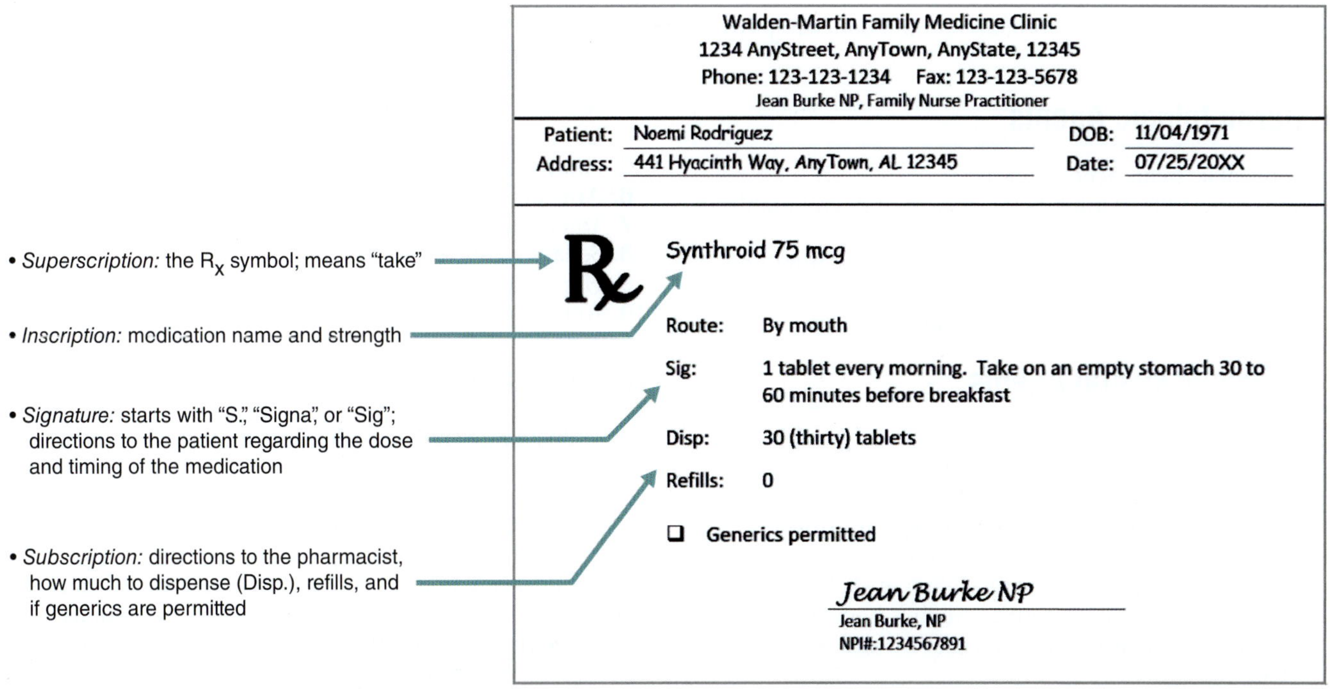

- *Superscription:* the R$_x$ symbol; means "take"
- *Inscription:* medication name and strength
- *Signature:* starts with "S.", "Signa", or "Sig"; directions to the patient regarding the dose and timing of the medication
- *Subscription:* directions to the pharmacist, how much to dispense (Disp.), refills, and if generics are permitted

Walden-Martin Family Medicine Clinic
1234 AnyStreet, AnyTown, AnyState, 12345
Phone: 123-123-1234   Fax: 123-123-5678
Jean Burke NP, Family Nurse Practitioner

Patient: Noemi Rodriguez   DOB: 11/04/1971
Address: 441 Hyacinth Way, AnyTown, AL 12345   Date: 07/25/20XX

Rx   Synthroid 75 mcg

Route: By mouth
Sig: 1 tablet every morning. Take on an empty stomach 30 to 60 minutes before breakfast
Disp: 30 (thirty) tablets
Refills: 0

☐ Generics permitted

Jean Burke NP
Jean Burke, NP
NPI#:1234567891

Fig. 22.1. Example of a prescription. (From Niedzwiecki B, et al: *Kinn's the medical assistant: an applied learning approach*, ed 14, 2020, Elsevier.)

7. Signature
   a. Sig (label)
   b. Patient instructions for taking the drug
8. Refill information: number of refills allowed for the prescription, if any
   a. Enter "0" or "none" if there are no refills allowed; do not leave blank
9. Practitioner's handwritten signature

C. Prescription Pads

1. Keep locked up except when being used
2. Never presign blank prescription forms
3. Never use blank prescription forms for scratch paper
4. Never leave blank pads in examination rooms

D. Electronic Prescribing

1. Electronic health record software includes program for electronic prescribing
2. The program can transmit electronically to pharmacy and also print out prescription
3. Provider enters medication information; program checks for patient's allergies as well as interactions with other drugs prescribed to patient; the medication is then recorded into the patient's electronic medical record

IV. Drug Classifications Based on Action

A. Antiinfectives

1. Antibiotic: destroys or inhibits the growth of microorganisms
2. Antifungal: kills or prevents the growth of fungi and yeast
3. Antiviral: prevents or treats viral infections
4. Antiparasitic: prevents or treats parasitic infections
5. Antiretroviral: manages human immunodeficiency virus (HIV) infections

B. Dermatologic Agents

1. Antiacneic: treats acne vulgaris
2. Antiseptic: kills or inhibits the growth of microorganisms
3. Antipruritic: relieves itching
4. Anesthetic: causes loss of sensation and local numbing
5. Emollient: soothes skin and mucous membranes
6. Keratolytic: causes sloughing of hardened skin

C. Musculoskeletal Agents

1. Antiarthritic: treats arthritis
2. Antigout: treats gout (gouty arthritis)
3. Antiinflammatory: decreases inflammation
4. Antispasmodic: relieves or prevents spasms from musculoskeletal injury or inflammation
5. Muscle relaxant: aids in the relaxation of skeletal muscles
6. Bone replacement therapeutics: inhibits bone reabsorption or promotes the use of calcium; prevent and treat osteoporosis
7. Osteoporosis agent: promotes bone mineral density

D. Cardiovascular and Hematologic Agents

1. Adrenergic blocking agent: controls hypertension
2. Angiotensin-converting enzyme (ACE) inhibitor: decreases blood pressure
3. Antianginal: reduces chest pain
4. Antiarrhythmic: regulates heart rhythm and rate
5. Anticoagulant: prevents or delays blood clotting
6. Antihyperlipidemic: decreases blood cholesterol levels
7. Antihypertensive: decreases blood pressure
8. Beta blocker: decreases blood pressure
9. Calcium channel blocker: decreases blood pressure
10. Cardiotonic: increases heart muscle strength
11. Hematinic: increases blood iron levels
12. Hemostatic: controls or stops bleeding
13. Hematopoietic: promotes red blood cell production
14. Thrombolytic: dissolves blood clots
15. Vasoconstrictor: constricts blood vessels, increases blood pressure
16. Vasodilator: dilates blood vessels, decreases blood pressure
17. Antiplatelet: prevents the function of platelets (formation of clots)

E. Endocrine Agents

1. Hypoglycemic: decreases blood glucose levels
2. Antihyperglycemic: reduces blood glucose levels
3. Thyroid: replaces thyroid hormones
4. Hormone replacement therapy (HRT): replaces hormones or compensates for deficiencies

F. Nervous System Agents

1. Anesthetic: produces insensibility to pain; can be local or general
2. Central nervous system (CNS) stimulant: increases brain and body activity
3. CNS depressant: decreases brain and body activity
4. Analgesic: relieves pain
   a. Narcotic agents: highly addictive
   b. Nonnarcotic agents
5. Antipyretic: reduces fever
6. Anticonvulsant: controls seizure activity
7. Tranquilizer: reduces anxiety; calms the patient
8. Sedative: produces relaxation
9. Hypnotic: induces sleep
10. Antiparkinsonian: treats Parkinson disease

G. Respiratory Agents

1. Antihistamine: relieves allergic symptoms; reduces secretions
2. Antitubercular: treats tuberculosis
3. Antitussive: suppresses cough
4. Bronchodilator: opens air passages (bronchi)
5. Decongestant: relieves congestion in respiratory tract
6. Expectorant: liquefies mucus; helps expel secretions
7. Mucolytic: breaks up thick mucus in respiratory tract
8. Smoking cessation aids: reduce nicotine levels while assisting with smoking cessation

H. Gastrointestinal (GI) Agents

1. Antacid: neutralizes stomach acid
2. Antiemetic: prevents nausea and vomiting
3. Antidiarrheal: controls or stops diarrhea
4. Cathartic, laxative: relieves constipation
5. Emetic: induces vomiting
6. Antispasmodic: prevents, controls spasms of the GI tract
7. Antiulcer: treats gastric or duodenal ulcers
8. Antiflatulant: relieves discomfort of gas
9. Anorexiant: reduces appetite for weight loss
10. Anticholinergic: reduces smooth muscle spasms
11. Proton-pump inhibitor: decreases stomach acid

I. Urinary Agents

1. Alpha-adrenergic inhibitor: relaxes smooth muscles in prostate
2. Diuretic: promotes or increases urination

J. Cancer Agents

1. Antineoplastic: inhibits growth of malignant cells
2. Antimetabolites: disrupts essential cell metabolic processes

K. Reproductive Agents

1. Abortifacient: terminates a pregnancy
2. Antiimpotence: alleviates erectile dysfunction
3. Contraceptive: inhibits conception
4. Emergency contraceptive: prevents pregnancy after unprotected intercourse
5. Ovulation stimulant: triggers ovulation
6. Spermicide: kills sperm

L. Eye and Ear Agents

1. Mydriatic: dilates the pupil
2. Miotic: constricts the pupil
3. Cerumenolytics: softens and emulsifies earwax

M. Mental Disorders and Substance Abuse Agents

1. Antianxiety: reduces anxiety and tension
2. Antidepressant: treats depression
3. Antimanic: treats manic/bipolar disorders
4. Antipsychotic: relieves symptoms of psychosis and severe neurosis
5. Alcohol cessation aid: treats alcoholism
6. Anti-Alzheimer: treats dementia, Alzheimer disease

N. Pain Relief/Inflammation

1. Analgesic: relieves pain
2. Corticosteroid: reduces inflammation

O. Common Drug Suffixes

(Table 22.1)

V. Herbal Therapies

A. General

1. Considered to be part of complementary and alternative medicine (CAM)
2. Limited studies on effectiveness but use is increasing
3. Medical assistant needs to ask about use when taking history

B. Herbal Products

1. Use of plant products as a medicine
2. Regulated by Dietary Supplement Health and Education Act (DSHEA) of the FDA
3. Can interact with conventional drugs

C. Commonly Used Herbal Products

1. Acai: weight loss; antiaging
2. Aloe vera
   a. Gel: burns; frostbite; cold sores; psoriasis
   b. Oral: fever; arthritis
3. Black cohosh: relieves symptoms of menopause; premenstrual syndrome; induction of labor
4. Cinnamon: lowers blood glucose levels
5. Echinacea: prevents colds, flu; stimulates immune system
6. Elderberry: stimulates immune system
7. Flaxseed: laxative; high cholesterol levels
8. Garlic: high cholesterol levels; hypertension
9. Ginger: stomach aches; nausea; diarrhea
10. Asian ginseng: boosts immune system; improves mental and physical performance; erectile dysfunction; lowers blood glucose; controls blood pressure
11. Gingko biloba: improves memory; prevents Alzheimer disease; tinnitus
12. Glucosamine: arthritis; joint pain
13. Green tea: improves mental alertness; relieves digestive symptoms; headaches; promotes weight loss; protective effects against heart disease and cancer
14. Melatonin: sleep disorders
15. Milk thistle: lowers cholesterol; reduces insulin resistance; liver health
16. Peppermint: relieves nausea
17. Saw palmetto: bladder disorders; urinary symptoms associated with enlarged prostate gland
18. St. John's wort: depression; anxiety; sleep disorders

VI. OTC Medications

A. General

1. Drugs that can be purchased without a prescription
2. Used for a wide variety of complaints
3. OTC classification determined by FDA
4. Standardized labeling that is easy to understand for consumers
5. OTC meds should also be charted
6. Can be abused

TABLE 22.1 Common Drug Suffixes

Suffix	Class	Clinical Use	Example
-afil	Phosphodiesterase inhibitors	Erectile dysfunction	Sildenafil
-ane	Inhaled anesthetics	Anesthesia	Halothane
-artan	Angiotensin receptor blockers	Hypertension	Losartan
-azepam; -zolam	Benzodiazepines	Anxiety	Lorazepam, Midazolam
-azine	Phenothiazines	Antipsychotic	Chlorpromazine
-azole	Azole antifungals	Antifungal	Ketoconazole
-barbital	Barbiturates	Anxiety	Phenobarbital
-caine	Local anesthetics	Anesthesia	Lidocaine
-cillin	Penicillin antibiotics	Antibiotic	Ticarcillin
-cycline	Tetracyclines	Antibiotic	Doxycycline
-etine	Selective serotonin reuptake	Depression	Fluoxetine
-feb, -fene	Selective estrogen response	Osteoporosis, breast cancer	Tamoxifen, Clomifene
-fine	Allylamine antifungals	Antifungal	Terbinafine
-floxacin	Fluoroquinolones	Antibiotics	Levofloxacin
-ide	Loop diuretics	Hypertension	Furosemide
-ipine	Calcium channel blockers	Hypertension	Nifedipine
-ipramine	Tricyclic antidepressants	Depression	Desipramine
-lukast	LTD4 receptor antagonist	Asthma	Montelukast
-navir	Protease inhibitor	Antiviral	Saquinavir
-olol	Beta blocker	Hypertension	Propranolol
-oxin	Cardiac glycoside	Arrhythmias	Digoxin
-phylline	Methylxanthine	Bronchodilator	Theophylline
-pril	ACE inhibitor	Hypertension	Lisinopril
-quine	Quinoline derivatives	Antimalarial	Chloroquine
-statin	HMG-CoA reductase inhibitors	Hyperlipidemia	Simvastatin
-terol	B2 agonist	Bronchodilator	Albuterol
-tidine	Second-generation antihistamine	Allergies	Cimetidine
-tropin	Pituitary hormone	Hormone deficiency	Somatotropin
-vaptan	Vasopressin receptor antagonist	Hypertension	Tolvaptan
-zosin	A1 antagonist	Hypertension, BPH	Terazosin

B. Commonly Used OTC Meds

(Table 22.2)

VII. 100 Most Prescribed Drugs of 2022 (Alphabetical) *ClinCalc DrugStats

(Table 22.3)

VIII. Calculation of Doses

A. Metric System

1. Basic units of measure
   a. Gram (g): used to measure solids
   b. Liter (L): used to measure liquids (volume)
   c. Meter (m): used to measure length
2. Metric conversion
   a. Length
      1) 1 m = 100 cm = 1000 mm
      2) 10 mm = 1 cm
   b. Weight
      1) 1 g = 1000 mg
      2) 1 mg = 1000 µg
      3) 1 kg = 1000 g
   c. Volume for solids
      1) 1000 mm^3 = 1 cc
      2) 1000 cc = 1 dm^3
      3) 1000 dm^3 = 1 m^3
   d. Volume for fluids
      1) 1 L = 1000 mL
      2) 1 mL = 1 cc
      3) 10 cm = 1 dL
      4) 10 dL = 1 L

TABLE 22.2   Commonly Used Over-the-Counter Medications

Brand Name	Generic/Ingredients	Indication
Abreva	Docosanol	Cold sore treatment
Advil	Ibuprofen	Analgesic (NSAID); fever reduction; antiinflammatory
Advil Cold & Sinus	Ibuprofen and pseudoephedrine HCl	Allergy and cold relief
Afrin	Oxymetazoline HCl	Nasal decongestant
Aleve	Naproxen sodium	Analgesic (NSAID)
Alli	Orlistat	Weight management
Anbesol	Benzocaine and phenol	Oral cavity analgesic
Azo Standard	Phenazopyridine HCl	Urinary analgesic
Aspirin	ASA	Analgesic (NSAID); fever reduction; antiinflammatory; anticoagulant
Benadryl	Diphenhydramine HCl	Allergy; cold relief; antipruritic
Benadryl Topical	Diphenhydramine and zinc acetate	Topical antipruritic
Bengay	Methyl salicylate and menthol	Topical analgesic
Bonine	Meclizine HCl and cyclizine HCl	Motion sickness
Bufferin	Aspirin with buffers	Analgesic (NSAID)
Capzasin	Capsaicin in emollient base	Topical analgesic
Cepacol	Benzocaine and menthol	Oral cavity analgesic in lozenge form
Citracal	Calcium citrate and vitamin D	Mineral replacement
Claritin	Loratadine DMD	Allergy and cold relief
Claritin-D	Loratadine DMD and pseudoephedrine sulfate	Allergy and cold relief
Colace	Docusate sodium	Stool softener
Compound W	Salicylic acid	Topical keratolytic
Cortaid	Hydrocortisone	Topical antipruritic
DayQuil	Acetaminophen, dextromethorphan HBr, and phenylephrine HCl	Cold relief
Delsym	Dextromethorphan polistirex	Cough suppression
Dimetapp	Brompheniramine maleate, phenylephrine HCl, and dextromethorphan HCl	Allergy and cold relief
Dramamine	Dimenhydrinate	Motion sickness
Dulcolax	Bisacodyl	Laxative
Emetrol	Phosphorated carbohydrates	Antiemetic
Estroven	Soy and black cohosh	Menopause support
Excedrin	Acetaminophen, aspirin, and caffeine	Analgesic
Imodium A-D	Loperamide HCl	Antidiarrheal
Lactaid	Lactase (enzyme)	Digestive aid
Lamisil	Terbinafine HCl	Topical antifungal
Lotrimin	Clotrimazole	Topical antifungal
Maalox	Aluminum hydroxide, magnesium hydroxide, and simethicone	Antacid; antiulcer agent
Metamucil	Psyllium husk	Laxative
Midol	Pyrilamine maleate, acetaminophen, and caffeine	Analgesic
Milk of Magnesia	Magnesium hydroxide	Laxative; antacid
Monistat Vaginal Cream	Miconazole nitrate	Vaginal antifungal
Motrin IB	Ibuprofen	Analgesic (NSAID)
Mucinex	Guaifenesin	Expectorant; antitussive

(Continued)

TABLE 22.2   Commonly Used Over-the-Counter Medications—cont'd

Brand Name	Generic/Ingredients	Indication
Mylanta	Aluminum hydroxide, magnesium hydroxide, and simethicone	Antacid; antiulcer
Naphcon A drops	Pheniramine maleate and naphazoline HCl	Ophthalmic antiallergy
Nasalcrom nasal solution	Cromolyn sodium	Allergy and cold relief
Neosporin	Polymyxin B sulfate, neomycin, and bacitracin	Topical antiinfective
NicoDerm	Nicotine	Smoking cessation aid
Nicorette	Nicotine polacrilex	Smoking cessation aid
Nix	Permethrin	Pediculicide
NoDoz	Caffeine	Analeptic
NyQuil	Doxylamine succinate, dextromethorphan HBr, and acetaminophen	Cold and allergy relief
Os-Cal	Calcium carbonate and vitamin D	Mineral replacement
Pepcid-AC	Famotidine	Acid reduction; antiulcer
Pepcid Complete	Famotidine, calcium carbonate, and magnesium hydroxide	Acid reduction; antiulcer
Pepto Bismol	Bismuth subsalicylate	Antidiarrheal
Peri-Colace	Docusate sodium and senna	Stool softener plus laxative
Pin-X	Pyrantel pamoate	Anthelmintic
Preparation H	Petroleum, mineral oil, shark liver oil, and phenylephrine HCl	Topical analgesic; hemorrhoid agent
Prevacid	Lansoprazole	Antacid; antiulcer agent
Prilosec OTC	Omeprazole magnesium	Antacid; antiulcer
Primatene Mist	Epinephrine, ephedrine, and guaifenesin	Bronchodilator
RID (shampoo)	Pyrethrin	Pediculicide
Robitussin	Guaifenesin	Cough relief
Rogaine	Minoxidil	Hair growth stimulant
Salivart	Sodium carboxymethylcellulose, sorbitol, sodium chloride, potassium chloride, calcium chloride dehydrate, magnesium chloride, hexahydrate, potassium phosphate, and dibasic	Saliva substitute
Senokot, Senokot-S	Senna	Laxative
Similasan	Chamomilla, mercurius, solubilis, and sulfur	Earache relief
Slow-Mag	Magnesium chloride and calcium chloride	Mineral replacement
Sudafed	Pseudoephedrine	Allergy and cold relief
Tums	Calcium carbonate	Antacid; antiulcer; mineral replacement
Tylenol	Acetaminophen	Analgesic
Unisom	Doxylamine succinate	Sleep aid
Zantac	Ranitidine HCl	Antacid; antiulcer
Zicam	Zincum gluconicum and zincum aceticum	Cold relief
Zilactin	Benzyl alcohol	Topical cold sore treatment
Zyrtec, Zyrtec-D	Cetirizine HCl, +pseudoephedrine in Zyrtec-D	Allergy and cold relief

ASA, Acetylsalicylic acid; *DMD*; *HBr*, hydrobromide; *HCl*, hydrochloric acid; *NSAID*, nonsteroidal antiinflammatory drug.

e. Weight conversion
   1) 1 kg = 2.2 lb
   2) 1 lb = 16 oz
   3) 1 oz = 0.028 kg
f. Temperature conversion
   1) $°C = (°F - 32) \times (5/9 \text{ or } 0.5556)$
   2) $°F = °C \times (9/5 \text{ or } 1.8) + 32$

B. Equivalents

1. 1 cc = 1 mL = 15 drops (gtt)
2. 5 mL = 5 cc = 1 teaspoon (tsp)
3. 15 mL = 15 cc = 1 tablespoon (T or tbsp)
4. 30 mL = 30 cc = 1 ounce (oz)
5. 240 mL = 240 cc = 1 cup = 8 oz

TABLE 22.3	100 Most Prescribed Drugs of 2022		
Trade Name	**Generic Name**	**Classification**	**Indication**
Abilify	Aripiprazole	Antipsychotic	Schizophrenia; bipolar disorder
Adderall	Dextroamphetamine	CNS stimulant	ADHD
Advair	Fluticasone propionate/salmeterol	Bronchodilator	Asthma
Allegra	Fexofenadine	Antihistamine	Allergic rhinitis; hay fever
Amaryl	Glimepiride	Antidiabetic	Type 2 diabetes
Amoxil	Amoxicillin	Antiinfective	Upper respiratory infections
Anaprox	Naproxen	NSAID	Arthritis
Aricept	Donepezil	Anti-Alzheimer	Alzheimer disease
Atarax	Hydroxyzine	Antihistamine	Nausea/vomiting; allergies; skin rash; hives; itching; treat anxiety/tension
Ativan	Lorazepam	Sedative	Anxiety; insomnia; alcohol withdrawal
Buspar	Buspirone	Antianxiety	Treat anxiety
Cardizem	Diltiazem	Calcium channel blocker	Dysrhythmia
Catapres	Clonidine	Adrenergic-inhibiting agent	Hypertension
Celebrex	Celecoxib	NSAID	Pain
Celexa	Citalopram hydrobromide	Antidepressant (SSRI)	Depression
Cipro	Ciprofloxacin HCl	Antiinfective	UTIs; lower respiratory infections; skin infections; bone and joint infections; acute sinusitis
Claritin	Loratadine	Antihistamine	Allergy
Concerta	Methylphenidate	CNS stimulant	ADHD
Coreg	Carvedilol	Beta blocker	HTN
Coumadin	Warfarin sodium	Anticoagulant	Embolism; MI
Crestor	Rosuvastatin	Antilipemic	Hyperlipidemia
Cymbalta	Duloxetine HCl	Antidepressant	Depression
Delestrogen	Estradiol	Hormone	Menopause
Deltasone	Prednisone	Analgesic; antiinflammatory	Pain relief; inflammation
Dyazide	HCTZ	Diuretic	Hypertension
Effexor	Venlafaxine HCl	Antidepressant	Depression
Elavil	Amitriptyline	Antidepressant	Depression
Eliquis	Apixaban	Anticoagulant	Treat/prevent blood clots
Flagyl	Metronidazole	Antibiotic	PID
Flexeril	Cyclobenzaprine HCl	Muscle relaxant	Muscle spasms
Flomax	Tamsulosin	Alpha-adrenergic blocker	BPH
Flonase	Fluticasone	Antiinflammatory; corticosteroid	Seasonal allergic rhinitis
Folvite	Folic acid	Vitamin replacement	Anemia
Fosamax	Alendronate	Osteoporosis treatment	Osteoporosis
Glucophage	Metformin	Antidiabetic	Type 2 diabetes
Glucotrol	Glipizide	Antidiabetic	Type 2 diabetes
HCTZ	Same	Diuretic	Edema; hypertension
Humalog	Insulin lispro	Antidiabetic	Treat diabetes
Humulin N	Insulin NPH	Insulin replacement	Diabetes mellitus
Hydrocodone/APAP	Same	Narcotic analgesic	Moderate to severe pain relief
Inderal	Propranolol HCl	Beta blocker	Hypertension; angina
Januvia	Sitagliptin	Antidiabetic	Lower blood sugar level

(Continued)

TABLE 22.3   100 Most Prescribed Drugs of 2022—cont'd

Trade Name	Generic Name	Classification	Indication
Jardiance	Empagliflozin	Antidiabetic	Lower blood sugar level
Keflex	Cephalexin	Antiinfective	Staph/strep infections; URI; bacterial infections
Klonopin	Clonazepam	Anticonvulsant	Seizure disorders
Lamictal	Lamotrigine	Anticonvulsant	Prevent/control seizures
Lanoxin	Digoxin	Cardiac glycoside; antiarrhythmic	Heart failure; atrial fibrillation
Lantus	Insulin glargine	Antidiabetic	Type 1 diabetes
Lasix	Furosemide	Diuretic	Edema; hypertension
Lexapro	Escitalopram oxalate	SSRI	Depression
Lipitor	Atorvastatin calcium	Antilipemic	High cholesterol
Lopressor	Metoprolol tartrate	Beta blocker	Hypertension
Lotensin	Benazepril	ACE inhibitor	Hypertension
Lyrica	Pregabalin	Anticonvulsant	Fibromyalgia; seizure disorders
Mevacor	Lovastatin	Antihyperlipidemic	Hypercholesterolemia
Mobic	Meloxicam	NSAID	Arthritis; rheumatoid arthritis
Neurontin	Gabapentin	Anticonvulsant	Seizure disorders
Nexium	Esomeprazole magnesium	Proton-pump inhibitor	Heartburn; gastroesophageal reflux disease
Norvasc	Amlodipine	Antianginal	Angina
OxyContin	Oxycodone HCl	Narcotic analgesic	Moderate to severe pain
Ozempic/ Wegovy/ Rybelsus	Semaglutide	Antidiabetic; antiobesity	Control type 2 diabetes
Paxil	Paroxetine HCl	Antidepressant	Major depressive disorder
Pepcid	Famotidine	Antacid	GERD; ulcers
Percocet	Oxycodone and acetaminophen	Opioid analgesic	Moderate to severe pain
Plavix	Clopidogrel bisulfate	Antiplatelet	Myocardial infarction; stroke; peripheral artery disease
Potassium	Potassium	Replacement	Hypokalemia
Pravachol	Pravastatin	Antilipemic	Hypercholesterolemia
Prilosec	Omeprazole	Proton-pump inhibitor	Duodenal and gastric ulcers; GERD
Prinivil	Lisinopril	ACE inhibitor	Hypertension
Propecia	Finasteride	Hormone blocker	PBH
Protonix	Pantoprazole	Acid reducer	GERD
Prozac	Fluoxetine HCl	Antidepressant	Depression
Pulmicort	Budesonide	Antiasthma	Asthma; CPOD
Ritalin	Methylphenidate	Stimulant	ADHD
Seroquel	Quetiapine fumarate	Antipsychotic	Bipolar disorder
Singulair	Montelukast sodium	Antiasthmatic	Asthma
Synthroid	Levothyroxine sodium	Hormone replacement	Hypothyroidism
Tenormin	Atenolol	Antihypertensive	Hypertension
Topamax	Topiramate	Antiseizure	Prevent/manage seizures
Tylenol#2	Acetaminophen (APAP)/codeine	Analgesic	Mild to moderately severe pain
Ultram	Tramadol HCl	Analgesic	Moderate to moderately severe pain
Valium	Diazepam	Antianxiety	Anxiety
Ventolin	Albuterol	Bronchodilator	Asthma
Vibramycin	Doxycycline calcium	Antiinfective	Respiratory tract infections; chlamydia infection

TABLE 22.3   100 Most Prescribed Drugs of 2022—cont'd

Trade Name	Generic Name	Classification	Indication
Vitamin D₂	Ergocalciferol	Replacement	Vitamin D deficiency
Vicodin	APAP	Analgesic (opioid)	Moderate to severe pain
Vyvanse	Lisdexamfetamine dimesylate	CNS stimulant	ADHD; binge eating disorder
Wellbutrin	Bupropion	Smoking cessation	Antidepressant; smoking cessation
Xanax	Alprazolam	Antianxiety	Anxiety
Xarelto	Rivaroxaban	Anticoagulant	Deep vein thrombosis; pulmonary edema; reduction of risk of stroke
Yasmin	Ethinylestradiol	Oral contraceptive	Prevent pregnancy
Zanaflex	Tizanidine	Antispasmatic	MS; CP; muscle spasticity
Zantac	Ranitidine HCl	Antiulcer	Ulcers; GERD
Zetia	Ezetimibe	Anticholesterol	Lower cholesterol levels
Zithromax (Z-Pak)	Azithromycin	Antiinfective	Infection
Zocor	Simvastatin	Antilipemic	Hypercholesterolemia
Zofran	Ondansetron	Antiemetic	Nausea and vomiting
Zoloft	Sertraline	Antidepressant	Depression; SAD; OCD; OMDD; PTSD
Zyloprim	Allopurinol	Antigout	Gout; lower uric acid
Zyprexa	Olanzapine	Antipsychotic	Schizophrenia; bipolar disorder
Zyrtec	Cetirizine HCl	Antihistamine	Allergy; hay fever; rhinitis

ACE, Angiotensin-converting enzyme; *ADHD*, attention deficit hyperactivity disorder; *APAP*, paracetamol/acetaminophen; *BPH*, benign prostatic hypertrophy; *CNS*, central nervous system; *COPD*, chronic obstructive pulmonary disease; *GERD*, gastroesophageal reflux disease; *HCl*, hydrochloride; *HCTZ*, hydrochlorothiazide; *MI*, myocardial infarction; *NSAID*, nonsteroidal antiinflammatory drug; *PID*, pelvic inflammatory disease; *SSRI*, selective serotonin uptake inhibitor; *URI*, upper respiratory infection; *UTI*, urinary tract infection.

6. 500 mL = 500 cc = 1 pint (pt) = 16 oz
7. 1000 mL = 1000 cc = 1 quart (qt) = 32 oz
8. 1 m = 39.372 inches (in) = 3.281 feet (ft)
9. 0.914 m = 3 feet = 1 yard
10. 0.3048 m = 12 inches = 1 foot
11. 2.54 cm = 1 inch

C. Adult Dose Calculation

1. Dose given is dose ordered divided by the available strength times the dose form:

dose ordered / available × form = dose given

   a. Dose given: amount administered to the patient to fill the practitioner's order
   b. Dose ordered: amount of drug the practitioner orders to be given to the patient
   c. Available strength: concentration of medicine on hand
   d. Dose form: number of tablets (or capsules) or amount of liquid that contains the available strength
2. Example: provider orders 500 mg amoxicillin; 250-mg/cap amoxicillin is available:

500 mg / 250 mg × 1 = two 250 – mg caps administered

D. Pediatric Dose Calculation

1. Young's rule
   a. Used for children younger than 12 years, based on age
   b. Formula: child's age divided by (child's age + 12) and multiplied by the average adult dose gives the amount administered to the child

2. Fried's rule
   a. Used for infants and children younger than age 2 years, based on age in months
   b. Formula: infant's age in months divided by 150 and multiplied by the average adult dose gives the amount administered to the child
3. Clark's rule
   a. Used for children younger than 12 years, based on weight in pounds
   b. Formula: (child's weight in pounds divided by 150) multiplied by the average adult dose gives the amount administered to the child

IX. Administration of Medications

A. Routes of Administration

1. Buccal: medication is placed between cheek and gum and dissolves
2. Oral: medication is administered by mouth and swallowed
3. Sublingual: medication is placed under the tongue and dissolves
4. Inhalation: medication is delivered to lungs by means of a nebulizer (inhaler unit)
5. Topical: medication is externally applied to skin, eyes, ears, nose, or mucous membranes
6. Vaginal: medication is inserted into, or applied to, the vagina
7. Rectal: medication is inserted into the rectum and absorbed
8. Parenteral: medication is administered through a needle

B. Nine Rules of Medication Administration

1. Right medication
2. Right dose
3. Right route
4. Right time
5. Right patient
6. Right education
7. Right to refuse
8. Right techniques
9. Right documentation

C. Safety

1. Three "befores": read the drug label three times when preparing the medication:
   a. Before removing the medication from storage
   b. Before preparing the medication for administration
   c. Before replacing the medication back in storage
2. Be familiar with the drug; use references
3. Prepare medication in a clean, quiet, well-lit area, away from distractions
4. Do not use a medication that does not appear normal (changes in color, odor, or appearance of sediment in the medication)
5. Check the expiration date; never administer a date-expired medication
6. Verify the patient's identity before administering (call by name; ask patient his or her name)
7. Always check for allergies
8. Correctly chart the procedure: include date, time, medication, dose, route, patient reactions, and medical assistant's initials

D. Considerations

1. Age: children and older adults require smaller doses than younger adults
2. Sex: females require smaller doses than males
3. Weight: smaller patients require smaller doses than larger persons
4. Tolerance: a patient who has taken this medication over a long period may require a larger dose for required results
5. Condition of the patient: physical and psychological conditions
6. Route: parenteral medications are absorbed more quickly than oral medications
7. Timing: medications are absorbed more quickly on an empty stomach

E. Undesirable Effects of Drugs

1. Adverse reaction: unintended or undesirable effect of a drug; secondary to the therapeutic effect; can be harmless (side effect) or harmful
2. Drug interactions: drugs taken at the same time may produce undesirable effects; all meds should be charted
3. Idiosyncratic reaction: abnormal or peculiar response that is unexplained and unpredictable

F. Allergic Reactions

1. Mild reaction: rash, pruritus, and rhinitis
2. Severe reaction (anaphylaxis): pruritus, edema, dyspnea, cyanosis, and shock; untreated, a severe reaction can lead to coma or death
3. Prevention
   a. Monitor the patient after administration of the drug
   b. Observe the patient for signs and symptoms
   c. Notify the practitioner immediately of any reaction
   d. Be prepared to provide emergency assistance

X. Parenteral Administration

A. Equipment

1. Syringe (Fig. 22.2)
   a. Parts
      1) Barrel: holds medication; calibrated for measuring (cc/mL and minims)
      2) Flange: rim at the end of the barrel; place to put the fingers while depressing the plunger; keeps the syringe from rolling off a flat surface
      3) Plunger: fits inside the barrel; brings the medication into and out of the barrel
      4) Tip: end of the barrel where the needle attaches
   b. Types (Fig. 22.3)
      1) Regular hypodermic
         a) Most commonly calibrated in 2, 3, 5, and 10 cc
         b) May be disposable (plastic) or nondisposable (glass)
         c) May come with needle attached or without needle
      2) Tuberculin (TB)
         a) Small syringe calibrated in 0.1 cc
         b) Holds up to a total volume of 1 cc
      3) Insulin
         a) Calibrated in units (U40, U80, U100)

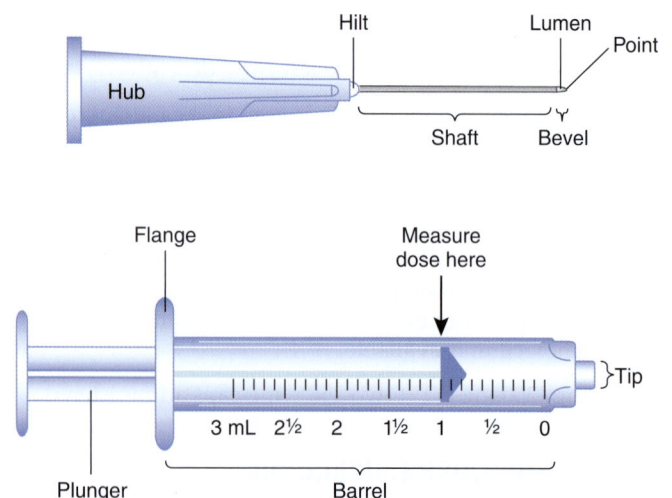

Fig. 22.2. Diagram of a needle and syringe. (From Bonewit-West K: *Clinical procedures for medical assistants*, ed 10, 2019, Saunders.)

b) Used for insulin injections
c) Syringe must correspond to type of insulin prescribed
4) Tubex, Carpuject
   a) Closed injection system
   b) Disposable medication cartridge-needle unit fits into a reusable plastic or metal holder
2. Needle
   a. Parts
      1) Hub: part of the needle that connects to the syringe
      2) Shaft: length of the needle; inserted into the body
      3) Point: sharpened end of the shaft

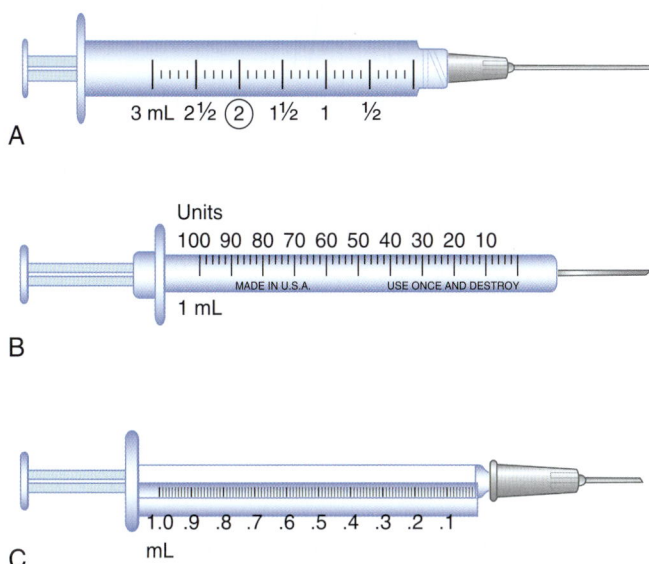

A

B

C

Fig. 22.3. Various syringes used to administer injections. (A) Hypodermic syringe; (B) insulin syringe; (C) tuberculin syringe. (From Bonewit-West K: *Clinical procedures for medical assistants*, ed 10, 2019, Saunders.)

4) Lumen: inside opening of the shaft
5) Bevel: slant of the point
b. Measured by
   1) Gauge: size of the lumen
      a) The smaller the gauge, the larger the needle
      b) 13–27 G
   2) Length
      a) Varies according to use
      b) ¼–6 inches

B. Administration

1. Intradermal (ID) (Figs. 22.4 and 22.5)
   a. Needle and syringe size
      1) Syringes: TB (1 cc)
      2) Needle gauge: 26–27 G
      3) Needle length: ⅜–½ inch
   b. Sites
      1) Anterior forearm
      2) Middle back
      3) Upper chest
   c. Uses of route
      1) Allergy skin testing (includes skin prick or scratch test)
      2) TB skin testing medication (Mantoux/purified protein derivative [PPD])
   d. Injection angle: 10–15 degrees (with bevel facing up)
   e. Goal of injection: formation of a wheal or bleb
   f. Amount given: 0.01–0.2 cc
2. Intramuscular (IM) (Figs. 22.6 and 22.7)
   a. Needle and syringe size
      1) Syringe: 3–5 cc (depending on amount administered)
      2) Needle gauge: 22–25 G (depending on area of the body and consistency of the medication)
      3) Needle length: ⅓–2 inches (depending on size of the patient and consistency of the medication)

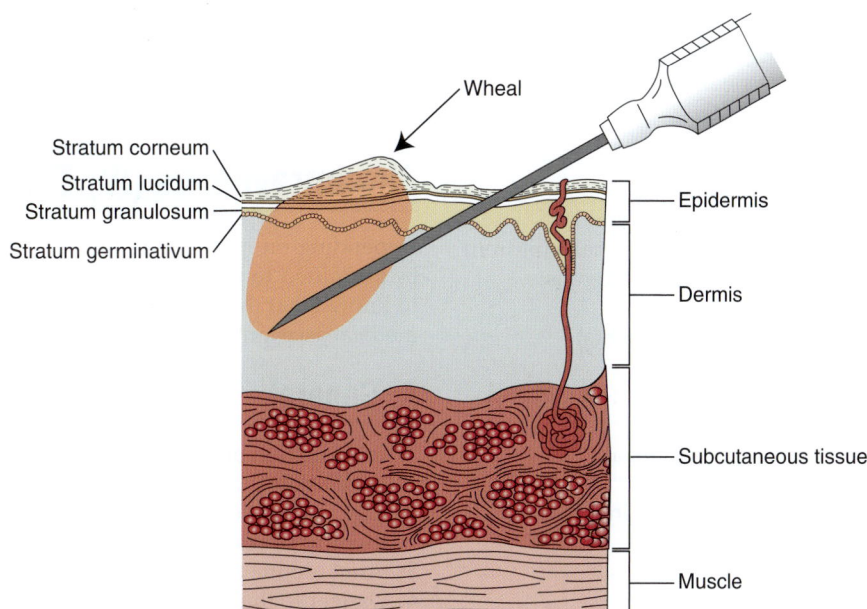

Fig. 22.4. Intradermal injection is administered just under the epidermis. (From Niedzwiecki B, et al: *Kinn's the clinical medical assistant: an applied learning approach*, ed 14, 2020, Elsevier.)

ANTERIOR   POSTERIOR

Upper arm   Upper back
                                      Upper arm

Forearm

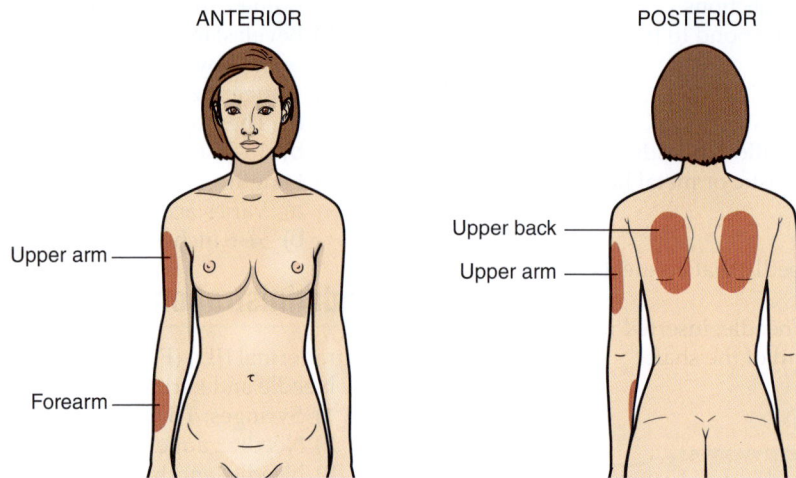

Fig. 22.5. Sites recommended for intradermal injections. (From Niedzwiecki B, et al: *Kinn's the clinical medical assistant: an applied learning approach*, ed 14, 2020, Elsevier.)

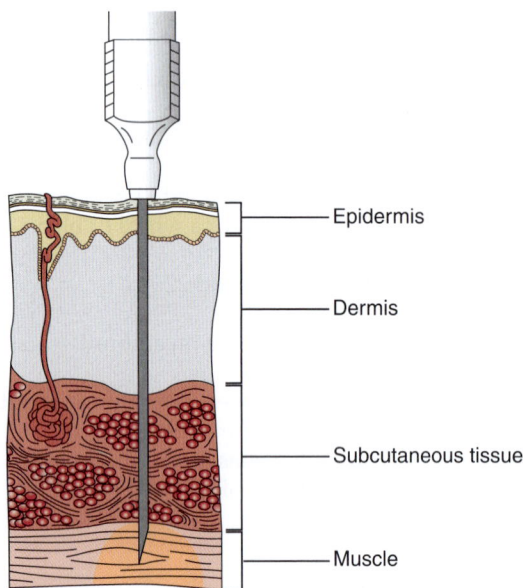

Epidermis

Dermis

Subcutaneous tissue

Muscle

Fig. 22.6. Anatomic illustration of the intramuscular injection. (From Niedzwiecki B, et al.: *Kinn's the clinical medical assistant: an applied learning approach*, ed 14, 2020, Elsevier.)

b. Sites
   1) Deltoid (not for infant or small child)
   2) Dorsogluteal (not for infant or small child)
   3) Vastus lateralis (used for infants and small children)
      a) Rectus femoris (medial to vastus lateralis; self-injection)
      b) Ventrogluteal (side of hip; all patients)
c. Uses of route
   1) Adult and childhood immunizations (deltoid and vastus)
   2) Thick or oil-based medications (gluteal)
d. Injection angle: 90 degrees
e. Goal of injection: to deliver medication into muscle tissue
f. Amount given
   1) Less than 2 cc (deltoid and vastus)
   2) 2–5 cc (gluteal)

3. Subcutaneous (SC, SQ, subq, subcut) (Figs. 22.8 and 22.9)
   a. Needle and syringe size
      1) Syringe: insulin, TB, or 2–3 cc syringe
      2) Needle gauge: 25–27 G
      3) Needle length: ⅜–1 inch
   b. Sites
      1) Upper arm (under deltoid, back of arm)
      2) Thigh
      3) Back
      4) Abdomen
      5) Any area where a fat surface exists
   c. Uses of route
      1) Insulin (rotate injection sites; do **not** aspirate, given at 90-degree angle)
         a) Only use insulin syringes for insulin
      2) Allergy injections
      3) Mumps, measles, and rubella (MMR) immunization
      4) Epinephrine
   d. Injection angle: 45 degrees
   e. Goal of injection: delivery of medication into subcutaneous (fatty) tissue
   f. Amount given: less than 2 cc

XI. Intravenous (IV) Therapy

Depending on location, a medical assistant may or may not be permitted to legally administer IV therapy. It is important to know what the scope of practice is for the state in which a medical assistant resides.

A. General

1. Introduction of therapeutic fluids directly into the venous circulation
2. Can be used for maintenance therapy, replacement therapy, or restoration therapy
3. Strict aseptic techniques must be used at all times
4. Danger to the patient can be great: medical assistant must be able to follow provider's orders exactly

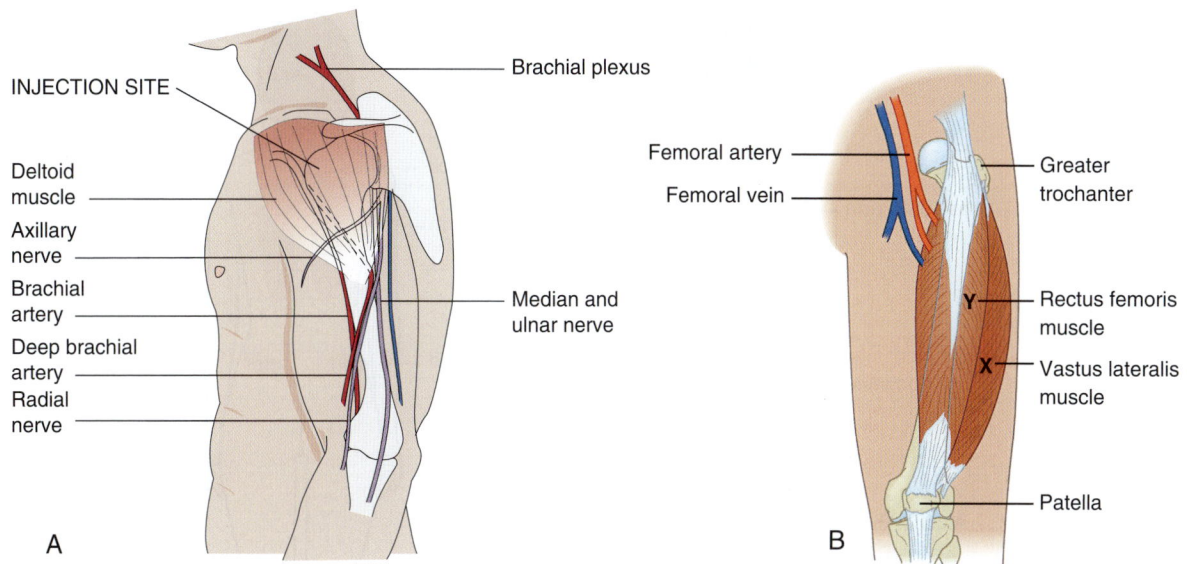

Fig. 22.7. Muscles commonly used for intramuscular injections. (From Niedzwiecki B, et al: *Kinn's the clinical medical assistant: an applied learning approach*, ed 14, 2020, Elsevier.)

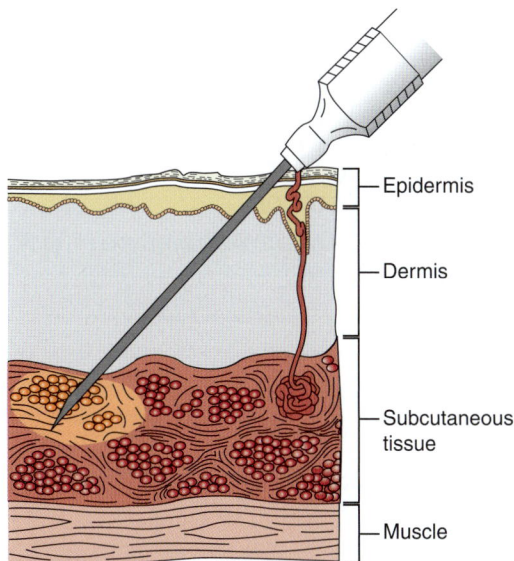

Fig. 22.8. Subcutaneous injection is administered into subcutaneous tissue. (From Niedzwiecki B, et al: *Kinn's the clinical medical assistant: an applied learning approach*, ed 14, 2020, Elsevier.)

B. Advantages and Uses of IV Therapy

1. Advantages
   a. Entire amount of a medication is distributed in the bloodstream immediately after administration
   b. No tissue barriers to cross
   c. Route may be indicated for patients who cannot take oral or parenteral medications
   d. Medications are not altered by GI tract
   e. Medications may be given to patients who are unconscious, vomiting, or uncooperative
   f. Useful in emergency situations
2. Uses
   a. Maintenance therapy
      1) Provides necessary requirements for water, electrolytes, and nutrition
      2) Amount given depends on patient's age, height, weight, and amount of body fat
      3) Used for patients who have little or no intake of fluids by mouth; require supplements
   b. Replacement therapy
      1) Replaces fluid and electrolyte deficits
      2) Indicated for vomiting and diarrhea, starvation, and hemorrhage
      3) Most common in ambulatory care settings
      4) Patient must be carefully monitored
   c. Restorative therapy
      1) Daily restoration of fluids and electrolytes
      2) Fluids are physiologically the same as fluids being lost
      3) Several types of fluids are often given
      4) Done more often in inpatient settings

C. Dangers of IV Therapy

1. Possible introduction of microorganisms into the bloodstream
   a. Aseptic technique must be followed
2. Infection at site
   a. Site care and bandaging using medical and surgical asepsis must be used
3. Hypertonic and hypotonic solutions may destroy red blood cells (RBCs)
   a. Can cause an embolus
4. Fluid overload
   a. Physician's order for amounts and rate must be carefully followed
5. Introduction of medications into IV fluids cannot be reversed
   a. Medications immediately travel throughout body once administered
6. Infiltration into tissue surrounding the needle site can cause pain, swelling, and possibly tissue damage

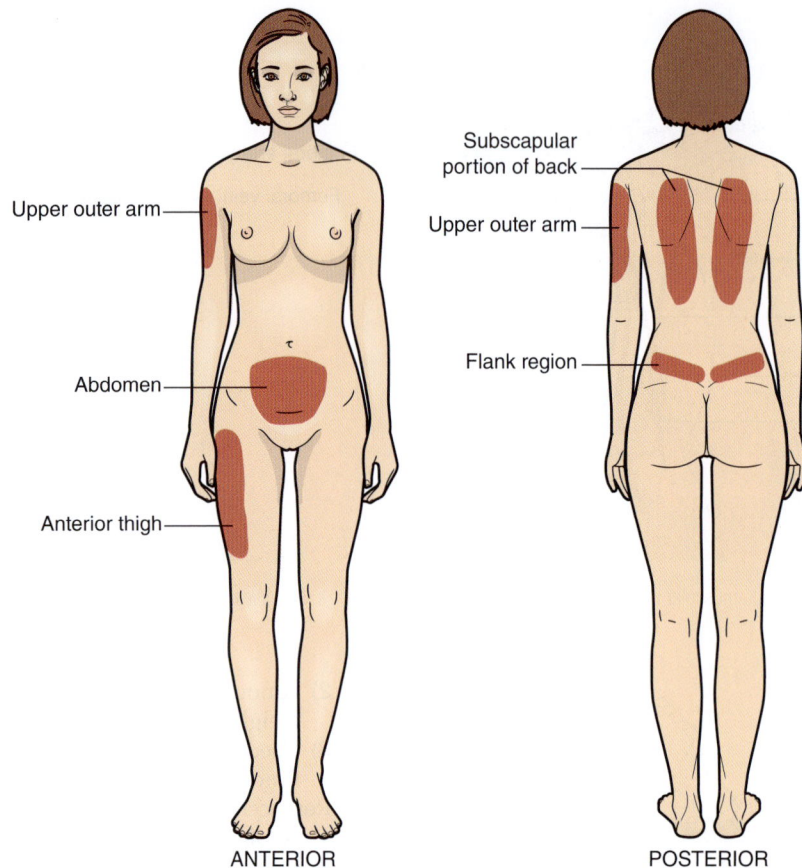

Fig. 22.9. Areas of the body used for subcutaneous injections. (From Niedzwiecki B, et al: *Kinn's the clinical medical assistant: an applied learning approach*, ed 14, 2020, Elsevier.)

D. Types of IV Therapy

1. 0.9% sodium chloride
   a. Normal saline
   b. Isotonic
   c. Maintains body fluid levels
2. Glucose
   a. Dextrose 5% in water (D5W)
   b. Saline (D5NS)
   c. Supplies nutritional needs or part of daily caloric requirement
3. Multiple electrolyte solution
   a. Ringer's and lactated Ringer's
   b. Contains sodium, calcium, chloride, and potassium
   c. Usually does not supply calories
4. Hypotonic solution
   a. Causes the flow of water into the cell
   b. Hydrates cells leading to depletion in amount of fluid in circulation
   c. Lowers blood pressure
5. Hypertonic solution
   a. Causes the flow of water out of the cell
   b. Increases blood volume
   c. Used to replace electrolytes
   d. Must be given slowly
6. Isotonic solution
   a. Similar to body fluids
   b. Can cause circulatory overload
7. Additions
   a. Drugs
   b. Supplements
   c. Fat emulsions
   d. Fluids
8. Maintenance solutions (i.e., Normosol, Plasmalyte)

E. Equipment

1. Usually found in kits containing all necessary supplies
2. Administration sets
   a. Primary administration sets (Fig. 22.10)
      1) Puts medications directly into bloodstream
      2) Used for infusion in ambulatory care
      3) Gravity or infusion pumps
      4) Macrodrip (8–20 drops/mL) and microdrip (50–60 drops/mL)
   b. Secondary infusion sets: used to add intermittent medications through secondary tubing
   c. Blood administration sets: used to administer blood and blood products
3. Tubing
   a. Varies in length
   b. Has a sharp spike at the top for insertion into the fluid bag
   c. May have injection port that acts as an access point for the addition of other fluids or secondary infusion sets

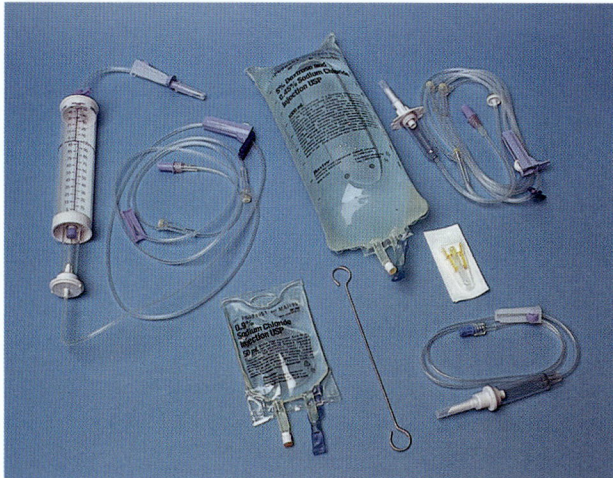

Fig. 22.10. Intravenous administration set. (From Williams PA: *deWit's fundamental concepts and skills for nursing*, ed 5, 2018, Saunders.)

4. Vent
   a. Located under spike
   b. Allows air to displace the fluid
5. Drip chamber
   a. Under vent
   b. Holds the fluids before infusion
   c. Opening of drip chamber contains the drop orifice, which determines the size and shape of fluid drops
6. Flow control clamp
   a. Compresses the tubing to allow fluid to flow through tubing
   b. Can be a roller or screw
7. Fluid containers
   a. Usually made of plastic
   b. Bag collapses as fluid infuses
8. Transparent dressing to cover IV site
9. Needles (Fig. 22.11)
   a. Winged-tip (butterfly)
      1) Used for short-term therapy
      2) 17–25 G
      3) 0.5–1 inch
      4) Patient needs to remain inactive so the tip of the needle does not puncture the vein

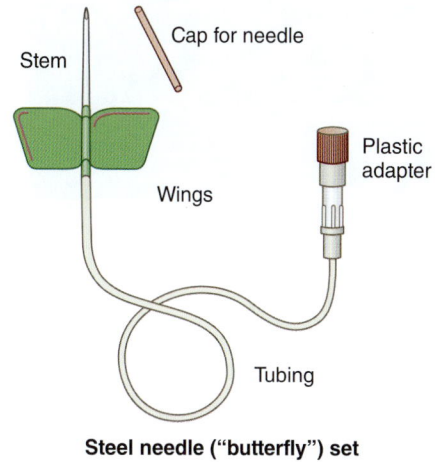

Steel needle ("butterfly") set

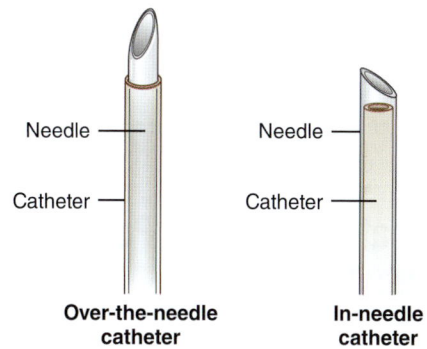

Fig. 22.11. Intravenous cannulas.

   b. Over-the-needle catheters
      1) Plastic sheath covers the distal point of the needle
      2) Needle is used to enter the vein and guide the catheter
      3) After entering the vein, the catheter is threaded off the needle and left in place
      4) Catheter comes in lengths of 0.5–2 inches
      5) 22–24 G

23

Minor Surgery

I. Surgical Procedures Performed in the Medical Office

A. General

1. No general anesthesia
2. Provider explains nature of the procedure and risks to patient; answers questions
3. Medical assistant is responsible for patient preparation and obtaining signature on consent form

II. Assisting With Surgical Procedures

A. Patient Preparation

1. Patient may need psychological and physical support
2. Allow patient to ask questions and voice concerns
3. Have all consent forms ready to sign
4. Make sure to check for any allergies
5. Give patient necessary preoperative instructions
   a. Instruct patient to bring or supply any needed equipment after procedure (e.g., crutches)
6. Instruct patient to bring someone to drive him or her home afterward

B. Informed Consent

1. Provider must have written informed consent before procedure
2. Provider is responsible for explaining the procedure and answering any patient questions
3. Must include a discussion of what will happen so that the patient can make an informed decision
4. Discussion and form put into patient's record

5. Patient should not be under the influence of sedation when the form is signed

C. Positioning

1. Patient undresses to expose surgical the site completely (be sure to use proper draping techniques to ensure patient privacy)
2. Patient positioned as comfortably as possible
3. Consider where medical assistant and provider will stand, instruments will be placed, and other equipment will be located

D. Skin Preparation

1. Skin cleansed with surgical soap and antiseptic; area shaved if needed
2. Patient may be instructed to cleanse area himself or herself at home before the procedure

E. Room Preparation

1. Know the procedure, provider's care preferences, and materials needed
2. Sterile supplies opened just before the procedure; opened materials exposed more than 1 hour are considered nonsterile
3. Once supplies are opened, sterile field should be covered with sterile drape and monitored until the procedure begins

F. Assisting the Provider

1. Sort and place instruments on the sterile field
2. Medical assistant stands opposite the provider
3. Protect the sterile field from contamination
4. Pass instruments and supplies to the provider as needed

G. Specimen Collection

1. Specimen collected during the procedure placed in appropriate container, labeled date, time, and initial, and sent to the laboratory for analysis
   a. Verify patient's identity prior to labeling

H. Postoperative Responsibilities

1. Disinfect the room, table, Mayo stand, back table, and any equipment
2. Instruments removed for sterilization or disposed of properly if disposable

I. Postoperative Care of Patient

1. Patient allowed to rest after the procedure; patient recovers from sedative
2. Explain any medications to patient and caregiver
3. Explain warning signs or changes that need medical attention: redness at site, bleeding from the wound, fever, swelling, or severe pain
4. Teach wound care and dressing change
5. Make follow-up appointment
6. Instructions may be preprinted forms with checkboxes

III. Surgical Instruments

A. General (Fig. 23.1)

1. Have clearly identifiable parts for visual identification
2. Classified according to use

B. Cutting and Dissecting Instruments

1. Scissors
   a. Used to cut tissue and sutures
   b. Blades touch at the tip; can be curved or straight
   c. Blade combinations
      1) Sharp/sharp (S/S)
      2) Blunt/blunt (B/B)
      3) Sharp/blunt (S/B)
   d. Bandage scissors
      1) Blunt probe tip for easy insertion under bandage
      2) Used to remove bandages and dressings
   e. Operating scissors
      1) Metzenbaum scissors: dissects tissues
      2) Mayo scissors: cuts and dissects fascia and muscle
      3) Iris scissors: general use
   f. Gauze shears: used to cut gauze, tubing, and adhesive
   g. Stitch (or suture) scissors (Littauer)
      1) One blade has a hook to slide under sutures
      2) Used to remove sutures
2. Scalpel (see Fig. 23.1)
   a. Surgical knife used to make incision
   b. May be reusable or disposable
   c. Parts
      1) Handle
         a) Holds the blade
         b) Many sizes and shapes (#3 is the standard)
      2) Scalpel blade
         a) Disposable
         b) Fits onto handle
         c) Different sizes and shapes (#15 is the standard)

C. Grasping and Clamping Instruments (Fig. 23.1)

1. Used to retract, clamp, hold, or manipulate tissue, other instruments, or sterilized materials
   a. Hemostat forceps (hemostats)
      1) Jaws may or may not be serrated
2. Used to clamp small vessels or hold tissue
   a. Kelly hemostats
   b. Mosquito hemostats
3. Needle holders (needle pushers)
   a. Jaws shorter and look stronger than hemostats
   b. Used to grasp suture needles
4. Splinter forceps
   a. Fine tip for foreign body retrieval or removal
   b. Various designs and construction
5. Thumb forceps (dressing forceps)
   a. Serrated jaws with teeth
   b. Used to insert packing into a wound or to remove objects from cavities
6. Allis tissue forceps
   a. Blunt teeth
   b. Used to grasp tissue, muscle, or skin surrounding a wound
7. Adson thumb forceps (tissue forceps)
   a. Teeth for grasping tissue
   b. Used to grasp tissue and in suturing
8. Bayonet forceps
   a. Smooth tipped
   b. Used to insert or remove objects from the nose and ear
9. Towel clamps (forceps)
   a. Very sharp hooks
   b. Various lengths
   c. Used to hold drapes in place during surgery
10. Transfer forceps
    a. Many sizes and lengths
    b. Sterile forceps used to arrange objects on the sterile field

D. Retracting Instruments (Fig. 23.1)

1. Holds tissue away from surgical incision
2. Rake retractor: has pronged end
3. Senn retractor
   a. Pronged end may be sharp or dull
   b. Flat end is blunt retractor
4. Skin hook: sharp point is used to retract small incisions or to secure skin edge for suturing
5. Ribbon retractor (Crile malleable retractor): used to hold back tissues and organs in large wounds

E. Probing and Dilating Instruments

1. Used for surgery and examinations
2. Probes search a cavity or wound

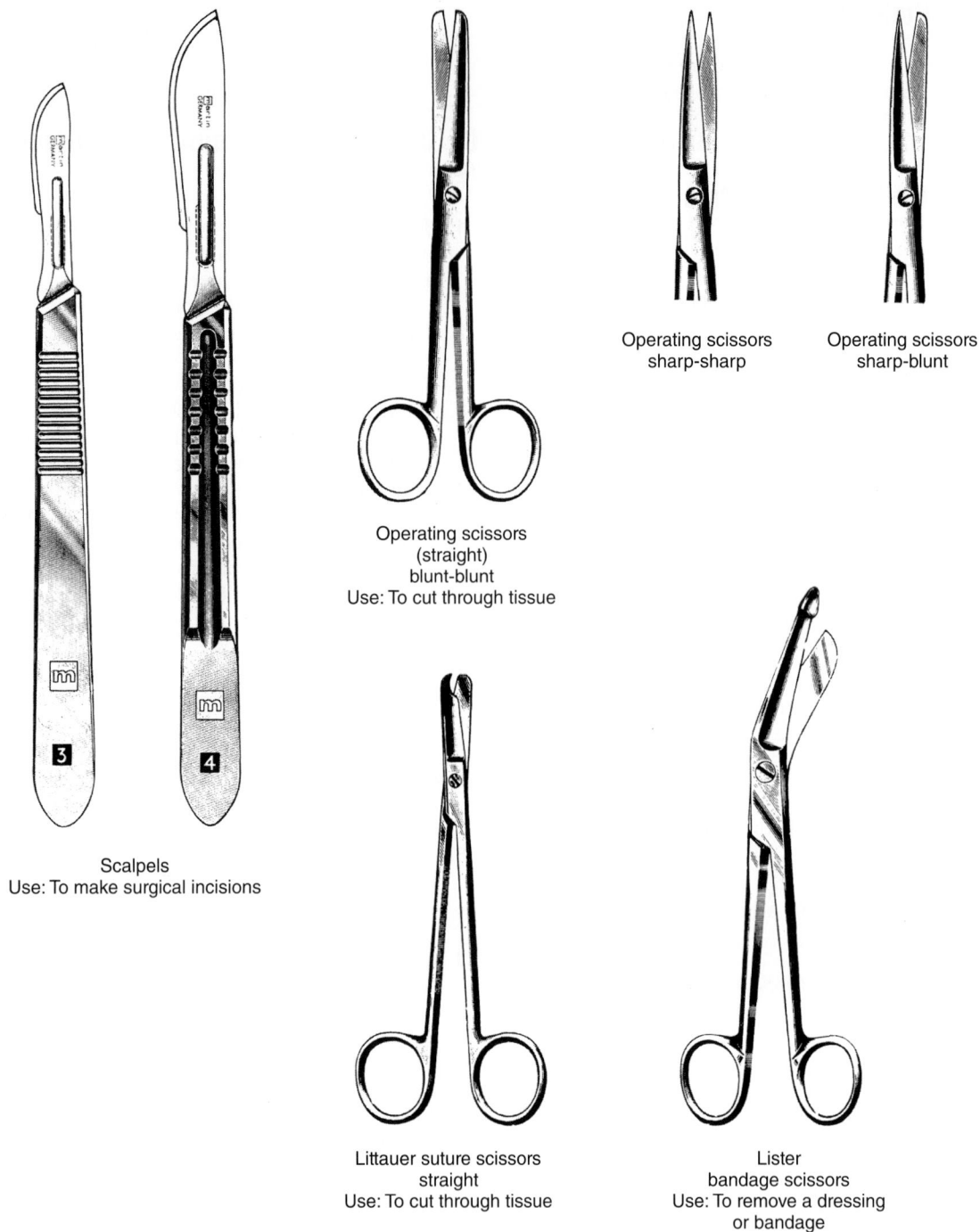

Scalpels
Use: To make surgical incisions

Operating scissors
(straight)
blunt-blunt
Use: To cut through tissue

Operating scissors
sharp-sharp

Operating scissors
sharp-blunt

Littauer suture scissors
straight
Use: To cut through tissue

Lister
bandage scissors
Use: To remove a dressing
or bandage

Fig. 23.1 Instruments used in minor office surgery. (Courtesy Elmed, Addison, Ill.)

3. Dilators used to stretch a cavity or opening
   a. Specula
      1) Most common dilator used
      2) Valves spread apart and dilate the opening
      3) Includes vaginal, nasal, rectal, and ear specula
   b. Trocars and obturators
      1) Sharply pointed instrument (trocar) contained within an outer tube
      2) Used to withdraw fluids from cavities or for draining and irrigating with a catheter

   c. Probes
      1) Different lengths (4–12 inches)
      2) Used to enter body cavities
   d. Sound: long, slender probe

F. Specialty Instruments

1. Four main categories: cutting/dissecting, grasping/clamping, retracting, and probing/dilating
2. Specific for particular examinations in a specialty

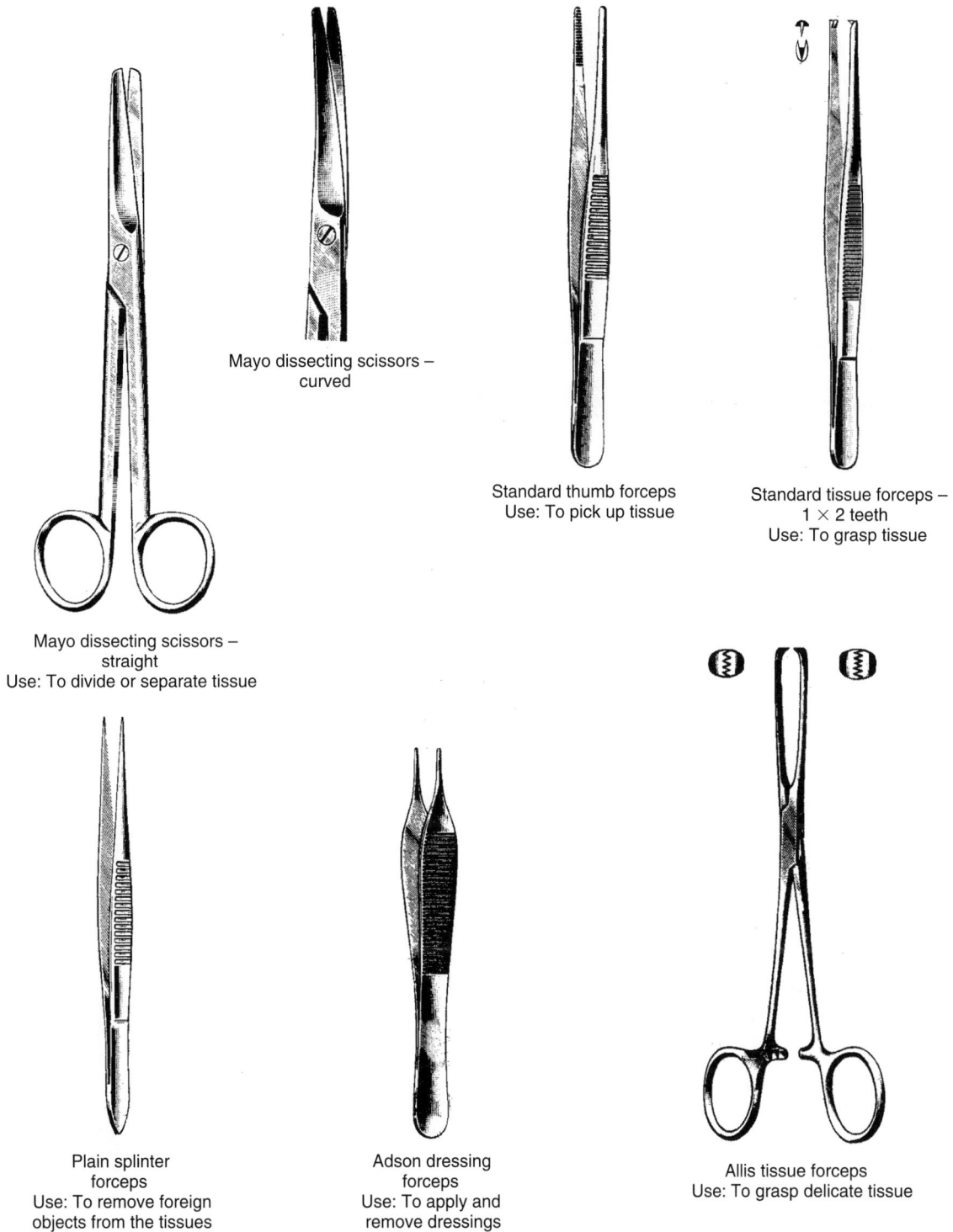

Mayo dissecting scissors –
curved

Standard thumb forceps
Use: To pick up tissue

Standard tissue forceps –
1 × 2 teeth
Use: To grasp tissue

Mayo dissecting scissors –
straight
Use: To divide or separate tissue

Plain splinter
forceps
Use: To remove foreign
objects from the tissues

Adson dressing
forceps
Use: To apply and
remove dressings

Allis tissue forceps
Use: To grasp delicate tissue

Fig. 23.1, cont'd

a. Gynecology
　1) Sponge forceps: used the way dressing forceps are used
　2) Uterine dressing forceps
　　a) Can reach the cervix and vagina
　　b) Used to swab an area or to apply medications
　3) Curettes (endocervical and uterine Sims)
　　a) Hollow and spoon shaped
　　b) Used to remove polyps, secretions, and tissue
　4) Schroeder tenaculum forceps
　　a) Sharp, pointed tips
　　b) Used to hold tissue or the cervix while obtaining specimen
　5) Hegar uterine dilators: used to dilate the cervix for dilation and curettage (D&C)
b. Ophthalmology and otolaryngology
　1) Krause nasal snare
　　a) Wire loop on tip
　　b) Used to remove polyps
　2) Alligator ear forceps: used to remove foreign bodies

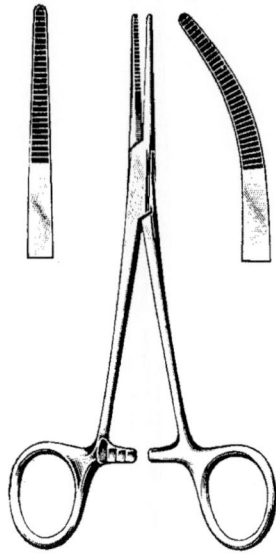

Kelly hemostatic forceps –
straight or curved
Use: To clamp off blood vessels

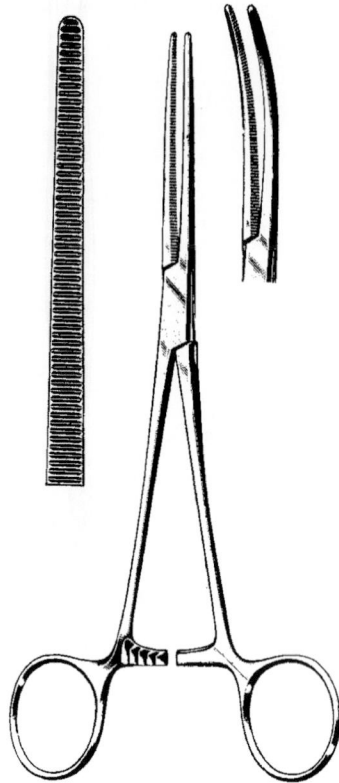

Rochester-Pean hemostatic forceps –
straight or curved

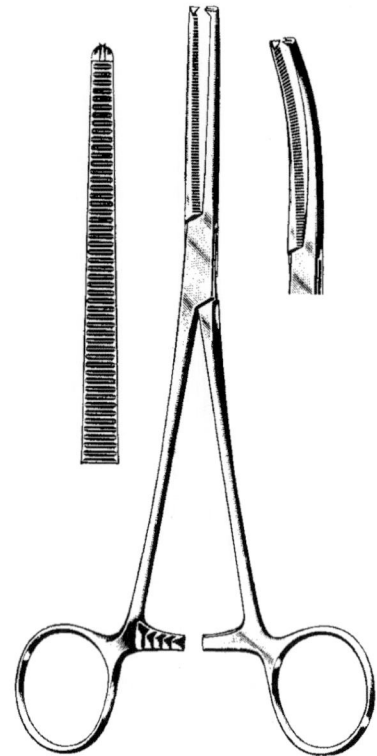

Ochsner-Kocher hemostatic forceps –
straight or curved,
1 × 2 teeth

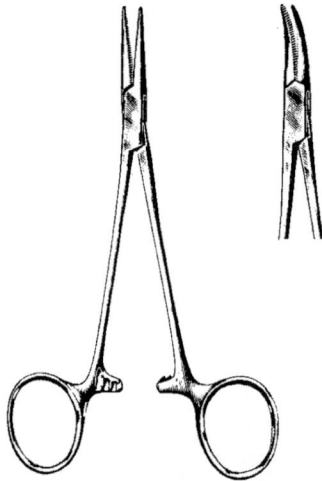

Halsted mosquito hemostatic forceps –
straight and curved
Use: To hold delicate tissue or to
clamp off small blood vessels

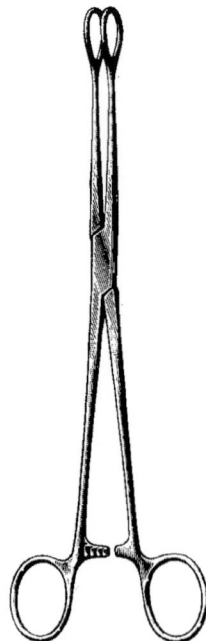

Foerster
sponge forceps
Use: To hold a sponge

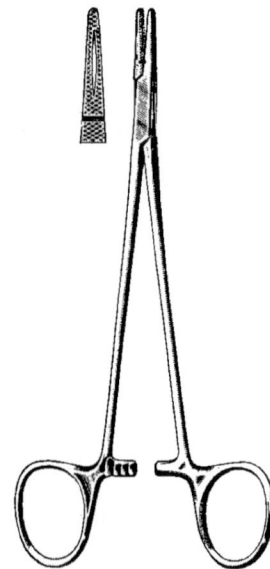

Crile-Wood needle holder
Use: To grasp a curved needle

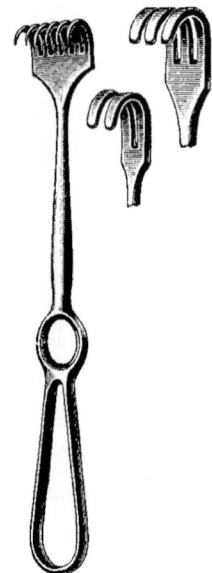

Volkmann rake retractor
Use: To hold tissue aside

Fig. 23.1, cont'd

GYNECOLOGIC INSTRUMENTS

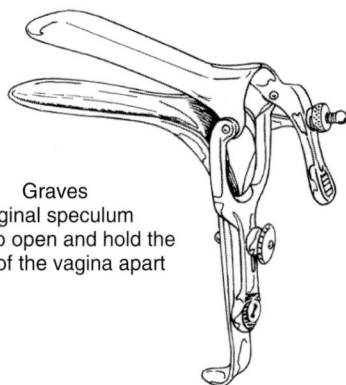

Graves
vaginal speculum
Use: To open and hold the
walls of the vagina apart

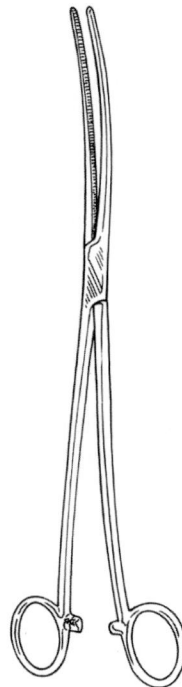

Uterine dressing forceps
Use: To hold dressings for procedures
involving the vagina, cervix, or uterus

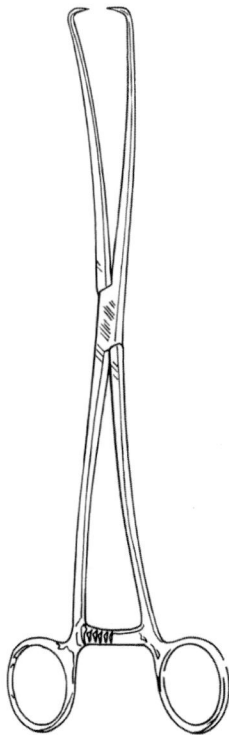

00

0

Sims
sharp

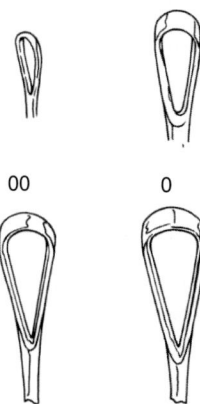

2
Uterine
curette
Use: To remove material from the
wall of a cavity or other surfaces

Duplay
uterine
tenaculum
Use: To grasp and hold the cervix

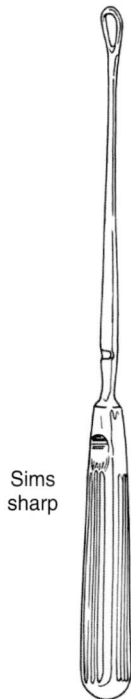

Fig. 23.1, cont'd

3) Laryngeal mirror
  a) Various sizes
  b) Used to examine larynx and postnasal area
4) Buck ear curette
  a) Sharp or blunt scraper end
  b) Used to remove foreign matter from ear canals
c. Biopsy
  1) Cervical biopsy forceps: used to obtain specimens
  2) Punch biopsy: used to remove tissue specimens
  3) Biopsy needle: works on the same principle as an obturator
  4) Abscess needle
    a) Used to withdraw fluids or pus from a cyst or abscess
    b) Usually disposable
d. Genitourinary: Foley catheter
  1) Manufactured in sizes 8–32 (French)
  2) Used as an indwelling catheter
e. Endoscopes
  1) Hollow, cylindrical instruments
  2) Used to visualize the interior of a cavity or opening
    a) Sigmoidoscope: used to visualize the sigmoid colon
    b) Proctoscope: used to visualize the rectum
    c) Anoscope: used to visualize the superficial rectum
    d) Bronchoscope: used to visualize the larynx, trachea, and bronchi
    e) Otoscope: used to visualize the external and middle ear
    f) Cystoscope: used to visualize the urinary bladder
    g) Laparoscope: used to visualize the peritoneal and abdominal cavities

IV. Sutures and Needles

A. General

1. Suture: act of stitching or sewing together
2. Material used to stitch or sew
3. May also be used to ligate (tie off)

B. Suture Types

1. Absorbable
   a. Dissolves and is absorbed by enzymes in the body
   b. Used in deep incisions and where suture removal may be difficult
   c. Types
     1) Surgical catgut (surgical gut)
       a) Used in tissues that heal rapidly
       b) Obtained from sheep, cattle, or pig intestines
       c) Packaged in alcohol to keep it pliable
     2) Chromic
       a) Catgut coated with chromic salts
       b) Delayed absorption of up to 80 days
     3) Vicryl
       a) Synthetic suture made of polyglactin
       b) Takes up to 11 weeks to absorb

2. Nonabsorbable
   a. Left in the body, where it embeds in scar tissue or must be removed when healing is complete
   b. Used frequently in minor office surgeries
   c. Types
     1) Silk
       a) Strong
       b) Easy to tie and remove
     2) Cotton: not used much (polyester more common)
     3) Polyester fiber: strongest of all suture material

C. Sizing

1. Diameter of strand determines the size
2. Sized from 6–0 (smallest) to 4 (largest)
3. Lengths of strands are precut (into 18-, 24-, 54-, and 60-inch lengths)
4. 2–0 to 6–0 most common

D. Suture Removal

1. Physician determines the length of time sutures remain in place
2. Must always be left in place long enough for proper healing to take place
3. General length of time until suture removal
   a. Skin sutures in head and neck: remove in 3–5 days
   b. Skin sutures in other areas: remove in 7–10 days

E. Needles

1. Chosen according to area used
2. Classified by
   a. Shape
     1) Straight
     2) Curved (more easily manipulated)
   b. Type of point
     1) Tapered (for delicate tissue)
     2) Cutting (for skin)
   c. Eye
     1) Eyelet (have to thread the needle)
     2) Eyeless (suture material attached to the needle; atraumatic)

F. Adhesive Skin Closures

1. Sterile, nonallergenic tape
2. Available in various widths and lengths
3. Used when not much tension exists on the skin edges
4. Applied transversely across the incision line
5. Eliminate the need for sutures and anesthetic
6. Easily applied and removed
7. Less scarring
8. Example: Steri-Strips

G. Surgical Skin Staples

1. Fastest method of closure for long incisions
2. Reduces trauma to tissue
3. Inserted using a skin-stapling device
4. Removed with a staple remover

H. Skin Glue

1. Special type of medical adhesive that joins the edges of a wound together
2. Can be used for children and adults
3. Usually used for simple cuts or wounds
4. Example: Dermabond

V. Drapes

A. General

1. Sterile paper or cloth material placed over or around the operative site
2. Used to maintain sterility

B. Types

1. Plain
2. Fenestrated
   a. Contains precut opening
   b. Opening is placed over the operative site
3. Incisional
   a. Adhesive-backed plastic
   b. Drape adheres directly to skin
   c. Incision is made through drape

VI. Anesthesia

A. General Information

1. Injected into the surgical site to prevent the sensation of pain
2. Medications used for anesthesia end in the suffix "-cain(e)"
3. Example of anesthesia medication: lidocaine (Xylocaine) and procaine (Novocain)
4. May contain epinephrine
   a. Enhances the effect of the anesthesia
   b. Minimizes bleeding at the operative site
5. Takes effect in 5–15 minutes; effective for 1–3 hours

B. Types of Local Anesthesia

1. Infiltration: solution is injected under the skin to anesthetize nerve endings
2. Nerve block: solution is injected into an accessible main nerve
3. Topical: a solution is painted (or sprayed) directly onto the skin or mucous membranes

VII. Surgical Asepsis (Table. 23.1)

A. General

1. Destruction of organisms before they enter the body
2. Used whenever skin or mucous membranes are punctured, pierced, or incised

TABLE 23.1   How to Distinguish Between Medical and Surgical Asepsis

	Medical Asepsis	Surgical Asepsis
Definition	Destruction of organisms after they leave the body	Destruction of organisms before they enter the body
Purpose	Prevent reinfection of patient; avoid cross infection from one person to another	Care for open wounds; used in surgery
Technique	Universal blood and body-fluid precautions; isolation techniques	Sterile technique
Procedure	Clean objects kept from contamination	Objects must be sterile
	Clean gloves and clean barriers used	Sterile gloves and articles used
	Objects disinfected as soon as possible after contact with patient	Objects must be sterilized before contact with patient
When used	For examinations that do not involve open wounds or breaks in the skin or mucous membranes but do involve patient blood or body fluids; isolating infected persons from others	Surgery, biopsy, wound treatment, and insertion of instruments into sterile body cavities
Handwashing technique	Hands and wrists washed for 1–2 minutes; soap, water, and plenty of friction used to remove oil and microorganisms from fingers	Hand and forearms scrubbed for 3–10 minutes; surgical soap, running water, friction, and sterile brush used; fingernails must be cleaned
	Hands held downward, running water allowed to drain off fingertips; hands dried with paper towels	Hands held up, under running water, to drain off elbows; hands dried with sterile towels

B. Basic Rules

1. Clean with clean
2. Dirty with dirty
3. Sterile with sterile
4. When in doubt, throw it out

C. Surgical Scrub

1. Hands and forearms scrubbed for 3–10 minutes
2. Use surgical soap with a brush
3. Clean under fingernails

4. Hands held up; rinsed from fingertips to elbows
5. Dry with sterile towels
6. Glove immediately

D. Sterile Gloves

1. Used whenever the patient needs to be protected from microorganisms (all surgical procedures)
2. Used when handling sterile instruments or sterile supplies
3. Gloving procedure
   a. Select proper glove size
   b. Open package
   c. With the nondominant hand, lift the glove for the dominant hand by the folded edge of the cuff
   d. Put on glove, keeping it above your waist
   e. Pick up the second glove by placing the gloved fingers under the cuff; insert the hand; adjust the cuffs and fingers
   f. Always keep gloved hands above your waist and away from your body

E. Sterile Field

1. Any surface on which sterile items are placed
2. Created by draping sterile towels over a Mayo stand
3. Sterile field is also a draped surgical site after the patient's skin is prepared and draped
4. Any item placed below the waist is considered contaminated

5. The 1-inch edge around the entire sterile field is considered nonsterile
6. Edges of all wrappers, packs, and towels are nonsterile
7. Sides of containers are nonsterile
8. Moisture carries bacteria from nonsterile to sterile surfaces

F. Handling Instruments and Supplies

1. Sterile forceps are used to handle sterile instruments or sterile supplies when sterile gloves are not being worn
   a. Lift forceps out of the container without touching the sides of the container
   b. Touch the tips of the forceps to sterile gauze to dry
   c. Always keep the forceps tips facing down
2. Lids removed from containers are placed face up on surfaces; hold face down if not placed on surfaces
3. Pour solutions to avoid splashing; avoid touching the rim of a sterile receptacle with the bottle
4. Do not reach over the sterile field
5. Cover the setup with a sterile towel if it is not to be used immediately

G. Skin Preparation

1. Skin cannot be sterilized
2. Resident and transient bacteria must be completely removed
3. Skin preparation is performed by a gloved assistant

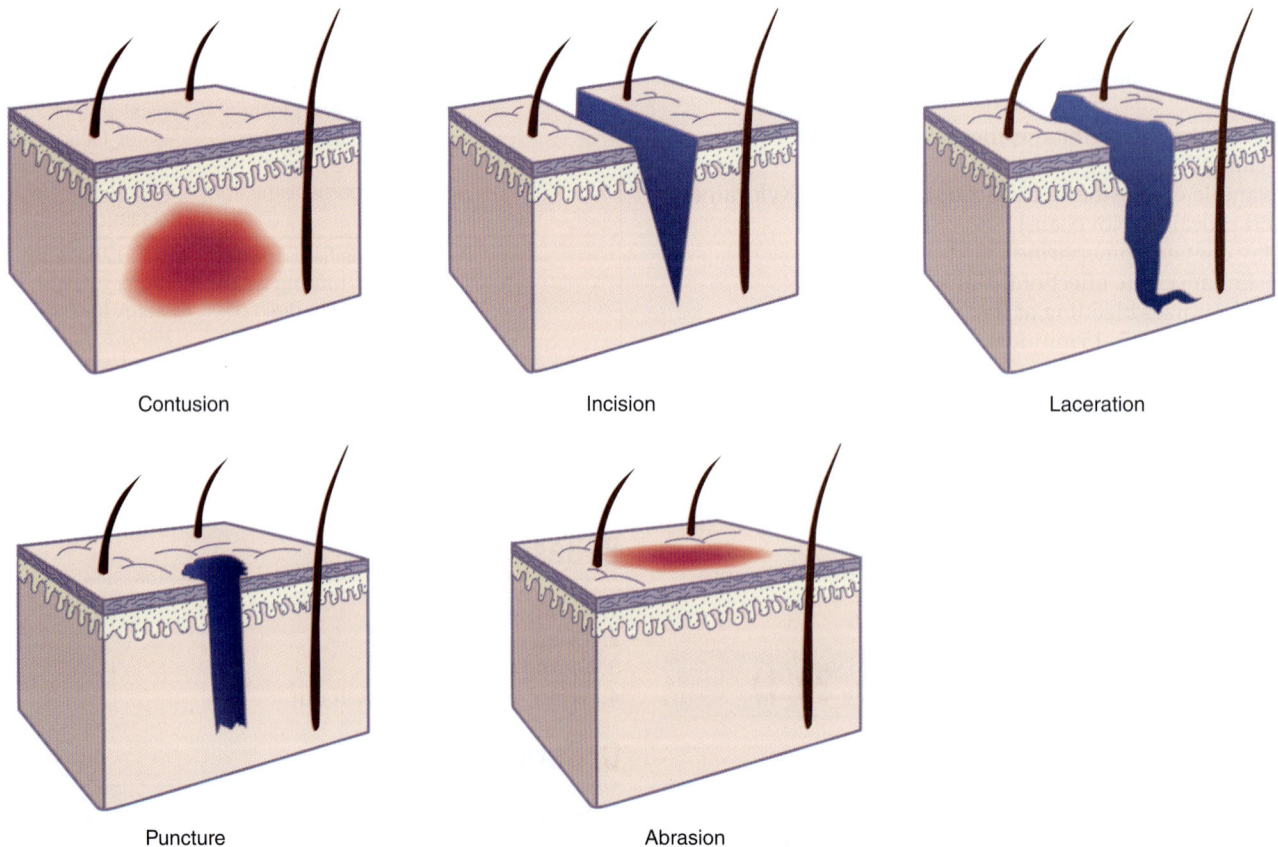

Contusion   Incision   Laceration

Puncture   Abrasion

Fig. 23.2 Types of wounds. (From Bonewit-West K: *Clinical procedures for medical assistants*, ed 10, 2018, Saunders.)

4. Make sure that the patient is not allergic to the surgical scrub solution used (e.g., povidone-iodine [Betadine], iodine)
5. Area is cleansed in a circular motion from the inside of the circle out; repeat the cleansing with a new sponge; dry with sterile, dry sponges

VIII. Wounds

A. Definition

1. Interruption in continuity of internal or external body tissues

B. Types of Wounds (Fig. 23.2)

1. Closed wound
   a. Nonpenetrating
   b. No outward opening
   c. Underlying tissue is damaged
2. Open wound
   a. Skin is broken
   b. Underlying tissue is exposed

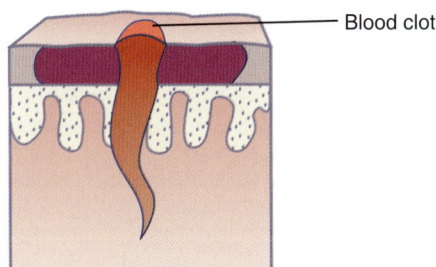

Phase 1: Inflammatory Phase

Blood clot

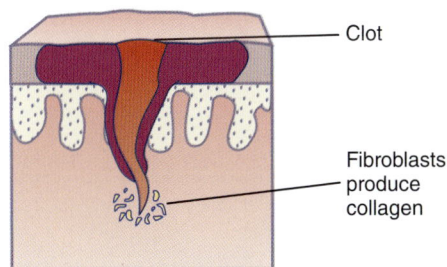

Phase 2: Proliferative Phase

Clot

Fibroblasts produce collagen

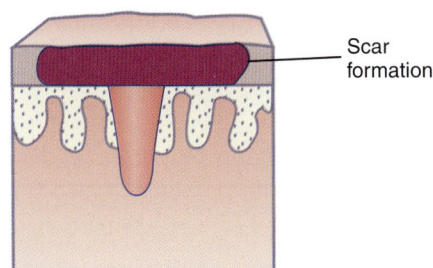

Phase 3: Maturation Phase

Scar formation

Fig. 23.3 Phases of wound healing. (From Bonewit-West K: *Clinical procedures for medical assistants*, ed 10, 2018, Saunders.)

c. Classified according to the appearance of the opening
   1) Laceration: jagged, irregular, breaking, or tearing of tissues
   2) Puncture: skin is pierced by a pointed object (e.g., pin, nail, and splinter)
   3) Abrasion: superficial wound; scraping of the skin
   4) Avulsion: tissue is torn away or separated
   5) Surgical incision: neat, clean cut
   6) Contusion: closed, nonpenetrating wound; blood from broken vessels accumulates in the tissues

C. Wound Healing (Fig. 23.3)

1. All wounds go through healing (repair)
2. Three phases
   a. Lag phase
      1) Blood vessels contract to control bleeding
      2) Platelets form a plug
      3) Fibrin is released to begin clotting (dried clot becomes the scab)
      4) White blood cells arrive at the site to clear away debris
      5) Within 1–4 days, fibrin threads contract and pull the edges of the wound together under the scab
   b. Proliferation phase
      1) Lasts 5–20 days
      2) Tissues repair themselves
      3) Wound continues to contract and seal
   c. Remodeling phase
      1) Beginning on day 21
      2) Scar tissue forms
      3) Scar tissue is not true skin; very strong and nonelastic
      4) Scar tissue is connective tissue without blood or nerve supply

D. Classification of Wound Repair

1. First intention
   a. Minimal tissue damage and scarring
   b. Wound may be sutured closed
2. Second intention
   a. Wound edges are not sutured or approximated
   b. Heals slowly from bottom up
   c. Large amount of scarring
3. Third intention: infected wound requires reopening

E. Wound Drainage (Exudate)

1. Serous
   a. Consists mainly of serum
   b. Clear and watery
2. Sanguineous
   a. Consists of red blood cells
   b. Bright red (fresh bleeding) or dark red (older bleeding)
3. Purulent
   a. Contains pus
   b. Thick; unpleasant odor; can be white, pink, green, or yellow
4. Serosanguineous
   a. Serum and blood mixed together
   b. Pink color; occurs postoperatively

IX. Dressings and Bandages

A. Dressings

1. Sterile covering placed over wound
2. Protect wound from injury or contamination
3. Maintain constant pressure on the wound
4. Help hold wound edges together
5. Control bleeding
6. Absorb drainage and secretions
7. Hide temporary disfigurement
8. May need to be removed periodically so that the wound can be checked for healing or suture removal
9. Always note amount and odor of any drainage in chart

B. Bandages

1. Nonsterile material used to hold dressings in place
   a. Splints and protects injured tissue
   b. Maintains pressure on the wound
   c. Aids in circulation
2. Made up of different materials and different sizes
   a. Gauze roller bandage
   b. Kling (self-adhering)
   c. Elastic cloth (Ace)
   d. Adhesive bandage (Band-Aid)
   e. Seamless tubular gauze (Tubegauze and Surgitube)

X. Patient Education

A. General

1. Instruct patient to contact the practitioner immediately to report
   a. Excessive bleeding at the wound site
   b. Fever
   c. Redness, swelling, or streaking around the wound site

24

Clinical Laboratory

I. Introduction to the Clinical Laboratory

A. Laboratory Tests

1. Provide essential information for accurate diagnosis and management of a patient's condition
2. Purpose of testing
   a. Assist in diagnosis of pathologic disease
   b. Confirm clinical diagnosis
   c. Assist in differential diagnosis
   d. Obtain information regarding patient's condition
   e. Evaluate patient's progress
   f. Establish a baseline
3. Reference range; normal range; acceptable range for chemical and physical body substances

B. Types of Clinical Laboratories

1. Physician's office laboratory: performs common and required testing; waived testing
2. Outside laboratories: include hospital and privately owned facilities; specimen collected in the office and sent to outside facility

C. Laboratory Request

1. Printed form that contains list of laboratory tests
2. Required when specimen is collected in the office and sent to outside or when patient is sent to outside laboratory for collection
3. Completed manually or computerized
4. Required information
   a. Provider's name and address
   b. Patient's name and address
   c. Patient's age and gender
   d. Date and time of collection of specimen
   e. Tests desired
   f. Source of specimen
   g. Diagnosis
   h. Medications the patient is taking
5. Request must be placed with the correct specimen

D. Laboratory Reports

1. Provide results of laboratory tests ordered
2. Usually in the form of computer printout or entire report generated by a computer
3. Patient results and normal range for each test reported
4. Provider reviews results; report filed in a chart

E. Patient Preparation and Instructions

1. Medical assistant (MA) responsible for instructing the patient for correct specimen collection
2. Fasting: abstaining from food and fluids for 12–14 hours before collection
3. Medications: usually discontinued 48–72 hours before collection only if the patient can be safely taken off medication

F. Occupational Safety and Health Administration (OSHA) Standards

1. Hazard communication standard
   a. Employer must provide information and training to employees who are exposed to hazardous agents (chemicals, noise, radiation, infectious agents)
   b. Standards must be in writing and include
      1) Training outline
      2) List of hazards and Safety Data Sheet (SDS) forms
      3) Warning and labeling system
      4) Method of informing employees

c. SDS
   1) Must be kept for each hazardous substance on site
   2) Prepared by the manufacturer
   3) Describes chemical and physical properties, hazards, precautions, and first aid
   4) Signs posted in laboratory
d. All hazardous agents must be labeled showing
   1) Name of hazardous substance
   2) Specific product warnings
   3) Name and address of manufacturer
2. Bloodborne pathogen standard
   a. Disease-causing microorganisms transmitted through blood and body fluids
   b. The Occupational Safety and Health Administration requires employers to ensure the safety of employees and provide training about exposure
   c. Bloodborne pathogens transmitted when contaminated blood or body fluids come into contact with nonintact skin or mucous membranes of another person
   d. Prevention
      1) Engineering controls: structural and mechanical devices that minimize exposure (e.g., sharps containers, eyewash stations)
      2) Work practice controls: promotion of behaviors necessary to use the engineering controls properly
      3) Personal protective equipment (PPE): equipment that decreases exposure (e.g., gloves, masks, laboratory aprons)
      4) Standard precautions: concept that all bodily secretions should be treated as if they are contaminated
      5) Body secretions include
         a) Blood and body fluids containing blood
         b) Semen
         c) Cerebrospinal fluid (CSF)
         d) Saliva
         e) Sputum
         f) Vaginal secretions
         g) Feces
         h) Urine
         i) Sweat and tears
         j) Vomitus
         k) Unidentifiable body fluids

G. Laboratory Safety

1. Postevacuation routes
2. Postemergency telephone numbers (fire, police, poison control)
3. First-aid kit accessible and up to date
4. Safety equipment accessible and in working order, including
   a. Eyewash station
   b. Shower
   c. Fire extinguisher
5. Laboratory coats or aprons worn at all times; remove before leaving the laboratory
6. Hair is pulled back; only minimal jewelry is allowed; fingernails are short
7. Dispose of sharps and broken glass immediately in a puncture-resistant container
8. Observe hazard identification labels
9. Work under the hood in a well-ventilated area when working with chemicals
10. Never pipette by mouth
11. Close all reagent containers when not in use
12. Label all reagent containers with name, expiration date, date of preparation, and preparer's initials
13. Pour acids into water when preparing solutions
14. Properly ground all electrical equipment
15. Wash hands after handling specimens and before leaving the laboratory
16. Do not eat, drink, smoke, apply makeup, or handle contact lenses in the laboratory
17. Do not store food in the laboratory refrigerator
18. Do not recap, break, or bend contaminated needles
19. Cap all tubes before centrifuging
20. Dispose of all contaminated nonsharps in labeled biohazard containers (red trash can or red trash bag)
21. Do not use cell phone while in the laboratory

H. Clinical Laboratory Improvement Act of 1988 (CLIA '88)

1. Federal legislation developed to regulate testing of specimens to diagnose, prevent, and treat diseases and disorders
2. Operated by the Centers for Medicare and Medicaid Services (CMS)
3. Laboratory must be in compliance with CLIA (Clinical Laboratory Improvement Amendments) to receive Medicare and Medicaid reimbursement
4. Three main standards
   a. Personnel standards
      1) Identify qualifications of persons directing or performing testing
      2) Qualifications depend on the complexity levels of the testing
   b. Testing standards: identify the tests that fall into one of three levels of complexity
      1) Waived tests
         a) Not subject to personnel or quality assurance requirements
         b) Common in medical office (physician's office laboratory)
      2) Moderately complex tests
      3) Highly complex tests
   c. Quality assurance standards
      1) Identify quality assurance requirements for qualified laboratories
      2) Apply only to laboratories that perform moderately and highly complex testing
      3) Standards include
         a) Written policies and standards
         b) Documented personnel training and proficiency testing
         c) Procedure manual
         d) Maintenance and documentation of the maintenance of instruments
         e) Quality control documentation

II. Clinical Laboratory Equipment

A. Microscope

1. Precision magnifying instrument used to view objects too small to be seen with the naked eye (Fig. 24.1)
2. Use involves focusing and illumination
3. Microscopic analysis usually performed by the provider or trained personnel
4. Total magnification equals objective lens magnification times ocular lens magnification
5. Care
   a. Transport with one hand under the base, the other on the arm
   b. Wipe immersion oil off the objective lens immediately after use
   c. Store with 10 × objective over the stage; bring the stage to the lowest level and cover
   d. Lenses should be cleaned only with lens paper to decrease the possibility of scratches

B. Centrifuge

1. Machine used to separate solids from liquids by rapid spinning
2. Must be balanced with tubes of equal size and containing equal volume

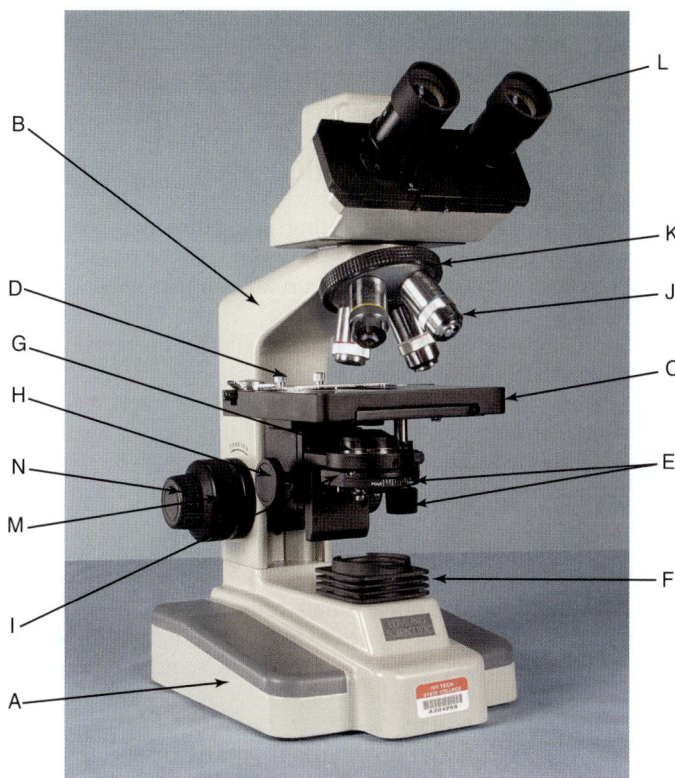

Fig. 24.1 Parts of a microscope. (A) Base; (B) arm; (C) stage; (D) slide holder; (E) mechanical slide controls; (F) light source; (G) condenser; (H) condenser adjustment; (I) diaphragm lever; (J) low-power objective; (K) nosepiece; (L) ocular lens; (M) coarse focus objective; and (N) fine focus adjustment. (From Garrels M: *Laboratory and diagnostic testing in ambulatory care: a guide for health professionals*, ed 4, 2019, Saunders.)

C. Incubator

1. Cabinets that maintain constant temperature
2. Used in microbiology to grow or incubate cultures

D. Autoclave

1. Instrument that uses steam under pressure at high temperatures
2. Used in the clinical laboratory to sterilize glassware and destroy specimens

III. Urinalysis

A. General

1. Physical, chemical, and microscopic examination of urine
2. Provides information about the conditions of the kidneys and urinary tract
3. Can help in the diagnosis of metabolic and systemic disorders

B. Collection of Specimens

1. Sterile liquid waste product easily obtainable
2. Volume needed is usually 25–50 mL
3. Should be analyzed within 30 minutes of collection but may be refrigerated for 8 hours
4. Specimen types
   a. First morning specimen
      1) Specimen of choice
      2) Most concentrated
   b. Random specimen: specimen collected at any time of the day
   c. Midstream specimen
      1) Used for routine urinalysis
      2) Patient is instructed to retract the foreskin or labia, void the first portion of the urine stream into the toilet, collect the midportion of the stream into a sterile container, and void the remaining portion of the stream into the toilet
      3) Properly label the container
   d. Clean-catch midstream
      1) Used for culture
      2) Patient is instructed to cleanse the glans penis or urethral meatus thoroughly with an antiseptic solution, continue with the midstream specimen collection technique, and collect in a sterile container
   e. 24-hour specimen
      1) Used to measure volume
      2) Used for quantitative analysis (amount) of chemicals
      3) Specimen requires a preservative and refrigeration (specimen container usually provided by laboratory)
      4) Patient is instructed to void first morning urine into the toilet; collect all urine into the same container for the next 24 hours, including the first morning specimen of the next day; and bring the entire specimen in the container to the laboratory

C. Physical Examination of Urine

1. Color
   a. Normal: yellow; color is due to urochrome pigment
   b. Pale (straw): dilute urine
   c. Dark yellow (amber): concentrated urine; may be seen in person with fever or dehydration
   d. Yellow-brown or green-brown: presence of bilirubin; foams when shaken
   e. Bright orange: seen in patients taking Pyridium; interferes with reagent strips
   f. Red: clear red may indicate hemoglobin (Hgb); cloudy red indicates the presence of red blood cells (RBCs) (hematuria)
   g. Dark brown or black: presence of melanin
   h. Pink, green, or blue: results from foods, dyes, chemicals, or vitamins
2. Appearance and clarity
   a. Normal: clear but becomes cloudy on standing
   b. Hazy: solid particles make urine appear hazy; print is not distorted when viewed through the sample
   c. Cloudy: solid particles make print difficult to see through the sample
   d. Turbid: solid particles make print impossible to see through the sample
   e. Normal cloudiness may be caused by
      1) Mucus
      2) Certain crystals
      3) Epithelial cells
      4) Sperm cells
   f. Abnormal cloudiness may be caused by
      1) Certain crystals
      2) White blood cells (WBCs) and RBCs
      3) Pus
      4) Epithelial cells
      5) Casts
      6) Fats
3. Specific gravity (SG)
   a. Measures amount of dissolved solids in urine
   b. Compares weight with an equal amount of distilled water
      1) Normal range: 1.005–1.035; usually 1.010–1.025; SG inverses with volume
      2) Low volume has high SG (concentrated urine)
      3) High volume has low SG (diluted urine)
   c. Methods of measuring SG
      1) Reagent strip
      2) Urinometer
      3) Refractometer
   d. Odor: may be noted if abnormal
      1) Normal: faintly aromatic; not unpleasant
      2) Ketones: sweet or fruity odor
      3) Ammonia: caused by bacterial growth that breaks down urea
      4) Food ingestion may cause strong odor

D. Chemical Examination

1. Chemical components are measured by the use of a reagent strip
2. Presence of a chemical causes a color change on the reagent pad on the strip
3. Tests are qualitative
4. Specimen should be well mixed before testing
5. Completely immerse the strip into the sample
6. Remove the strip and keep it in a horizontal position (avoids cross-contamination of pads)
7. Compare the color of the reagent pad with the color on the bottle or chart at the time specified
8. Quality control must be performed when each new bottle of strips is opened or question of reliability
9. Testing includes
   a. pH: measures acidity and alkalinity of urine; normal is 5–7
   b. Protein: significant for renal disease; normal is negative
   c. Blood: significant for kidney disease or hemorrhage in the urinary tract; normal is negative
   d. Nitrite: significant for urinary tract infection (UTI) (some bacteria convert nitrate to nitrite); normal is negative
   e. Leukocytes: significant for UTI; normal is negative
   f. Glucose: significant for diabetes mellitus; normal is negative
   g. Ketones: end product of metabolism; significant for diabetes mellitus and starvation; normal is negative
   h. Bilirubin: by-product of RBC destruction; significant for liver disease or bile duct obstruction; normal is negative
   i. Urobilinogen: result of the breakdown of bilirubin in the intestine; significant for anemias and malaria; normal is small amount
10. Automated (Clinitek) method
    a. Analyzer that automatically reads reagent strips
    b. Based on the principle of photometry
    c. Timing and color interpretation are consistent
    d. Results are printed out

E. Microscopic Examination

1. Consists of examining, counting, and categorizing solid material found in urine
2. Standardized method (KOVA urine sediment system) is used
3. Sample is centrifuged, supernatant (liquid portion) is poured off, and sediment is stained
4. MA may prepare the slide; the practitioner interprets the results; the lab has to be certified for this type of testing
   a. Examined under low power (10 ×)
   b. Examined under high power (40 ×) for cells and bacteria
   c. Examination includes
      1) RBCs: normal is zero to two per high-powered field (HPF); cells appear small, round, and clear
      2) WBCs: normal is zero to five per HPF; cells appear two to three times the size of RBCs and round with a grainy appearance
      3) Epithelial cells
         a) Squamous epithelial cells: normal; not significant unless a large quantity per HPF; appear approximately the same size as WBCs
         b) Renal epithelial cells: normal is zero per HPF; presence indicates renal tubule destruction; appear round and grainy, approximately twice the size of WBCs

4) Bacteria: normal is a few per HPF; more indicates UTI; appear as tiny grains
5) Yeast: normal is a few per HPF; more indicates yeast infection (*Candida albicans*); appear as round, clear bodies; some have buds (hyphae); may be confused with RBCs
6) Mucous threads: wavy, threadlike structures
7) Spermatozoa: appear as small oval bodies, with tail; normal in males after intercourse, indicate contamination in females
8) Casts: structures formed in nephron tubules; material solidifies in tubules and may contain cells, fats, and bacteria; normal is zero to two per low-powered field (LPF); appear as cylindrical bodies, longer than wide; types include
   a) Hyaline: colorless and semitransparent
   b) Fatty cast: contains fat globules
   c) RBC cast: orange-yellow in color
   d) WBC cast: contains WBCs
   e) Granular cast: sandlike granules
   f) Waxy cast: yellowish, wide cast with irregular edges
9) Crystals
   a) Normal crystals found in acidic urine
      (1) Uric acid: appears lemon shaped
      (2) Calcium oxalate: square shape with an "X"
   b) Normal crystals found in alkaline urine
      (1) Triple phosphate: coffin-lid shaped
      (2) Calcium phosphate: flat plates
   c) Abnormal crystals found in acidic urine
      (1) Cystine: hexagonal plates
      (2) Tyrosine: fine needles
      (3) Leucine: yellow spheres
      (4) Sulfonamides: large needles in rosettes
      (5) Cholesterol: large, flat, and hexagonal plates with notched corners

F. Urine Pregnancy Testing

1. Detects the level of human chorionic gonadotropin (HCG)
2. Immunoassay test: rapid, qualitative detection of HCG in a urine specimen; 5 minutes for results; observe for color change on test cassette
3. Guidelines for urine pregnancy testing
   a. Use clean, disposable collection containers
   b. Use first-voided specimen if possible; refrigerate specimen if collected at home or cannot be tested immediately
   c. Test specimen at room temperature

G. Ovulation Testing

1. CLIA-waived test to predict ovulation
2. Detects luteinizing hormone (LH) levels approximately 14 days before menstruation (LH surge)
3. Ovulation usually occurs within 2–3 days of the surge

H. Menopause Testing

1. CLIA-waived test to detect follicle-stimulating hormone (FSH) in urine
2. Rise in FSH (positive test) can indicate a female has entered menopause

I. Toxicology

1. Tests for poisonous substances and drugs
2. Can test for illegal drugs and alcohol (preemployment, insurance, or legal reasons)

IV. Phlebotomy and Hematology

A. General

1. Study of blood and blood components

B. Blood Components

1. Part of the circulatory system
2. Functions as transport mechanism for nutrients, waste, and defense agents to tissues and cells
3. Specimens collected by venipuncture (anticoagulated specimens) or capillary puncture
4. Plasma
   a. Liquid portion of circulating, unclotted blood
      1) If allowed to clot, the liquid portion is called serum; serum contains no clotting factors (formed clot)
      2) Appears clear and light yellow
   b. 55% of total blood volume made up of
      1) 90% water
      2) 10% solutes (proteins, hormones, vitamins, carbohydrates, enzymes, lipids, and salts)
5. Formed elements
   a. Blood cells
   b. 45% of total blood volume made up of
      1) Erythrocytes (RBCs)
      2) Leukocytes (WBCs)
      3) Thrombocytes (platelets)

C. Collection of Specimens

1. Sample can be separated into components by centrifuging or settling
   a. Plasma
      1) Liquid component of circulating blood
   b. Buffy coat: consists of WBCs and platelets
   c. RBCs
2. Blood collection: vacutainer collection system
   a. Vacuum tubes with color-coded stoppers (Fig. 24.2)
   b. Tube used depends on the test to be performed on the sample
      1) Yellow stopper
         a) Used for serum collection
         b) Contains no additive
         c) Tube is sterile and used for bacteriologic testing
      2) Red stopper
         a) Used for serum collection
         b) Contains no additives
         c) Tube must sit for 15 minutes to allow a clot to form, then centrifuge
         d) Used for samples for chemistry and serology
      3) Tiger-speckled serum separator tube (SST)
         a) Red-and-black mottled stopper or gold stopper
         b) Used to collect serum

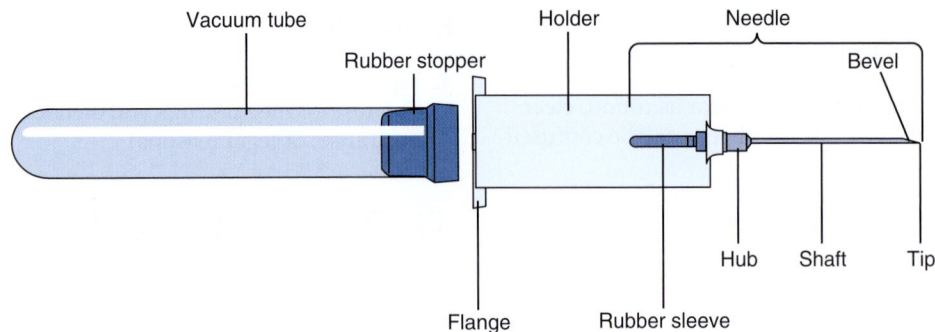

Fig. 24.2 Vacuum tube system. (Modified from Hunt SA: *Saunders fundamentals of medical assisting*, 2007, Saunders, revised reprint.)

Table 24.1 Vacuum Tube Table			
Colors of the Picture and the Plastic Vacutainer Tubes Placed in Order of Draw From Top to Bottom		**Additives**	**Laboratory Uses**
Blue sky	Blue topped	Citrate	Coagulation studies
Red rays and gold rays	Red-topped "clot tube"	Clot activator in plastic tubes (note: red glass tubes do not have clot activator)	Both yield serum commonly used for testing blood chemistry
	Gold-topped "SST tube"	Clot activator and gel	
Green grass	Green topped	Heparin (with lithium or sodium)	Special tests such as electrolytes
Lavender flowers	Lavender topped	EDTA	Hematology tests
Gray rocks	Gray topped	Oxalate	Glucose testing

EDTA, Ethylenediamine tetraacetic acid; *SST*, serum separator tube.
Modified from Garrels M: *Laboratory and diagnostic testing in ambulatory care: a guide for health professionals*, ed 4, 2019, Saunders.

c) Tube contains a silicon gel that creates a barrier between the serum and the clotted cells when centrifuged
d) Tube must sit for 15 minutes to allow a clot to form, then centrifuge
e) Used for the same purpose as red stopper
4) Lavender stopper
a) Used to collect plasma
b) Tube contains the anticoagulant ethylenediamine tetraacetic acid (EDTA)
c) Used for hematology
d) Tube must be gently mixed after collection
5) Blue stopper
a) Used to collect plasma
b) Contains anticoagulant sodium citrate
c) Used to perform coagulation testing
6) Green stopper
a) Used to collect plasma
b) Contains the anticoagulant sodium heparin
c) Used in chemistry for immediate (STAT) testing
7) Gray stopper
a) Contains the anticoagulant sodium fluoride
b) Used in chemistry for glucose testing and alcohol testing
3. Order of collection: when multiple tubes are to be collected, collect in the following order (Table 24.1)
a. Yellow stopper/blood culture bottle
b. Blue stopper
c. Red/SST stopper
d. Green stopper

e. Lavender stopper
f. Gray stopper
4. Venipuncture (phlebotomy) (Figs. 24.3 and 24.4)
a. Puncture of vein to withdraw blood sample
b. Usually performed on the median cubital vein in the antecubital area
1) Apply tourniquet approximately 3–4 inches above site; palpate and observe for the vein; release the tourniquet (do not leave the tourniquet on for >60 seconds)
2) Assemble all equipment
3) Reapply tourniquet
4) Glove; cleanse the site with an alcohol wipe, and allow it to dry
5) Anchor the vein; insert the needle at approximately 15 degrees, bevel up
6) Fill the syringe by slowly pulling back on the plunger or by inserting the vacuum tube onto the needle in the holder
7) As the blood fills, release the tourniquet
8) After collection is complete, place clean gauze over the site, and quickly withdraw the needle; instruct the patient to apply pressure to the site; apply a pressure dressing to the site
9) Label the specimen; dispose of the needle into a sharps container
5. Butterfly-winged infusion set
a. Used on small veins and for older adult and pediatric draws
b. Can be attached to a vacutainer collection system or syringe

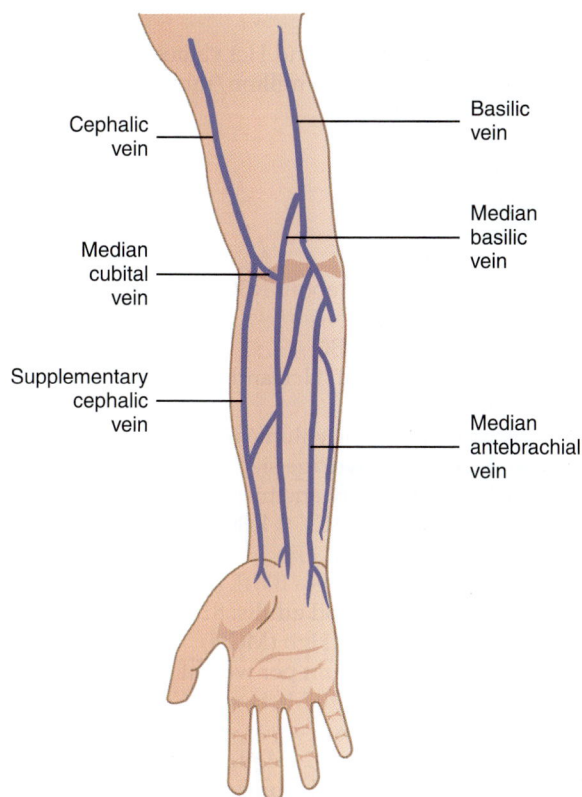

Fig. 24.3 Antecubital veins. (From Bonewit-West K: *Clinical procedures for medical assistants*, ed 10, 2019, Saunders.)

6. Syringe method
   a. Used on fragile veins that might collapse under the pressure of the vacutainer
   b. Same procedure as the vacutainer except the phlebotomist pulls back on the plunger to draw the blood into the syringe
   c. Blood can be seen entering the tip of the syringe as soon as the needle enters the vein (flash)
   d. Blood must be transferred into vacuum tubes quickly so it does not clot
7. Capillary puncture (Fig. 24.5)
   a. Used to collect small amounts of blood
   b. Sites include
      1) Middle or ring finger of nondominant hand
      2) Earlobe
      3) Heel or big toe on an infant
   c. Procedure
      1) Cleanse the site with alcohol, and allow it to dry
      2) Quickly puncture the skin with a lancet; wipe away the first drop of blood
      3) Collect a sample in the appropriate container

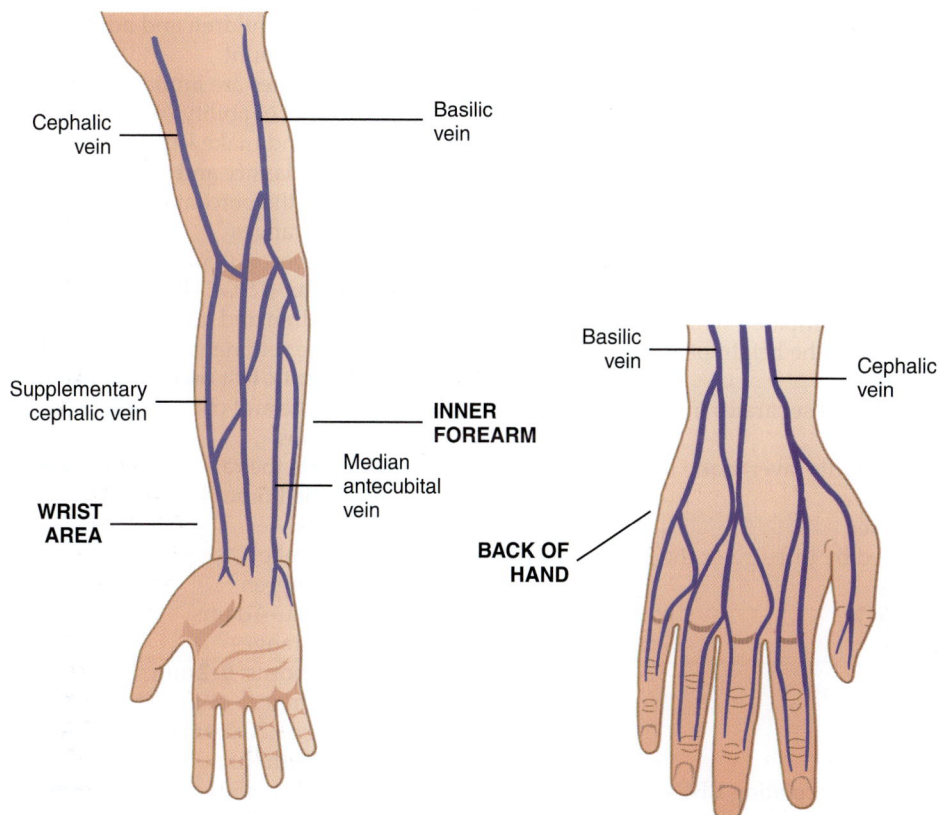

Fig. 24.4 Alternative venipuncture sites. (From Bonewit-West K: *Clinical procedures for medical assistants*, ed 10, 2019, Saunders.)

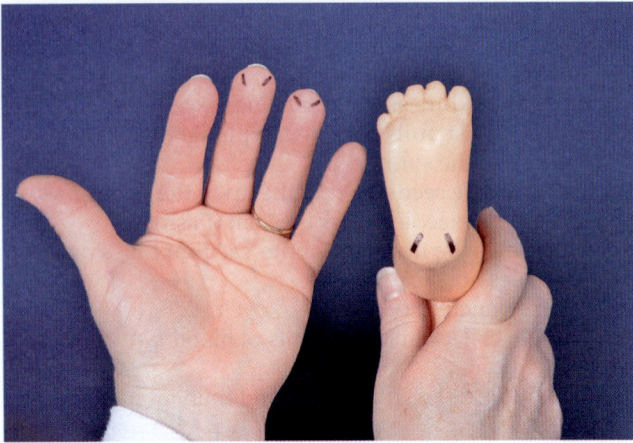

Fig. 24.5 Capillary puncture sites. (From Niedzwiecki B, et al: *Kinn's the clinical medical assistant: an applied learning approach*, ed 14, 2020, Elsevier.)

D. Testing on Erythrocytes

1. Hgb test
   a. Measures the total amount of Hgb in the blood
   b. Rapid indirect measurement of RBC count
   c. Evaluates patients with anemia
   d. Routine portion of complete blood count (CBC)
   e. Common CLIA-waived methods
      1) HemoCue
      2) Hgb meter
      3) i-STAT
   f. Normal Hgb ranges
      1) Newborns: 15–23 g/dL
      2) Infants: 9–14 g/dL
      3) Children: 10–15 g/dL
      4) Males: 15–18 g/dL
      5) Females: 12–16 g/dL
2. Hematocrit (Hct, microhematocrit, crit)
   a. Direct measurement of percentage of RBCs in total blood volume
   b. Indirect measurement of RBC number and volume
   c. Rapid measurement of RBC count
   d. Routine portion of CBC
   e. Height of RBC column is measured after the blood sample is centrifuged; compared with the height of the column of whole blood (the height of the column of whole blood is 100%)
   f. After centrifuging, blood separates into three layers
      1) Plasma (top) layer
      2) Buffy coat: thin middle layer made up of WBCs and platelets
      3) RBC (bottom) layer
   g. Hgb value multiplied by three gives the Hct value (±3)
   h. Normal Hct ranges
      1) Newborns: 44–64%
      2) Infants: 37–41%
      3) Children: 35–41%
      4) Males: 42–52%
      5) Females: 37–47%
3. RBC count
   a. Counts the number of circulating RBCs in 1 mm³ of peripheral venous blood

b. Routine portion of CBC
c. Closely related to Hgb and Hct values
d. Normal RBC ranges (in million/mm³)
   1) Newborns: 4.8–7.1
   2) Infants: 3.5–5.5
   3) Children: 4.5–4.8
   4) Males: 4.5–6
   5) Females: 4–5.5
4. Indices
   a. Provide information about RBC size, weight, and Hgb concentration
   b. Part of automated CBC
   c. Results of RBC count, Hct, and Hgb necessary to calculate indices
      1) Mean corpuscular volume (MCV)
         a) Measure of average size per volume of RBC
         b) Used to classify anemias
         c) Hct (%) × 10 MCV = RBC (in million/mm³)
         d) Normal ranges
            (1) Newborns: 96–108 fL (femtoliters)
            (2) Children and adults: 82–98 fL (femtoliters)
      2) Mean corpuscular Hgb (MCH)
         a) Measures amount per weight of Hgb within RBC
         b) Hgb (g/dL) × 10 MCH = RBC (in million/mm³)
         c) Normal ranges
            (1) Newborns: 32–34 picograms (pg)
            (2) Children and adults: 26–34 pg
      3) Mean corpuscular Hgb concentration (MCHC)
         a) Measure of average concentration per percentage of Hgb in single RBC
         b) Hgb (g/dL) × 100 Hct = g/dL or (%)
         c) Normal ranges
            (1) Newborns: 31–33 g/dL
            (2) Children and adults: 31–37 g/dL
5. Reticulocyte count
   a. Reticulocytes are immature RBCs
   b. Indication of ability of bone marrow to respond to anemia and make RBCs
   c. Used to classify and monitor anemia therapy
   d. Count is the percentage of the total number of RBCs
   e. Normal ranges
      1) Newborns: 0.5%–2% of total RBCs
      2) Infants: 0.5%–3.1% of total RBCs
      3) Children and adults: 0.5%–2% of total RBCs
6. Erythrocyte sedimentation rate (ESR; sed rate)
   a. Nonspecific test used to detect illnesses associated with acute and chronic infection, inflammation, and neoplasms
   b. Measures the rate at which RBCs settle in plasma over a specified time (1 hour)
   c. Methods
      1) Wintrobe
      2) Westergren
      3) Landau-Adams
   d. Normal ranges
      1) Newborns: 0–2 mm/hour
      2) Children: 0–10 mm/hour
      3) Males: <50 years = 0–15 mm/hour; >50 years = 0–20 mm/hr
      4) Females: <50 years = 0–2 mm/hour; >50 years = 0–30 mm/hour

E. Testing on Leukocytes

1. Mature cells vary in morphology depending on type
2. Neutrophil (segmented neutrophil [seg], poly, polymorphonuclear [PMN]): most numerous of granulocytes
3. Bands (stabs): immature form of segmented neutrophil
4. Eosinophil (eos): granulocyte
   a. Increase seen in allergic reactions, parasite infestation, and inflammation
5. Basophil (baso): granulocyte
   a. Increase seen in allergic reactions, radiation exposure, and after splenectomy
6. Monocytes (mono): agranulocyte
7. Lymphocyte (lymph): agranulocyte
   a. Increase seen in acute and chronic infections
8. Laboratory testing
   a. WBC count
      1) Measurement of the total number of WBCs
      2) Routine part of CBC
      3) Helps evaluate and diagnose infection, allergy, neoplasm, or immunosuppression
      4) Normal ranges
         a) Newborns: 9000–30,000/mm^3
         b) Children: 5000–13,000/mm^3
         c) Adults: 5000–10,000/mm^3
   b. Differential (diff)
      1) Measurement of different WBCs in a smear
      2) Can be performed manually or by automation
      3) Smear is stained with polychromatic stain (Wright stain)
      4) Preparation of smear
      5) Normal adult ranges
         a) Segs: 50–65
         b) Bands: 0–7
         c) Lymphs: 25–40
         d) Monos: 3–9
         e) Eos: 1–3
         f) Baso: 0–1

F. Thrombocytes

1. Platelet count test
   a. Actual count of the number of platelets in a cubic millimeter of blood
   b. Used to monitor the course of disease and therapy for thrombocytopenia and bone marrow failure
   c. Normal ranges
      1) Newborns: 140,000–300,000/mm^3
      2) Infants: 200,000–473,000/mm^3
      3) Children and adults: 150,000–400,000/mm^3
2. Bleeding time
   a. Measures platelet function by noting the length of time required for bleeding to stop
   b. Two methods
      1) Ivy method: small incision in the patient's arm
      2) Duke method: small incision in the patient's earlobe (not commonly performed)
      3) Normal range: 1–9 minutes for bleeding to stop
3. Prothrombin time (PT; also known as pro-time)
   a. Used to evaluate clotting mechanism
   b. Used to monitor warfarin (Coumadin) therapy
   c. Normal range: 11–12.5 seconds; international normalized ratio (INR) 2–2.5
4. Partial thromboplastin time (PTT)
   a. Used to evaluate the pathway to clot formation
   b. Used to monitor heparin therapy
   c. Normal range: 60–70 seconds

G. Complete Blood Count

1. Advanced concept
2. Consists of seven or more separate tests that reflect total count, analysis, and microscopic descriptions of the cellular elements of blood
3. Tests
   a. RBC count
   b. Hct
   c. RBC indices
   d. Hgb
   e. WBC count
   f. Differential smear
   g. Platelet count

V. Clinical Chemistry

A. General

1. Testing of the chemical analytes found in various liquid body specimens (urine, whole blood, serum, plasma, synovial fluid, pleural fluid, CSF)
2. Change in blood chemistry allows detection of confirmation of a diagnosis
3. Testing usually requires a serum sample
4. Tests may be ordered in groups (panels)

B. Lipids

1. Fats essential to the body
2. Before lipid testing, the patient should fast for 12–14 hours; the patient should consume no alcohol for 24 hours before the test; the patient should reduce fat intake for 2 weeks before the test
3. These tests can assess the risk of coronary and vascular disease
4. Lipid profile is made up of the following tests
   a. Cholesterol
      1) Fatty compound
      2) Necessary for production of sex hormones and bile
      3) Helps in the formation of cell membranes
      4) Normal reading: <200 mg/dL
   b. High-density lipoproteins
      1) "Good" cholesterol
      2) Removes excess cholesterol from cells and carries it back to the liver for excretions
      3) Normal reading: >50 mg/dL
   c. Low-density lipoproteins (LDLs)
      1) "Bad" cholesterol
      2) Picks up fat from liver and carries it in the blood
      3) Normal reading: <100 mg/dL
   d. Triglycerides
      1) Form fat in the bloodstream
      2) Transported in blood by LDLs

3) Make up most of the fat in the body
4) Normal reading: 30–150 mg/dL

C. Glucose

1. Simple sugar from the breakdown of carbohydrates
2. Provides energy for cells and tissues
3. Excess is stored as glycogen in the liver
4. Blood levels regulated by hormones produced by pancreas
   a. Glucagon: converts glycogen to glucose (increased blood levels)
   b. Insulin: transports glucose into cells (decreased blood levels)
5. Tests
   a. Fasting blood glucose (FBG)
      1) Testing done on blood sample of patient after fasting for 8–12 hours (water permitted)
      2) Test is commonly used in the diagnosis or evaluation of diabetes mellitus
      3) Normal range: 65–110 mg/dL
   b. Postprandial glucose (2-hour postprandial blood sugar [PPBS])
      1) Measures the amount of glucose in the patient's blood after a meal is ingested
      2) Blood level should return to the premeal range within 2 hours
      3) Normal range: 65–110 mg/dL
   c. Glucose tolerance test (GTT)
      1) Assists in the diagnosis of diabetes mellitus
      2) Patient's blood glucose levels are evaluated at fasting and 30, 60, 120, and 180 minutes after ingestion of a standard oral glucose solution
      3) Urine samples are evaluated at the same time
      4) Patient is to fast 12 hours before the test
      5) Fasting blood sugar is drawn
      6) Patient drinks 75 g of glucose solution
      7) Collect blood samples and urine samples 30, 60, 120, and 180 minutes (or any combination of these times) after the patient takes the glucose solution
      8) Patient may drink water during the test, but no coffee, tea, or tobacco permitted
      9) Normal glucose readings
         a) Fasting: 65–110 mg/dL
         b) 30 minutes: 200 mg/dL
         c) 1 hour: 200 mg/dL
         d) 2 hours: 140 mg/dL
         e) 3 hours: 65–115 mg/dL
6. Hgb A1c
   a. Glycosylated Hgb (sugar-coated Hgb)
   b. Provides an assessment of the average blood sugar during the 60–90 days before the test
   c. Performed every 3 months
   d. Normal range: 4%–5.6%

D. Electrolytes

1. Charged particles of the body
2. Includes
   a. Cation: positively charged ions
   b. Anion: negatively charged ions
3. Found in extracellular fluids

4. Body strives for neutrality (balance of anions and cations); if balance is not achieved, can be dangerous or fatal for the patient
5. Lungs and kidneys control the electrolyte balance
6. Functions of electrolytes
   a. Maintain water balance in the body
   b. Maintain pH of the body
   c. Help with blood coagulation
   d. Control neuromuscular excitability
7. Sodium (Na^+)
   a. Major extracellular cation
   b. Helps maintain osmotic pressure
   c. Low sodium level: hyponatremia
   d. High sodium level: hypernatremia
   e. Normal range: 135–146 mEq/L
8. Potassium (K^+)
   a. Major intracellular cation
   b. Influences muscle activity of the heart
   c. Works with sodium for acid-base balance
   d. Low K^+ level: hypokalemia
   e. High K^+ level: hyperkalemia
   f. Normal range: 3.5–5.3 mEq/L
9. Chloride (Cl^-)
   a. Major extracellular anion
   b. Counterbalances sodium for neutrality in body fluids
   c. Helps maintain osmotic pressure (water distribution between cells), plasma, and interstitial fluid
   d. Helps maintain acid-base balance
   e. Normal range: 98–108 mEq/L
10. Bicarbonate (HCO_3^-)
    a. Major anion
    b. Measured by blood carbon dioxide levels
    c. Works with Cl^-
    d. Normal range: 21–31 mEq/L

E. Bilirubin

1. Yellow pigment in bile
2. Comes from the heme portion of Hgb (heme is released when RBCs break down)
3. Two types
   a. Unconjugated (indirect): transported by albumin to the liver
   b. Conjugated (direct): becomes water soluble in the liver and enters the bile; transported to the small intestine, where it is converted into urobilinogen
4. Increased levels may indicate
   a. Destruction of RBCs
   b. Impaired liver function
   c. Obstruction of flow of bile
5. Exposure to ultraviolet light results in oxidation of bilirubin
6. Normal range: 0.1–1.2 mg/dL

F. Proteins

1. Make up muscles, enzymes, hormones, Hgb, and other important functional and structural substances in the body
2. Albumin
   a. Principal plasma protein

b. Found in the liver
c. Functions
  1) Maintenance of osmotic pressure
  2) Transportation of drugs, hormones, and enzymes
d. Can be a measure of nutritional status
e. Normal range: 3.5–5.0 g/dL
3. Globulin
  a. Building block of antibodies, lipids, and clotting factors
  b. Transport mechanism
  c. Can be a measure of nutritional status
  d. Normal range: 1.7–3.5 g/dL
4. Albumin-to-globulin (A/G) ratio
  a. Normal range: 1.1–2.5
5. Total protein
  a. Albumin plus globulin
  b. Component of osmotic pressure (keeps fluids within vascular system)
  c. Normal range: 6.0–8.5 g/dL

G. Nitrogenous Compounds

1. Forms of nitrogen in the body
2. Waste product of metabolism
3. Blood urea nitrogen (BUN)
  a. Main indicator of kidney function
  b. Urea is the main nonprotein nitrogen in blood
  c. Urea is formed in the liver and is the waste product of the breakdown of protein
  d. Normal range: 8–26 mg/dL
4. Creatinine
  a. End product of creatine metabolism in muscles
  b. Constantly being formed; the amount has a direct relationship to muscle mass
  c. Filtered by the kidneys and excreted in urine
  d. Reliable screening test for renal function
  e. Normal range: 0.7–1.4 mg/dL
5. Uric acid
  a. By-product of protein metabolism
  b. Blood levels from food metabolism (high-protein diet) and muscle tissue breakdown
  c. Normal range: 3.6–8.0 mg/dL in males; 2.5–6.8 mg/dL in females

H. Enzymes

1. Substances that speed up chemical reactions but remain unchanged themselves
2. Values expressed in international units (IU)
3. Always end with the suffix "-ase"
4. Can originate in cells, specific organs, or tissues
5. Release may be caused by damage or disease of tissues
6. Alanine aminotransferase (ALT)
  a. Formerly serum glutamic pyruvic transaminase (SGPT)
  b. Found in highly metabolic tissues (heart muscle, liver, skeletal muscles)
  c. Levels increase post–myocardial infarction (MI) (indication of MI)
  d. Normal range: 0–37 U/L in males; 0–31 U/L in females

7. Creatine phosphokinase (CPK, CK)
  a. Enzyme found in mitochondria of cells
  b. High concentration in the heart, skeletal muscles, and brain
  c. Useful in diagnosis of MI and muscle disease
  d. Normal range: 25–130 IU/L
8. Alkaline phosphatase (ALP)
  a. High concentration in the bone and liver
  b. Bone growth or liver disease can cause levels to increase
  c. Normal range: 117–390 U/L in children; 39–117 U/L in adults
9. Acid phosphatase
  a. Largest source is the prostate gland
  b. Elevated in prostate cancer
  c. Normal value: 0–0.8 IU/L

I. Minerals

1. Inorganic chemical elements needed in small amounts but essential for life
2. May be part of hormones or enzymes or work with vitamins
3. Calcium (Ca)
  a. Found in bone tissue
  b. Required for
    1) Bone development
    2) Cardiac function
    3) Blood clotting
    4) Transmission of nerve impulses
    5) Muscle contractions
  c. Normal range: 8.5–11.5 mg/dL
4. Phosphorus (P)
  a. Required for metabolism of protein, calcium, and glucose
  b. Combines with calcium
  c. Normal range: 2.5–4.5 mg/dL
5. Magnesium (Mg)
  a. Found in bone
  b. Binds with adenosine triphosphate (ATP) molecule for energy
  c. Required for
    1) Muscle action
    2) Nerve impulse transmission
    3) Calcium regulation
    4) Enzyme activity
  d. Normal range: 1.2–2.0 mEq/L

J. Thyroid

1. Triiodothyronine (T_3)
  a. Evaluates thyroid function (hyperthyroidism, hypothyroidism)
  b. Monitors thyroid replacement and suppressive therapy
  c. Normal range: 70–205 ng/dL
2. Thyroxine (tetraiodothyronine) (T_4)
  a. Initial test done for assessing thyroid function
  b. Used to diagnose thyroid function
  c. Used to monitor replacement and suppressive therapy
  d. Normal range: 4–12 µg/dL in males; 5–12 µg/dL in females

VI. Serology and Immunology

A. General

1. Tests done on serum to evaluate antigen-antibody reaction
2. Helps detect disease or amount of antibodies present (titer)
3. Some tests available in kit or rapid forms
4. Test reactions
   a. Precipitation: antigen-antibody complex visibly settles out of solution
   b. Agglutination: type of precipitation method that creates visible clumping

B. Infectious Mononucleosis

1. Disease caused by Epstein-Barr virus
2. Body produces heterophil antibodies in response
3. Tests (Monospot, QuickVue +) are designed to detect heterophil antibody

C. *Streptococcus*

1. Group A beta-hemolytic *Streptococcus* causes strep throat, rheumatic fever, and impetigo
2. Tests detect antibody antistreptolysin O (ASO)

D. Rheumatoid Factor

1. Group of proteins (autoantibodies)
2. Causes rheumatoid arthritis
3. Test detects antibodies against factor

E. Human Chorionic Gonadotropin

1. Hormone produced by the placenta
2. Test for hormone in blood and urine
3. Basis of pregnancy testing

F. Blood Groups

1. Blood cells are mixed with antisera; agglutination indicates the presence of antigens on RBCs
2. Can detect ABO group (A, B, AB, O)
3. Can detect Rh (Rh+, Rh−)

G. Syphilis

1. Antibody test for *Treponema pallidum*
2. Tests
   a. Rapid plasma reagin (RPR)
   b. Venereal Disease Research Laboratory (VDRL)

H. Systemic Lupus Erythematosus

1. Testing to detect antinuclear antibodies (ANA)

I. *Helicobacter pylori*

1. Spiral-shaped bacteria believed to be the cause of most peptic ulcers
2. QuickVue *H. pylori* gII test is performed from a finger stick

J. Human Immunodeficiency Virus (HIV)

1. Virus attacks and destroys T helper (CD4) lymphocytes
2. Enzyme-linked immunosorbent assay (ELISA) detects antibodies
3. Antibodies can also be detected in oral specimens (OraQuick)

K. Antibody Titer

1. Laboratory-based quantitative test to determine the amount of antibody in blood
2. Examples: rubella, hepatitis B, and varicella

VII. Microbiology

A. General

1. Study of microorganisms
2. Includes
   a. Bacteria
   b. Fungi
   c. Viruses
   d. Rickettsiae
   e. Mycobacteria
   f. Parasites
3. Main objective is to identify the organism so that the practitioner can treat the patient properly
4. Collection of most common specimens
   a. Throat culture
      1) Use a sterile swab and swab the back of the throat in a rainbow or figure-8 pattern
      2) Collect any material in the area
      3) Transport or send the specimen to the laboratory using a transport medium or streak immediately
   b. Urine culture
      1) Clean-catch specimen in a sterile container
      2) Use a sterile loop to streak the plate
   c. Genitourinary culture
      1) Collect a specimen using a sterile swab
      2) Roll the swab over the plate in a "Z" or "W" pattern
      3) Streak across the "Z" or "W," using a sterile loop
   d. Blood culture
      1) Collect a specimen in a yellow-stoppered tube
      2) Cleanse the skin with povidone-iodine (Betadine) before venipuncture
      3) Inject approximately 10 mL of the specimen into two separate blood culture bottles
   e. Wound culture
      1) Collect a specimen with a sterile swab
      2) Streak the plate using the "Z" or "W" method
5. Fecal culture
   a. Collect a specimen in a clean container
   b. Streak the plate with a sterile loop

B. Classification of Organisms

1. Scientific study of classification process is taxonomy
2. Simple, orderly method
3. Places organisms into categories according to similar morphologic and biochemical properties

a. Species: basic unit; based on reproduction (members of the same species can mate successfully)
b. Genus: share biologic likenesses
c. Family: similar genera
d. Order: related families
e. Class: related orders
f. Phylum: classes with common characteristics

4. Organisms in laboratory setting have two separate names
   a. Genus: name is capitalized; often abbreviated, using the first initial
   b. Species: name in lowercase
5. Both names are underlined or italicized when written

C. Bacteria (Bacteriology)

1. Characteristics: help with the identification of organisms in the laboratory (Fig. 24.6)
   a. Shape
      1) Cocci: round (singular: coccus)
      2) Bacilli: rod shaped (singular: bacillus)
      3) Vibrio: comma shaped
      4) Spirilla: spiral shaped (singular: spirillum)
   b. Arrangement
      1) Diplo: arranged in pairs
      2) Strepto: arranged in chains
      3) Staphylo: arranged in grapelike clusters
      4) Tetra: four cocci together in capsule
   c. Staining properties
      1) Gram stain
         a) Gram positive: stain blue or dark purple
         b) Gram negative: stain pink or red
      2) Acid-fast stain: type of stain used on bacteria that are difficult to stain with other stains
   d. Oxygen requirements
      1) Aerobic: requires oxygen to survive
      2) Anaerobic: requires no oxygen to survive
      3) Facultative: can survive in either environment
   e. Colony growth
      1) Size
      2) Color
      3) Shape
      4) Elevation
      5) Texture
      6) Margins
      7) Hemolysis (present or absent)

f. Chemical reactions: bacteria respond differently to chemical reagents

2. Bacterial growth requirements
   a. Nutrients: differ among species
   b. Temperature: usually thrive at normal body temperature (98.6°F [37°C])
   c. Oxygen: differs among species (aerobic or anaerobic)
   d. pH: human pathogens thrive at pH of 7 (neutral); blood, milk, and seawater are neutral
   e. Sterile: medium must be sterile and uncontaminated for use
   f. Moisture: most bacteria require some level of moisture

3. Culture and sensitivity (C&S)
   a. Determines an organism's susceptibility to selected antibiotics
   b. Streak the plate with culture; cover the entire plate, rotating 45 degrees between each streak
   c. Apply antibody disks using a dispenser or sterile forceps; make sure the disk is in contact with the medium
   d. Incubate; check after 24 hours
   e. Measure the zones of inhibition around each disk; compare with the chart provided by the manufacturer
   f. Report the results

D. Mycology

1. Study of fungus
2. Medical mycology fungal forms
   a. Molds
      1) Multicellular organisms made up of hyphae
      2) Produce powdery, fuzzy, or fluffy colonies on media
   b. Yeasts
      1) Single-cell organisms
      2) Multiply by budding
      3) Produce moist, creamy colonies on media
3. Identification methods
   a. Potassium hydroxide (KOH) preparation
      1) Place the specimen on a slide
      2) Mix KOH with the specimen and allow to sit for 15–20 minutes
      3) Observe under low power
   b. India ink
      1) Helps identify capsules
      2) Mix bodily fluid with ink on the slide

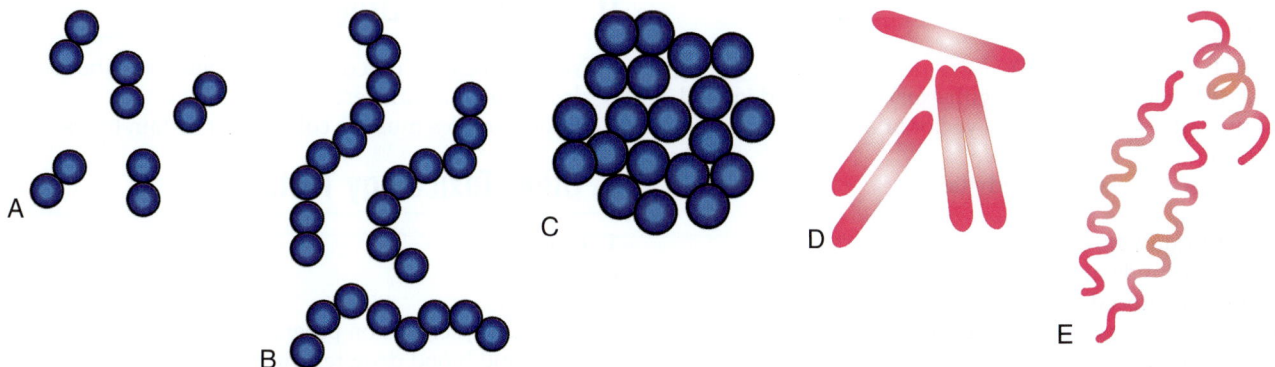

Fig. 24.6 Classification of bacteria by shape and grouping: (A) diplococci, (B) streptococci, (C) staphylococci, (D) bacilli, and (E) spirilla. (From Garrels M: *Laboratory and diagnostic testing in ambulatory care: a guide for health professionals*, ed 4, 2019, Saunders.)

3) Observe under low power
4) Cells appear to have halo around them

E. Virology

1. Study of viruses
2. Intracellular parasites that require a host to carry out their functions
3. Do not have cellular structure (nucleic acid and protein layer)
4. Reproductive by replication

F. Parasitology

1. Study of parasites
2. Organisms that live in or on a host and derive nourishment from the host
3. Can be one-celled (protozoa) or many-celled (helminths) parasites
4. Relationships
   a. Commensalism: neither organism harmed; one benefits
   b. Mutualism: both organisms benefit
   c. Parasitism: one organism benefits at the expense of the other
   d. Symbiosis: dependent relationship between two dissimilar organisms
5. Infection: invasion of microscopic parasites causing disease
6. Infestation: external or internal invasion of animal-like parasites
7. Classifications
   a. Protozoa: unicellular organisms
      1) Transmission
         a) Ingestion of cysts in fecally contaminated water or food
         b) Become adults after infection; they multiply in the intestine and are passed in feces
      2) Ameba
         a) Move by means of pseudopods (false foot)
      3) Flagellates
         a) Move by flagella
      4) Ciliates
         a) Move by cilia
      5) Sporozoans
         a) Have sexual and asexual reproductive cycles
   b. Helminths: parasitic worms
      1) Nematodes: roundworms
      2) Cestodes: tapeworms
      3) Trematodes (flukes)
   c. Arthropods: organisms with exoskeletons and jointed appendages; can serve as vector or as intermediate host
      1) Insects: head and body lice
      2) Fleas
      3) Mosquitoes
      4) Arachnids: itch mite
8. Diagnostic procedures
   a. Ova and parasites (O&P): examination of feces for ova and parasites
      1) Collect a sample in a clean, dry container; do not allow the specimen to touch water or urine

2) Scoop out an amount of specimen and place in the prepared specimen containers as directed by the manufacturer
   b. Cellophane-tape test
      1) Pinworm diagnosis
         a) Affix tape onto the end of a slide and drape over the slide so that the adhesive side faces outward
         b) Gently touch the anal area with the adhesive side of the tape
         c) Undrape the tape and stick it to the slide
         d) Send the slide with tape on it to the laboratory

VIII. Toxicology

A. General

1. Tests for levels of both therapeutic and drugs of abuse
2. May also test for other poisons (e.g., lead)
3. Testing performed on blood, urine, and stomach contents

B. Drug Screening

1. MA may collect specimens to be sent to the lab
2. Reasons for drug screenings may include
   a. Cause of symptoms in an emergency situation (drug overdose)
   b. Drug use in the workplace, schools, and preemployment
3. CLIA-waived drug screening tests available for in-office screening

C. Common Drugs of Abuse That Can Be Detected in Urine Drug Screening

1. Cocaine
2. Amphetamines
3. Methamphetamines
4. Marijuana
5. Methadone
6. Opiates
7. Oxycodone
8. Barbiturates
9. Benzodiazepines
10. Lysergic acid diethylamide
11. Phencyclidine

D. Therapeutic Drug Monitoring

1. Measures effects of a drug on the patient or the levels of drug being administered to the patient
2. Blood samples must be collected at certain times

E. Other Toxicology Tests

1. Lead
2. Iron
3. Mercury
4. Urine drug screens on pregnant females
5. Urine and blood drug testing on employees for on-the-job injuries to rule out impairment; may also test for other poisons (e.g., lead) of abuse

IX. Other Specimen Collection

A. Cerebrospinal Fluid

1. Fluid that surrounds the brain and spinal cord
2. Normal CSF is clear and colorless
3. Collected by lumbar puncture procedure between L3, L4, and L5
4. Fluid may be cultured for bacteria, analyzed for chemical components (glucose and protein), or tested for the presence of blood cells

B. Serous Fluids

1. Include pericardial, pleural, and peritoneal fluids
2. Normal fluids appear clear or light yellow
3. May be tested for chemical components, cultured and smeared for bacteria, or tested for cell counts

C. Synovial Fluid

1. Fluid that lines and lubricates joints
2. Normal fluid appears yellow and viscous
3. Collected through joint puncture
4. May be cultured, analyzed for cells and crystals, and tested for glucose and protein

D. Feces

1. Collected in a clean container
2. Avoid contamination from water or urine
3. Tests
   a. Occult blood (stool guaiac test)
      1) Detects hidden blood
      2) Helps diagnosis of cancer or bleeding
      3) Hemoccult; ColoScreen
   b. O&P: detects eggs and parasites in the intestinal tract
   c. Culture: detects microorganisms

E. Sputum

1. Secretions of trachea and bronchi
2. Avoid contamination with saliva and nasal secretions
3. Patient is instructed to cough deeply into the container for the culture

F. Other Secretions

1. Collected with sterile swabs for cultures
   a. Wound secretions
   b. Throat secretions
   c. Genital secretions

X. Reference Values for Common Laboratory Tests

A. Normal Urine Reference Values

1. Volume (mL/24 hours)
   a. Newborns: 20–350 mL
   b. Children: 300–1500 mL
   c. Adults: 750–2000 mL
2. Physical and chemical components
   a. Color: straw to amber, light to dark
   b. Turbidity: clear to slightly hazy
   c. SG: 1.005–1.030
   d. pH: 4.6–8.0
   e. Protein: negative to trace
   f. Glucose: negative
   g. Ketone: negative
   h. Bilirubin: negative
   i. Blood: negative
   j. Urobilinogen: 0.1 EU/dL
   k. Bacteria (nitrates): negative
   l. Leukocytes: negative
3. Urine: sediment
   a. RBCs/HPF: rare
   b. WBCs/LPF: 0–4
   c. Epithelial cells/HPF: occasional
   d. Casts/LPF: occasional
   e. Bacteria: negative
   f. Mucus: negative to 2+
   g. Crystals: only cystine, leucine, and tyrosine are significant

B. Normal Blood Chemistry Reference Values

1. ALT (SGPT): 4–36 U/L
2. Albumin: 3.5–5 g/dL
3. ALP: 30–120 U/L
4. Aspartate transaminase (or serum glutamate-oxaloacetate transaminase): 0–35 U/L
5. Bicarbonate: 21–28 mEq/L
6. Bilirubin (total): 0.3–1 mg/dL
7. BUN: 10–20 mg/dL
8. Calcium: 9–10.5 mg/dL
9. Cholesterol: <200 mg/dL
10. Creatinine: 0.5–1.2 mg/dL
11. C-reactive protein: <1 mg/dL
12. Gamma-glutamyl transferase: 8–38 U/L
13. Glucose: 70–105 mg/dL
14. Iron: 60–180 μg/dL
15. Phosphorus: 3–4.5 mg/dL
16. Potassium: 3.5–5 mEq/L
17. Sodium: 136–145 mEq/L
18. T_3: 75–220 μg/dL
19. T_4: 4–12 μg/dL
20. Total protein (albumin/globulin): 6.4–8.3 mg/dL
21. Uric acid: 2.7–8.5 mg/dL

C. Normal Hematology Reference Values

1. Hgb
   a. Adult males: 14–18 g/dL
   b. Adult females: 12–16 g/dL
2. Hematocrit
   a. Adult males: 42%–52%
   b. Adult females: 37%–47%
3. WBC count
   a. Adults: 5000–10,000/mm^3

4. RBC count
   a. Adult males: 4.7–6.1 million/mm^3
   b. Adult females: 4.2–5.4 million/mm^3
5. RBC indices
   a. MCV: 80–90 μm^3/cell
   b. MCH: 27–31/RBC
   c. MCHC: 32%–36%
6. Platelet count
   a. Adults: 150,000–400,000/mm^3
7. ESR: Wintrobe
   a. Adult males: 0–9 mm/hour
   b. Adult females: 0–20 mm/hour

8. PT: 11–12.5 seconds
9. PTT: 25–38 seconds
10. Bleeding time (Ivy): 1–9 minutes
11. Differential leukocyte count
    a. Neutrophil: 55%–70%
    b. Eosinophil: 1%–4%
    c. Basophil: 0.5%–1%
    d. Monocyte: 2%–8%
    e. Lymphocyte: 20%–40%

25

First Aid and Office Emergencies

I. First Aid

A. General

1. Immediate, temporary care given to a person who has been injured or suddenly taken ill
2. A medical assistant, in emergencies, is covered by Good Samaritan laws at the scene of an accident
3. Keep emergency telephone numbers near telephones in the office
4. As an employee of a medical facility, keep cardiopulmonary resuscitation (CPR) and first-aid cards current
5. Do not provide care beyond your scope of training or beyond your abilities
6. Call for help or 911 when needed

II. Guidelines for Providing Emergency Care

A. General

1. Know your limits and do only what is in your scope of practice
2. Stay calm; speak in a normal tone of voice; explain what has happened
3. Practice standard precautions and follow Occupational Safety and Health Administration (OSHA) blood-borne pathogens standards
4. Assess the situation quickly; check for possibilities of life-threatening injuries
   a. Use the ABC method to assess patient
      1) Airway
      2) Breathing
      3) Circulation
5. Know how to contact emergency response (911)
6. Do not move the patient unless he or she is in harm's way
7. Keep the patient warm
8. Look for medical alert tags
9. Move bystanders away from the patient
10. Do not leave the patient until emergency medical personnel have arrived and taken over; provide information from your observations

III. Common Emergencies in the Medical Office

A. Fainting (Syncope)

1. Lay or sit the patient with the patient's head lower than the heart
2. Loosen the patient's tight clothing
3. Maintain an open airway
4. Apply a cool cloth to the patient's head
5. Pass aromatic spirits of ammonia under the patient's nose
6. Keep the patient supine for 10 minutes after consciousness is regained

B. Choking

1. Do not interfere if the patient can speak, cough, or breathe
2. Use the Heimlich maneuver if the victim cannot speak, cough, or breathe
3. If the patient becomes unconscious, position the patient on his or her back; call for help
4. Begin CPR after removing the foreign body

C. Chest Pain

1. Sit the patient down
2. Keep the patient quiet and warm
3. Loosen the patient's tight clothing
4. Take the apical and radial pulse
5. Administer oxygen if the practitioner orders
6. Bring the emergency (crash) cart into the room
7. If cardiac arrest occurs, perform CPR

D. Cerebrovascular Accident (CVA)

1. Call for help
2. Protect the patient against injury while waiting for transport
3. Keep the patient lying down
4. Maintain an open airway
5. Do not give food or water

E. Poisoning

1. Ask what was taken, how much was taken, how long ago, and whether vomiting has occurred
2. Call the Poison Control Center
3. Induce vomiting (unless a corrosive had been ingested) or dilute with 1 to 2 cups of water or milk; give 1 tablespoon of syrup of ipecac (or follow specific directions given by the Poison Control Center)

F. Animal Bites

1. Thoroughly wash the wound with soap and water
2. Report the bite to the authorities

G. Insect Bites and Stings

1. Remove the stinger by brushing it off or using tweezers
2. Apply ice to the bite area
3. Be aware of patient allergy to insect bites or stings
4. If the patient is allergic and shows signs of shock or difficulty breathing, a true emergency exists

H. Shock

1. Ensure and maintain an open airway
2. Call 911
3. While waiting for transport, place the patient on his or her back with legs elevated above the heart
4. Loosen the patient's tight clothing
5. Cover the patient with a blanket to maintain warmth

I. Asthma Attack

1. Assist the patient with an inhaler
2. Encourage and assist the patient to relax
3. Patient may breathe into a paper bag if hyperventilating

J. Seizures

1. Lay the patient on his or her back
2. Loosen the patient's tight clothing
3. Do not restrain the patient

4. Do not place anything between the patient's teeth
5. Protect the patient's head from injury
6. Give the patient nothing by mouth
7. Let the patient rest after the seizure subsides

K. Sprain

1. Begin treatment within 10–20 minutes of the injury
2. RICE
   a. *R*est the injured area
   b. *I*ce the area
   c. *C*ompress the area by wrapping it with an elastic bandage
   d. *E*levate the injured area

L. Fractures

1. Make the patient as comfortable as possible
2. Prevent movement of the injured area
3. Apply ice
4. Control bleeding, if applicable
5. Assist the health care provider

M. Burns

1. Remove the patient's clothing from the burned area
2. Stay with the patient
3. Assist the health care provider

N. Lacerations

1. Keep the patient as calm as possible
2. Cover the area with a sterile dressing using standard precautions
3. Apply direct pressure to the wound to control bleeding using standard precautions
4. Elevate the injured area above the level of the patient's heart
5. Ask the patient about when the last tetanus injection was given
6. Cleanse the wound if it is not bleeding severely
7. Assist the health care provider

O. Nosebleed (Epistaxis)

1. Keep the patient quiet and in a sitting position
2. Apply direct pressure to the affected nostril by pinching

P. Hemorrhage

1. Apply direct pressure over the area; do not remove the original pad when it becomes saturated; add additional pads
2. Elevate the injured part above the patient's heart
3. Apply pressure over the area's pressure point
4. As a last resort, apply a tourniquet as directed by the health care provider
5. Assist the health care provider

Q. Head Injuries

1. Lay the patient flat
2. Do not move the patient if a neck injury is suspected

3. Do not give the patient anything by mouth
4. Keep the patient warm and quiet
5. Watch the patient's pupils for changes
6. Assist the health care provider

R. Diabetic Emergencies

1. For hypoglycemia (insulin shock): give juice, candy, or soda (a sugar source)
2. For hyperglycemia (diabetic coma): if the patient is conscious, administer fluids; if you are uncertain whether this is insulin shock or diabetic coma, give the patient a sugar source
3. Assist the health care provider

S. Foreign Body in the Eye

1. Place the patient in a darkened room
2. Apply a cool, wet compress to the affected eye; do not apply pressure
3. Assist the health care provider

IV. Basic Medical Office Emergency Cart (Crash Cart)

A. Equipment and Supplies (Fig. 25.1)

1. Defibrillator: automated external defibrillator (AED) (Figs. 25.2 and 25.3)
2. Oxygen tank, tubing, mask, and nasal cannula
3. Airways
4. Ambu bag
5. Intravenous supplies
6. Intravenous fluids
7. Gloves (sterile, nonsterile)
8. Scissors (bandage, operative)
9. Syringes and needles
10. Biohazard containers
11. Sterile gauze squares (2×2 inches, 4×4 inches)
12. Penlight
13. Pen and paper
14. Pocket mask
15. Kling dressings
16. Blood pressure cuff and stethoscope

B. Medications

1. Adenosine
2. Aminophylline
3. Atropine
4. Albuterol

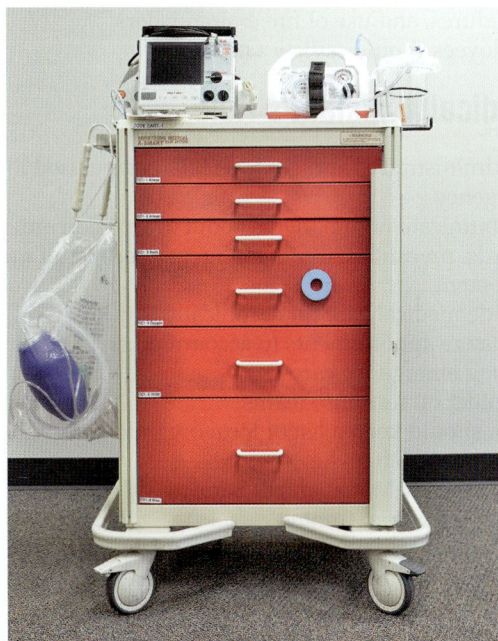

Fig. 25.2 Fully automated external defibrillator.

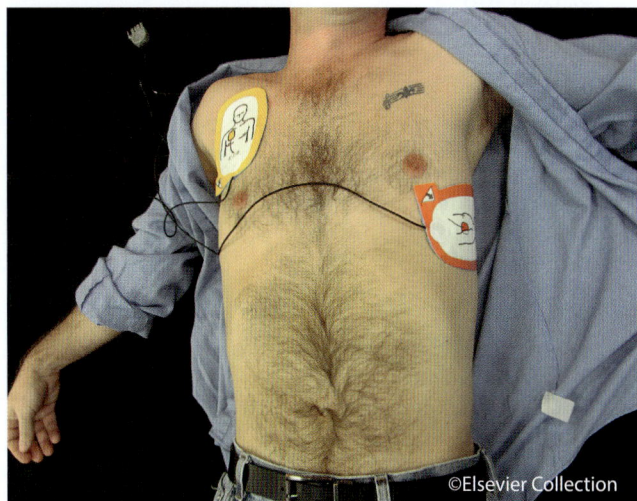

Fig. 25.1 Office emergency cart with defibrillator. (From Niedzwiecki B, et al: *Kinn's The medical assistant: an applied learning approach*, ed 14, 2020, Elsevier.)

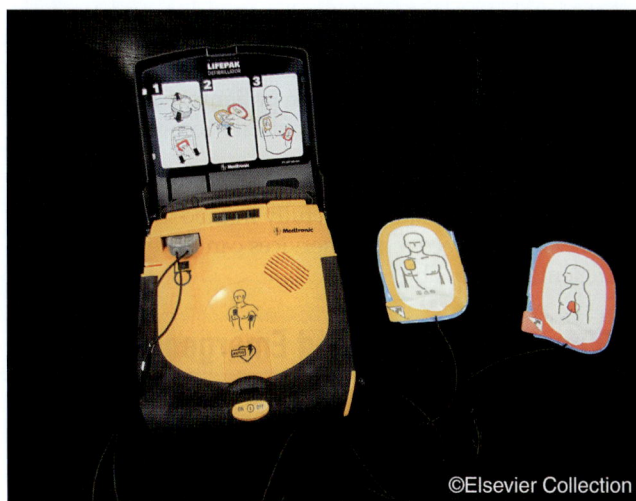

Fig. 25.3 Connect the adhesive pads to the automatic external defibrillator and apply them to the patient.

5. Diazepam
6. Digoxin
7. Benadryl
8. Dopamine
9. Adrenalin
10. Lasix
11. Lidocaine
12. Narcan
13. Solu-Medrol
14. Dilantin
15. Sodium bicarbonate
16. Activated charcoal
17. Ammonia inhalants
18. Glucose or glucagon

V. Emergency Preparedness

A. Definition

1. Act of making plans to prevent, respond to, and recover from emergencies
2. Coordinated actions to meet the needs of a community
3. May cause damage or threaten patients, employees, and buildings with harm or inability to provide usual services
4. Each facility will have its own requirements and expectations; staff should be fully trained
5. Goal: facilitate recovery so services can be restored as efficiently as possible

B. Types of Disasters and Emergencies

1. Natural disasters
   a. Results from a natural hazard that occurs with or without warning
   b. Can cause significant damage to the environment
   c. Examples
      1) Earthquakes
      2) Floods
      3) Heat waves
      4) Hurricanes
      5) Tornadoes
      6) Winter storms
      7) Wildfires
2. Man-made disasters
   a. Serious damage caused either directly or indirectly by negligent or intentional human actions or failure of a man-made system
   b. Includes
      1) Crimes
      2) Fires
      3) Structural collapse
      4) Power outage
      5) Chemical contamination
      6) Radiation hazards
      7) Terrorism

C. Psychological Effects of Serious Emergencies

1. Stress
   a. Body's response to change or threat
   b. Four-part general adaptation syndrome (GAS): alarm reaction, resistance, recovery, and exhaustion
2. Anxiety
   a. Feeling of uneasiness or worry triggered by an event with an uncertain outcome
   b. Can manifest as an anxiety attack: hyperventilation, rapid heart rate, and unresponsiveness
3. Posttraumatic stress disorder (PTSD)
   a. Emotional disturbance that develops after a traumatic/catastrophic event

D. Emergency Management

1. Mitigation: prevent or minimize emergencies
2. Preparedness: actions taken to enable future responses
3. Response: plans put into action
4. Recovery: activities to help a community return to normal

E. Emergency Action Plan

1. Written emergency action plan required by OSHA
2. Plan must include
   a. Means of reporting fires
   b. Evacuation procedures and escape routes
   c. Procedures for employees who remain
   d. Way to account for all employees after evacuation
   e. Destination of medical and rescue duties
   f. Secure location to store essential records

F. Training Employees

1. Orientation at hiring
2. Should include evacuation plan, alarm systems, reporting procedures, and use of fire extinguishers
3. Employees should review annually

G. Medical Assistant's Role

1. All administrative and clinical skills can be used in an emergency
2. Communicate with patients about evacuation orders, hazards, precautions, and emergency sources of medical equipment
3. Provide medical care for chronically ill patients
4. Rearrange appointments to accommodate patients needing emergency care
5. Volunteer on response teams
6. Office should keep a list of local organizations with telephone numbers for
   a. Emergency Management Services (911)
   b. Poison Control Center
   c. Telephone numbers of local hospitals
   d. Telephone numbers of local and state health departments
   e. Telephone number for HAZMAT team

Posttest

Directions: Select the *best* response.

1. An agent that prevents the growth, development, or proliferation of malignant cells is an:
   A. Antitussive
   B. Antineoplastic
   C. Anticoagulant
   D. Antidepressant

2. Which of the following is most likely to reduce patient satisfaction with a medical practice?
   A. Explaining the risks and benefits of a procedure
   B. Discussing fees
   C. Overbooking
   D. Taking notes while interviewing the patient

3. If a patient refuses to consent to treatment, the medical assistant should:
   A. Schedule the patient for another appointment
   B. Force treatment on the patient
   C. Force the patient to consent
   D. Delay treatment and inform or consult with the physician

4. Which of the following telephone calls should be given immediately to the physician?
   A. Another physician
   B. An angry patient
   C. A patient's family member
   D. An insurance company

5. Blood that is low in oxygen exits the heart through the:
   A. Aorta
   B. Pulmonary artery
   C. Pulmonary vein
   D. Inferior vena cava

6. Which of the following is a segment of the large intestine?
   A. Pylorus
   B. Cecum
   C. Duodenum
   D. Jejunum

7. Personality differences are due to:
   A. Experience
   B. Heredity
   C. Environment
   D. All of the above

8. The combining form for uterus is:
   A. Vagin/o
   B. Hyster/o
   C. Salping/o
   D. Oophor/o

9. Professionalism may best be displayed by:
   A. Displaying emotions
   B. Staying calm when dealing with angry patients
   C. Showing no consideration for other members of the team
   D. Referring all problems to the physician

10. Legally, a physician:
    A. May refuse to provide follow-up care after initial treatment
    B. Must provide a diagnosis to a patient's employer if requested
    C. Must provide a medical history to the patient's insurance company if the insurance company requests it
    D. May refuse to accept a patient if he or she chooses

11. These tiny projections on the surface of the small intestines increase the surface area and allow for greater absorption of nutrients.
    A. Rugae
    B. Villi
    C. Diverticula
    D. Omenta

12. The alpha cells in the pancreas are responsible for the production of:
    A. Insulin
    B. Glucagon
    C. Hydrochloric acid
    D. Pepsin

13. Release of a patient's medical records without proper authorization might result in charges of:
    A. Abandonment
    B. Invasion of privacy
    C. Defamation of character
    D. Negligence

14. *Res ipsa loquitur* is best illustrated by which of the following?
    A. A physician accidentally amputates the wrong finger from a patient
    B. A physician diagnoses lung cancer, but the patient continues to smoke
    C. A physician prescribes the wrong medication for a patient
    D. A physician terminates care of a patient but does notify him or her in writing

15. Which of the following is an example of an open-ended question?
    A. "Have you been staying on your diet?"
    B. "Did you have a nice trip?"
    C. "Are you single or married?"
    D. "Can you tell me more about that?"

16. A failure of bone marrow to produce red blood cells results in which type of anemia?
    A. Aplastic
    B. Hemolytic
    C. Pernicious
    D. Microcytic

17. According to Maslow's hierarchy of needs, which of the following is the primary motivation for human behavior?
    A. Survival
    B. Safety
    C. Love
    D. Self-actualization

18. The bone located in the posterior of the skull is the:
    A. Frontal
    B. Ethmoid
    C. Temporal
    D. Occipital

19. Spermatozoa are produced in the:
    A. Epididymis
    B. Seminiferous tubules
    C. Prostate gland
    D. Vas deferens

20. Which of the following is the most effective way of communicating with a patient who does not speak English?
    A. Speaking slowly and loudly
    B. Encouraging nonverbal communication
    C. Maintaining eye contact with the patient
    D. Putting messages in writing

21. A mucous membrane:
    A. Lines closed cavities of the body
    B. Covers the lungs
    C. Lines the abdominal cavity
    D. Lines body cavities that open to the outside of the body

22. Which of the following punctuation marks is used to indicate the exact words of the patient?
    A. Semicolon
    B. Comma
    C. Quotation marks
    D. Colon

23. Tingling in the hands, numbness in the arm, and frequent episodes of blurred vision are characteristic of:
    A. Epilepsy
    B. Tourette syndrome
    C. Lou Gehrig disease
    D. Transient ischemic attack

24. A patient whose husband recently died comes into the office because of malaise. She is unkempt and weepy. She tells the medical assistant that she wishes she were dead. Which of the following would be the most sensitive response to this patient?
    A. "Please tell me more about those feelings."
    B. "Why is that?"
    C. "You need to talk to the doctor about this."
    D. "It's natural to feel that way after the death of a spouse."

25. Ischemia is:
    A. An irregular heartbeat
    B. Dilation of the aorta
    C. Lack of blood flow to tissue
    D. Infection of the myocardium

26. The best method for transmitting confidential information from one medical practice to another is by:
    A. Fax
    B. E-mail
    C. Cellular telephone
    D. Answering machine

27. "Have you had this problem in the past?" is an example of which of the following types of questions?
    A. Leading
    B. Open-ended
    C. Closed-ended
    D. Nonleading

28. Which of the following agencies regulates licensure for physicians?
    A. Local hospital boards
    B. Federal government
    C. Medical colleges
    D. State government

29. A 75-year-old female with emphysema continues to smoke and to miss appointments against the orders of her physician. What is the most appropriate next step?
    A. Notify the patient that her medical care is being terminated
    B. Instruct her family how to change her behavior
    C. Accept her behavior and adjust her treatment
    D. Refer her to a psychiatrist

30. Which of the following would be the most appropriate first step when dealing with a patient who is distraught and angry?
    A. Escort the patient to a private area
    B. Ask the patient to calm down
    C. Inform the patient that the physician will see him or her shortly
    D. Ask the patient to have a seat in the waiting room

31. In which of the following situations can a patient's medical record be released without a signed authorization?
    A. The patient's attorney makes a request
    B. The patient is human immunodeficiency virus (HIV) positive
    C. An insurance company makes a request
    D. Another physician makes a request

32. Which of the following documents applies to donation of anatomic gifts?
    A. Advance directive
    B. Uniform Anatomical Gift Act
    C. Living will
    D. Durable power of attorney

33. An elderly patient wishes to move into a facility where she can remain autonomous. To which of the following might the medical assistant refer this patient?
    A. An assisted living community
    B. A retirement complex with individual apartments
    C. An extended care facility
    D. A rehabilitation hospital

34. How often must employee payroll taxes be reported to the Internal Revenue Service?
    A. Weekly
    B. Monthly
    C. Annually
    D. Quarterly

35. Which of the following is the most appropriate first step in correcting a misspelled word in a patient's medical record?
    A. Apply a thin covering of correction fluid over the error
    B. Circle the misspelled word in red
    C. Draw a single line through the misspelled word
    D. Completely erase the misspelled word

36. Which of the following allows data that are saved on a compact disk to be read but not altered?
    A. Clipboard
    B. Save As
    C. Write-protect
    D. Read-only memory

37. "Radial pulses are present bilaterally." When entering this information in the medical record, under which of the following headings should it be entered?
    A. Reflexes
    B. Head and neck
    C. Extremities
    D. Axilla

38. An illness that existed before an insurance policy is written is known as a(n):
    A. Special risk
    B. Exclusion
    C. Preexisting condition
    D. Prior authorization required

39. A spreadsheet would be commonly used for which of the following?
    A. Word processing
    B. Appointment scheduling
    C. Electronic mailings
    D. Accounting

40. Which of the following taxes are paid entirely by the employer?
    A. Social security
    B. Health insurance
    C. Federal income tax
    D. Unemployment tax

41. When selecting the E&M code for CPT coding, which of the following elements is required for all levels of the history?
    A. Chief complaint
    B. Family history
    C. Social history
    D. Review of systems

42. Which is not an indexing rule?
    A. Unit 1 is the surname
    B. A hyphen is disregarded
    C. Initials come after complete names
    D. Apostrophes are disregarded

43. Which of the following is the purpose of records management?
    A. Storage
    B. Arranging
    C. Classifying
    D. All of the above

44. The correct way to indicate an enclosure notation is:
    A. encl:
    B. Enclosure
    C. enclosure
    D. enc

45. Which of the following circumstances would waive the need for a written release of medical records?
    A. A subpoena
    B. Attorney request
    C. Hospital request
    D. Insurance company request

46. According to CPT, E&M codes begin with which of the following two digits?
    A. 93
    B. 95
    C. 97
    D. 99

47. Which of the following is considered to be capital equipment?
    A. Coffee maker
    B. Laboratory coats
    C. Photocopier
    D. Trash cans

48. The scheduling system based on scheduling similar appointments or procedures together is called:
    A. Wave
    B. Modified wave
    C. Grouping
    D. Double-booking

49. The record of the proceedings of a meeting is the:
    A. Agenda
    B. *Robert's Rules of Order*
    C. Itinerary
    D. Minutes

50. Which of the following forms indicates an employee's withholding allowance?
    A. 1099
    B. W-2
    C. W-3
    D. W-4

51. In the double-entry accounting system, an asset would be:
    A. The amount owed to a creditor
    B. Properties owned by the business
    C. Money owed to the practice by patients
    D. The amount by which liabilities exceed the equity

52. Which of the following telephone calls from a patient should not be charted?
    A. A request for a change in appointment time
    B. A request for a prescription renewal
    C. A request for a referral to a specialist
    D. Patient reports that symptoms have disappeared

53. When creating an office policy manual, it should begin with:
    A. The dress code
    B. The hierarchy chart
    C. Office hours
    D. The mission statement
54. Which of the following is an example of an indirect filing system?
    A. Alphabetic
    B. Chronologic
    C. Numerical
    D. Subject
55. The amount of federal tax withheld is based on the employee's exemptions, pay period, and:
    A. State income tax
    B. Employee's marital status
    C. Benefits offered by the employer
    D. Disability of the employee
56. A patient has had a left thyroid lobectomy performed. In preparing the insurance claim form, coding for which of the following body systems should be selected?
    A. Sensory
    B. Integumentary
    C. Endocrine
    D. Nervous
57. A tickler file is:
    A. A guide for processing insurance claims
    B. A list of procedures for equipment maintenance
    C. A type of color coding
    D. Future events arranged in chronological order
58. When is the most appropriate time to discuss payment arrangements with a new patient?
    A. When the patient calls to make an appointment
    B. When the insurance form is processed
    C. When statements are sent out
    D. At the time of the first visit
59. Which of the following may be used to replace a medical record that has temporarily been removed from the filing cabinet?
    A. 3 × 5 card
    B. An OUTguide
    C. A yellow Post-it note
    D. An empty file folder
60. When the word "Confidential" is to be typed on the envelope, it should be placed:
    A. In the lower right corner
    B. In the lower left corner
    C. Below the return address
    D. Both B and C
61. The date must be changed daily on which of the following?
    A. Computer
    B. Transcriber
    C. Fax machine
    D. Postage meter
62. The file folder label for Jennie Holmes-Mathis should be:
    A. Jennie, Holmes-Mathis
    B. Mathis, Jennie Holmes
    C. Holmes-Mathis, Jennie
    D. Mathis, Jennie (nee Holmes)

63. What is the monthly net income for a medical practice whose expenses are $8500, revenue is $14,130, total assets are $263,000, and liabilities are $53,000?
    A. $5630
    B. $22,630
    C. $39,000
    D. $210,000
64. Which of the following devices has the ability to digitize and convert images into an electronic format?
    A. A keyboard
    B. A monitor
    C. A printer
    D. A scanner
65. Which needle length and gauge would the medical assistant choose to administer an intramuscular injection?
    A. 1 inch, 25 gauge
    B. 1½ inch, 22 gauge
    C. 1 inch, 18 gauge
    D. ½ inch, 22 gauge
66. Warfarin (Coumadin) and heparin are classified as:
    A. Anticoagulants
    B. Diuretics
    C. Vasoconstrictors
    D. Vasodilators
67. To set up for an examination of a patient with vaginitis, all of the following would be used *except:*
    A. Vaginal speculum
    B. Microscope slide
    C. Potassium hydroxide (KOH)
    D. Cytologic fixative
68. When performing an electrocardiogram, which of the following chest leads would be placed on the fifth intercostal space at the midclavicular line?
    A. V_1
    B. V_2
    C. V_3
    D. V_4
69. During a Snellen visual acuity test, the patient should stand how many feet from the chart?
    A. 5
    B. 10
    C. 15
    D. 20
70. Which of the following terms refers to the total amount of air that is exhaled from fully inflated lungs?
    A. Forced vital capacity
    B. Forced expiratory flow
    C. Forced expiratory volume in 1 second
    D. Tidal volume
71. Which of the following methods is used to listen to heart, lung, and bowel sounds?
    A. Manipulation
    B. Auscultation
    C. Mensuration
    D. Percussion
72. A sphygmomanometer is used to perform which of the following procedures?
    A. Assess hearing
    B. Examine the rectum
    C. Evaluate vision
    D. Measure blood pressure

73. Which of the following results on a urinalysis is abnormal?
    A. Color: yellow
    B. pH: 5.2
    C. Specific gravity: 1.005
    D. Leukocytes: ++
74. Which of the following additives should be used when drawing a specimen for a differential smear?
    A. EDTA
    B. Heparin
    C. Potassium oxalate
    D. Sodium citrate
75. The drug order "2 gtt AU q4h prn" is translated as:
    A. Two drops in both ears every 4 hours as needed
    B. Two drops in both eyes every 4 hours as desired
    C. Two drops in both ears four times a day
    D. Two drops in the left eye every 4 hours if needed
76. Which of the following is the most effective method to clean a drop of blood from a countertop?
    A. Iodine and sterile gauze
    B. 1:10 bleach solution
    C. Alcohol and sterile cotton ball
    D. Surgical soap and water
77. The first group of leads to be recorded on an electrocardiogram consists of:
    A. Leads I, II, and III
    B. aVR, aVL, and aVF
    C. Leads V_1 through V_3
    D. Leads V_1 through V_6
78. A patient in the medical office has a nosebleed. What would be the most appropriate first action to be taken by the medical assistant?
    A. Apply ice to the patient's nose
    B. Call 911
    C. Tell the patient to lie down
    D. Tilt the patient's head forward
79. The correct injection technique used to place a tuberculin (Mantoux) skin test is:
    A. Intradermal
    B. Intramuscular
    C. Intravenous
    D. Transdermal
80. The abbreviation for both eyes is:
    A. OS
    B. OD
    C. OU
    D. BE
81. On a Gram stain, Gram-negative bacteria appear:
    A. Blue
    B. Pink or red
    C. Green
    D. Purple
82. Which of the following substances in urine may indicate liver dysfunction?
    A. Albumin
    B. Glucose
    C. Ketones
    D. Urobilinogen

83. This term is used to describe a variation in the size of erythrocytes.
    A. Anisocytosis
    B. Poikilocytosis
    C. Polychromic
    D. Leukocytosis
84. Which of the following instructions should be given to a patient who needs to collect stool specimens for occult blood screening?
    A. Eat a high-carbohydrate diet for 48 hours before collection
    B. Fast for 12 hours before the collection
    C. Do not eat red meat for 48 hours before the collection
    D. Do not eat fats for 12 hours before the collection
85. Controlled substances that are considered to be illegal and of no medical use are classified as:
    A. Schedule I
    B. Schedule II
    C. Schedule III
    D. Schedule IV
86. Albuterol (Proventil) is classified as a(n):
    A. Antiinflammatory
    B. Antihistamine
    C. Antihypertensive
    D. Bronchodilator
87. Which of the following injuries is classified as a closed wound?
    A. Puncture
    B. Laceration
    C. Ecchymosis
    D. Avulsion
88. During manual audiometry, the patient should be positioned:
    A. Facing away from the examiner
    B. Behind the examiner
    C. Facing the examiner
    D. Next to the examiner
89. Sanitization:
    A. Destroys all pathogenic microorganisms
    B. Destroys most pathogenic organisms
    C. Reduces the number of contaminants to a safe level
    D. Replaces defective instruments with new instruments
90. The body's reaction to a issue injury is called:
    A. Inflammation
    B. Cancer
    C. Ecclymosis
    D. Emesis
91. Which of the following materials is not acceptable for wrapping items to be autoclaved?
    A. Cotton
    B. Disposable autoclave paper
    C. Muslin
    D. Aluminum foil
92. Forceps is an instrument used to:
    A. Cut
    B. Grasp
    C. Hold back
    D. Suture

93. Which of the following is used to measure the oxygen saturation of the blood?
    A. Stethoscope
    B. Spirometer
    C. Oxygenator
    D. Oximeter
94. In the medical office setting, sharps are:
    A. Used once and discarded in a sharps container
    B. Thrown away in regular waste receptacle
    C. Sanitized, sterilized, and used again
    D. Sterilized separately from other instruments
95. Before Pap smear is taken, the patient should be instructed to:
    A. Douche
    B. Not douche
    C. Insert a lubrication jelly
    D. Use vaginal cream
96. Which of the following methods is used in listening with a stethoscope?
    A. Auscultation
    B. Inspection
    C. Palpation
    D. Percussion

97. By the end of 1 year, a normal, healthy, infant should have:
    A. Doubled in length and tripled in weight
    B. Doubled in length and gained 10 to 15 pounds
    C. Tripled in length and doubled in weight
    D. Tripled in weight and grown 10 to 12 inches in length
98. Which of the following injections are administered subcutaneously?
    A. HBV and DTaP
    B. Hib and MMR
    C. MMR and HBV
    D. MMR and VarEating
99. Using a blood pressure cuff that is too small for the patient's arm:
    A. Can cause an incorrect low blood pressure reading
    B. Can cause an incorrect high blood pressure reading
    C. Makes no difference in the blood pressure reading
    D. None of the above
100. A type of drug that increases urinary output is a(n):
    A. Emetic
    B. Diuretic
    C. Miotic
    D. Cathartic

General

1. **A** "arthr/o"
   RATIONALE: "arthr/o" is the correct combining form for "joint"
2. **B** OS
   RATIONALE: The correct abbreviation for "left eye" is "OS" (oculis sinister)
3. **E** All of the above
   RATIONALE: Functions that the liver performs include: production and secretion of bile, synthesis of plasma proteins, storage of glycogen, lipid metabolism, and detoxification.
4. **C** Resondeat Superior
   RATIONALE: "Respondeat Superior" is a legal doctrine whereby the Employer is liable for the negligent acts of the Employee so long as the Employee follows practice protocols.
5. **B** Hyperglycemia
   RATIONALE: "hyper-" is excessive; "glyc/o"is sugar; and "-emia" is blood.
6. **A** Contract
   RATIONALE: The patient-provider relationship ia a contractual relationship. Each party has rights and responsibilities in the relationship.
7. **C** Emphysema
   RATIONALE: Emphysema causes the terminal bronchioles to become plugged with mucus.
8. **E** All of the above.
   RATIONALE: Nonverbal communication is all types of communication that occur without using words.
9. **E** Bulemia
   RATIONALE: Bulimia is an eating disorder character-ized by episodes of binge eating followed by self-in-duced vomiting.

10. **C** Septum
    RATIONALE: The wall-like septum separates the atrium and ventricle on the right side from those on the left side of the heart.
11. **E** Mole on the inside of the elbow
    RATIONALE: A nevus is a mole. The antecubital area is located on the inner aspect of the elbow.
12. **D** Arthritis
    RATIONALE: The root word "arth-" means joint. The suffix "-itis" means inflammation.
13. **C** Smelling
    RATIONALE: The olfactory nerve, cranial nerve I, is one of two pairs of nerves associated with the sense of smell.
14. **D** Physical, mental, and social well-being
    RATIONALE: Health is the condition of physical, mental, and social well-being and the absence of disease and other abnormal conditions. It is not static. Constant change and adaptation results in homeostasis.
15. **A** Urticaria
    RATIONALE: Urticaria is a pruritic skin eruption characterized by wheals (hives) of various shapes and sizes. This condition can be caused by allergic reactions to drugs, insect bites, and foods.
16. **B** Excretion of nitrogen-containing waste
    RATIONALE: The skin is the largest organ of the body. Its main functions are sensory perception, temperature regulation, protection, excretion of nonnitrogen wastes, and synthesis of vitamin D.
17. **C** Pericardium
    RATIONALE: The pericardium is the serous membrane that surrounds the heart.
18. **D** Lines body cavities that open to the outside
    RATIONALE: A mucous membrane lines body cavities or spaces of the body that open to the outside, including the mouth, digestive tract, respiratory tract, and genitourinary tract.

19. **C** Abdominal
   RATIONALE: The abdominal cavity is part of the ventral cavity of the body. It contains the stomach, small and large intestines, spleen, liver, gallbladder, and pancreas.

20. **C** Adduction
   RATIONALE: Adduction moves a bone or limb toward the midline of the body. The opposite is abduction, which moves away from the midline. Supination moves a part to face upward. Pronation moves a part to face downward. Rotation moves a bone on its own axis.

21. **A** Can follow a viral illness in children
   RATIONALE: Reye syndrome is an acute and sometimes fatal illness characterized by fatty invasion of internal organs and swelling of the brain. The cause is unknown, but the condition has been linked to the use of aspirin and viral illnesses in children.

22. **C** Lumbar
   RATIONALE: The vertebral column is divided into five sections: (1) cervical (neck), (2) thoracic (chest), (3) lumbar (lower back), (4) sacral (below the lumbar), and (5) coccygeal (tailbone).

23. **D** Occipital
   RATIONALE: The occipital bone of the skull is located at the back of the skull. It articulates with the two parietal bones and contains the foramen magnum (opening for the spinal cord).

24. **E** 31
   RATIONALE: The peripheral nervous system is made up of the motor and sensory nerves and ganglia located outside the brain and spinal cord. It consists of 12 pairs of cranial nerves and 31 pairs of spinal nerves.

25. **A** Brainstem
   RATIONALE: The brainstem is the portion of the brain made up of the midbrain, pons, and medulla. It performs sensory, motor, and reflex functions. Vital centers that regulate internal body functions are located here.

26. **A** Aplastic
   RATIONALE: Aplastic anemia results from a failure of blood cell production caused by the failure of bone marrow to produce cells. The cause is unknown.

27. **C** Hiatal hernia
   RATIONALE: A hernia is the abnormal protrusion of an organ or tissue through the structures that normally contain it. A hiatal hernia is the protrusion of the upper portion of the stomach upward through the esophageal opening in the diaphragm.

28. **D** Eardrum
   RATIONALE: The tympanic membrane is the membrane between the external and middle ear. It is commonly called the eardrum.

29. **D** Aorta
   RATIONALE: The aorta is the main trunk of the systemic arterial circulation. Blood is pumped out of the left ventricle through the aortic valve into the aorta. The aorta then branches and carries blood throughout the body.

30. **C** Is the pacemaker of the heart
   RATIONALE: The sinoatrial node of the heart is located in the right atrium. The electrical impulse that initiates the heartbeat originates here.

31. **B** Radius and ulna
   RATIONALE: The radius is the lateral lower arm bone in line with the thumb. The ulna is the medial lower arm bone.

32. **E** All of the above
   RATIONALE: Involuntary (smooth) muscle is muscle that is not under a person's conscious or voluntary control. Involuntary muscle actions involve muscles of the heart and muscles of the intestines, stomach, and other visceral organs.

33. **A** Liver
   RATIONALE: The right upper quadrant of the abdominopelvic area contains the liver, gallbladder, part of the pancreas, and parts of the small and large intestines.

34. **D** Phrenic
   RATIONALE: The diaphragm is stimulated by the phrenic nerve from the cervical plexus. The diaphragm aids in respiration by moving up and down.

35. **C** Scoliosis
   RATIONALE: Scoliosis is a lateral curvature of the spine commonly seen in children. Unequal heights of hips and shoulders may be a sign of this condition.

36. **B** Glucagon
   RATIONALE: Glucagon is a hormone produced by the alpha cells in the islets of Langerhans in the pancreas. It stimulates the conversion of glycogen to glucose in the liver.

37. **C** 4 to 12 feet
   RATIONALE: 4 to 12 feet is considered social personal space for the US culture and is most often observed. 12 to 15 feet is public space; touching to 1 ½ feet is intimate space; 1½ to 4 feet is personal space.

38. **D** 32
   RATIONALE: The deciduous (baby) teeth are replaced by 32 adult (permanent) teeth. These adult teeth include four central incisors, lateral incisors, cuspids, first and second premolars, first molars, second molars, and third molars (wisdom teeth).

39. **E** May refuse to accept a patient if he or she chooses
   RATIONALE: Physicians have the right to determine whom they will accept as patients. Patient load may be as large as one person can adequately care for, and the decision may be made to limit new patients.

40. **B** Staying calm when dealing with angry patients
   RATIONALE: Professional qualities that a medical assistant must have include a friendly and pleasant attitude, ability to maintain confidentiality, courtesy, ability to control temper, consideration, respect and kindness, dependability, and accuracy.

41. **B** The physician
   RATIONALE: The physician owns the medical record, but the patient owns the information contained in the record.

42. **A** Denial
RATIONALE: Denial is the unconscious avoidance of the reality of an unpleasant or disturbing situation.

43. **E** All of the above
RATIONALE: Personality is the pattern of behavior each person develops as a means of adapting to a particular environment and its standards. Age, life experiences, heredity, and environment all play a part in this development.

44. **E** All of the above
RATIONALE: Adaptability, flexibility, friendliness, compassion, courtesy, loyalty, and attitude are all professional characteristics required of a health care professional.

45. **E** Young children react differently to stressful situations
RATIONALE: Stereotyping is a preconceived generalized belief. Young children do react differently to adults to stressful situations.

46. **C** The patient must sign a release form
RATIONALE: The patient must sign a release of information form before information from the medical record can be released to anyone. This precaution preserves the patient's confidentiality.

47. **E** Human immunodeficiency virus (HIV)
RATIONALE: The physician has a legal duty to report communicable diseases to the county health department. This requirement helps the state provide for the public's health, safety, and welfare.

48. **E** Implied contract
RATIONALE: When the physician accepts the patient, an implied contract exists. An implied contract is indicated by actions rather than words.

49. **A** Another physician
RATIONALE: A call from another physician or professional colleague should be transferred to the physician immediately.

50. **C** Social need
RATIONALE: Maslow believed that lower level needs must be satisfied before higher level needs can be satisfied. These levels, from lowest to highest, include physiologic needs, safety needs, social needs, self-esteem needs, and self-actualization needs.

51. **D** Delay treatment and inform or consult with the physician
RATIONALE: A physician must have consent to treat a patient even though this consent is usually implied. A physician who fails to secure some formal type of consent might be charged with assault and battery or trespass.

52. **E** All of the above
RATIONALE: A contract is an agreement that creates an obligation. To be valid or enforceable, the contract must have four basic elements: (1) an offer and acceptance, (2) consideration, (3) capacity, and (4) legality.

53. **E** All of the above
RATIONALE: Blood is pumped by the heart and carried through vessels. It carries nutrients, ions, water, oxygen, carbon dioxide, waste products, and hormones. It regulates water content of cells and body pH. It is made up of cells suspended in a liquid matrix.

54. **D** Posterior
RATIONALE: The anterior of a structure is the front of the structure. The posterior of a structure is the back of the structure.

55. **E** All of the above
RATIONALE: Informed consent must be obtained from the patient when a complex procedure is to be performed. Informed consent implies an understanding of what is to be done, why it should be done, the risks involved, the expected outcomes, alternative treatments, and consequences of failure to treat.

56. **E** Providing atypical care
RATIONALE: The license to practice medicine may be revoked or suspended under certain circumstances. Grounds for revoking or suspending a license generally fall within one of three categories: (1) conviction of a crime, (2) unprofessional conduct, and (3) personal and professional incapacity.

57. **C** Nucleus
RATIONALE: The nucleus is the control center of every cell. It contains DNA, which is the genetic material.

58. **E** All of the above
RATIONALE: The subcutaneous tissue is a layer of connective tissue found between the skin and the deep fascia. It contains a fatty layer. Hypodermic injections into this tissue are usually on the upper arm, thigh, or abdomen.

59. **B** Humerus
RATIONALE: The humerus is the largest bone of the upper arm. The femur is the bone of the thigh; the tibia and fibula make up the lower leg; the metatarsals form the arch of the foot.

60. **A** Deltoid
RATIONALE: The deltoid is a large, thick, triangular muscle that covers the shoulder.

61. **E** Setting standards for employees with disabilities
RATIONALE: The Americans with Disabilities Act (ADA) was established to prevent individuals with physical or mental disabilities from discrimination from employment.

62. **E** Alveoli
RATIONALE: The alveoli are small saclike structures at the terminal ends of the bronchioles. They are the functional units of respiration and are composed of a single layer of epithelium, which allows oxygen and carbon dioxide to be easily exchanged with the surrounding capillaries.

63. **E** All of the above
RATIONALE: The liver is the largest gland of the body. Its main functions include production of bile, detoxification of toxins and wastes, metabolism of proteins and carbohydrates, storage of vitamins and glycogen, production of heparin, and recycling of worn-out red blood cells.

64. **A** Cerebrum
    RATIONALE: The cerebrum is the largest portion of the brain. It is divided into two hemispheres, which are further divided into lobes. Its outer surface (cortex) is made up of gray matter.

65. **E** 31
    RATIONALE: There are 31 pairs of spinal nerves that are connected to the spinal cord. They are numbered according to the vertebra from which they emerge.

66. **A** Mouth
    RATIONALE: The gustatory sense is the sense of taste. The receptors are located on the tongue within papillae (taste buds).

67. **D** Decreases blood sugar levels
    RATIONALE: Insulin is a hormone manufactured by the beta cells in the pancreas. Its main function is to move glucose into cells for metabolizing, thus reducing blood glucose levels.

68. **E** Leukopenia
    RATIONALE: Leukopenia is an abnormal decrease in the number of white blood cells to less than 5000 cells/mm^3 of blood. The root word "leuko-" means white, or white blood cell. The suffix "-penia" means a decrease.

69. **B** Stat
    RATIONALE: The term STAT is the abbreviation for *statim*, meaning immediately.

70. **E** All of the above
    RATIONALE: The physician has a legal duty to report information that may have an effect on the health, safety, or welfare of the public. This information includes births, deaths, communicable diseases, abuse, criminal acts, and professional misconduct.

71. **A** Slow
    RATIONALE: The prefix "brady-" means slow.

72. **C** Deep
    RATIONALE: Superficial pertains to the skin or another surface. Deep refers to away from the surface.

73. **C** An advance directive
    RATIONALE: An advance directive is a legal document that gives persons the right to determine what medical procedures they want to be provided if they become unable to make those decisions.

74. **C** Myoblast
    RATIONALE: The root word "myo-" means muscle. The suffix "-blast" means immature cell, form.

75. **B** Denial
    RATIONALE: Unconscious defense mechanisms help protect the mind from guilt or anxiety. Denial is the unconscious avoidance of the reality of an unpleasant or disturbing feeling, thought, or event.

76. **A** An open-ended statement
    RATIONALE: An open-ended statement or question helps the patient decide what is relevant. It also encourages the patient to continue the discussion.

77. **D** Lecturing
    RATIONALE: Techniques for interacting with an adolescent successfully include allowing for privacy (asking the parent to leave), including the adolescent in the decision-making process, explaining procedures, and answering questions. Lecturing is a roadblock to communication.

78. **E** All of the above
    RATIONALE: Nonverbal communications are messages conveyed without the use of words. They are transmitted by body language. Body language involves grooming, dress, eye contact, facial expression, hand gestures, space, tone of voice, posture, and touch.

79. **B** An eating disorder
    RATIONALE: Bulimia is an insatiable craving for food characterized by binge eating and self-induced vomiting.

80. **C** Breast
    RATIONALE: A mammogram is an x-ray film of the soft tissue of the breast. The root word "mammo-" refers to breast. The suffix "-gram" refers to a record (x-ray).

81. **D** Stroke
    RATIONALE: A cerebrovascular accident, or brain attack, is an abnormal condition of the blood vessels of the brain characterized by an occlusion that results in ischemia of the brain tissue. Paralysis, weakness, speech defect, aphasia, or death may occur.

82. **C** Never allow yourself to make value judgments
    RATIONALE: Interaction with persons of another culture requires trust, empathy, respect, and active listening. Effective communication requires one to recognize personal biases and prejudices and put them aside.

83. **C** Trichomoniasis
    RATIONALE: Trichomoniasis is a vaginal infection caused by the protozoan *Trichomonas vaginalis*. It is transmitted by sexual intercourse.

84. **B** Emphysema
    RATIONALE: Emphysema is an abnormal condition of the pulmonary system. It is characterized by overinflation and destructive changes of the alveoli, which results in a loss of lung elasticity and decreased gas exchange.

85. **B** Serous
    RATIONALE: A serous membrane lines the walls of body cavities that do not open to the outside.

86. **E** Compound fracture
    RATIONALE: An open or compound fracture is one in which the broken end of the bone tears open the skin.

87. **C** Control their own health care decisions
    RATIONALE: The Patient Self-Determination Act includes the advance directive giving patients the right to be involved in their health care decisions.

88. **B** Adipose tissue
    RATIONALE: Adipose tissue is made up of fat cells arranged in globules. It is found under the skin and serves as a reserve energy source and for insulation.

89. **D** Anterior
    RATIONALE: The ventral area of the body is toward the front of the body (anterior).

90. **A** Impetigo
    RATIONALE: Impetigo is an infection of the skin caused by staphylococci, streptococci, or a combination of the two. The lesions usually begin around the mouth and nose and spread locally. The lesions blister and crust.

91. C Cholecystectomy

RATIONALE: The root word "cholecyst-" means gallbladder. The suffix "-ectomy" means surgical removal.

92. B Empathy

RATIONALE: Empathy is the ability to recognize the emotions and state of mind of another person.

93. C Leaving records on counters where other patients may see them

RATIONALE: Protected health information (PHI) of the patient must be protected under the Health Insurance Portability and Accountability Act (HIPAA). Medical records should be safeguarded against disclosure of this information.

94. B Palliative

RATIONALE: Palliative treatment reduces the effects of a disease or condition but does not remove the disease itself.

95. B Examination by the provider

RATIONALE: After checking in at the reception desk, the patient is seen by the provider to ascertain the chief complaint and medical history and for examination to be performed. Diagnostic testing, medications, and follow-up care depend on the findings of the provider's examination.

96. E All of the above

RATIONALE: MDs, DOs, nurse practitioners, and physician assistants are health care providers who are licensed to practice medicine in the state where they are employed.

97. C Diagnosing the patient

RATIONALE: An advocate is one who intercedes on another's behalf. This would include assisting the patient. A medical assistant never diagnoses.

98. E All of the above

RATIONALE: Confidentiality restrictions apply to any information documented in the patient's medical record. If the law does not require it, providers should allow minors to consent to care and should not notify parents/guardians without the minor's consent.

99. A A contract

RATIONALE: The physician-patient relationship is a contractual relationship. Each party has certain responsibilities and rights under the relationship.

100. B The patient must sign a release form

RATIONALE: The patient must sign a "Release of Information" form or otherwise give consent for his/her medical records to be released.

Pretest 2 Answer Key

Administrative

1. **B** Date of birth
   RATIONALE: Demographic information is the routine personal data of the patient that includes name, gender, date of birth, marital status, home address and phone number, and occupation.

2. **C** Copayment
   RATIONALE: The copayment is payment of a specified amount required when seen by the provider. It is collected before the patient is seen.

3. **B** Patient confidentiality
   RATIONALE: Health Insurance Portability and Accountability Act (HIPAA) requires the adoption of privacy and security standards to protect an individual's identifiable health information.

4. **C** Electronic health record (EHR)
   RATIONALE: The patient's EHR is a combination of multiple sources of patient records into one source.

5. **E** All of the above
   RATIONALE: An electronic medical record software program creates, stores, edits, and retrieves patient data. If all data are entered correctly, the computer software can find the chart, store inputted information, and allow more than one person to access the information.

6. **E** All of the above
   RATIONALE: Information must be entered into the EHR. This can be accomplished by the patient completing the questionnaire on a computer, the patient completing the history in paper form and the office staff scanning it into the computer, or the medical assistant entering the information directly into the computer while interviewing the patient.

7. **E** All of the above
   RATIONALE: Medical records, whether paper or electronic, are a crucial part of a medical practice. They are legal documents that provide an ongoing record of patient treatment and care. They are a source of communication between members of the health care team.

8. **B** As a separate procedure
   RATIONALE: The Current Procedural Terminology (CPT) code manual provides both a narrative description and a five-digit code for each procedure or service a provider performs on the patient. The Medicine section of the CPT manual gives codes for noninvasive diagnostic and treatment services.

9. **D** To decide whether the care being given corresponds to the patient's disease
   RATIONALE: Procedure codes are a means of classifying the type of care given to patients. Procedure codes justify medical services by correlating procedures to diagnosis.

10. **A** The primary care provider
    RATIONALE: In a managed care system, the patient selects a primary care provider. The provider is considered to be the gatekeeper and must provide a referral for specialist care.

11. **D** If the physician accepts assignment of benefits
    RATIONALE: Assignment of benefits is authorization for insurance reimbursement to be made to the provider of services rather than the insured individual.

12. **E** Grouping
    RATIONALE: Grouping is the practice of scheduling patients with the same type of examination (e.g., complete physicals), conditions (e.g., pregnancy), or procedures (e.g., Papanicolaou [Pap] smears) within a certain time frame.

13. **E** All of the above
    RATIONALE: A computer has the ability to process data according to a program to produce desired results. Computers perform tasks quickly and accurately, are versatile, and can perform the same task repeatedly while maintaining accuracy.

14. **B** Absence of punctuation after the salutation and a comma after the complimentary close
    RATIONALE: Open punctuation style uses no punctuation at the end of any line outside of the body of the letter unless the line ends with an abbreviation. This type of punctuation is used with the simplified block letter style.

15. **D** Medicaid
    RATIONALE: Medicaid is a federally funded insurance program that was set up by the federal government in 1965 to provide for the medically indigent. It is regulated by each state.

16. **B** An alphabetic cross-reference
    RATIONALE: Numeric filing involves filing records, correspondence, or cards by number. It is an indirect filing system and requires the use of an alphabetic cross-reference to find a given file.

17. **D** Holmes-Mathis, Jennie
    RATIONALE: Hyphenated elements of a name, whether first name, middle name, or surname, are considered as one unit.

18. **C** Physician, patient, and insurance company
    RATIONALE: A third-party payer is some entity other than the patient, spouse, or parent who is responsible for paying all or part of the patient's medical costs.

19. **E** All of the above
    RATIONALE: If a claim form is not sufficiently detailed, complete, and accurate, the insurance company may reject the claim. Reasons for claim rejection include missing or incomplete diagnosis; incorrectly coded diagnosis; charges not itemized; patient's group, member, or policy number missing; patient's signature missing; patient's date of birth missing; dates missing or incorrect; and physician's signature missing.

20. **A** Identify the practice and himself/herself
    RATIONALE: The telephone is usually the first contact between the medical office and the patient. Identifying the office and one's self is a good telephone courtesy practice.

21. **A** Very truly yours
    RATIONALE: The complimentary close is the writer's way of saying "good-bye." The words used are determined by the formality used in the salutation.

22. **D** Insurance information
    RATIONALE: The patient's insurance information is obtained at the time of the first visit to the office. Necessary information includes the patient's name, telephone number, reason for coming to the office, and times available for the appointment.

23. **B** Conference call
    RATIONALE: A conference call allows more than two people to participate in a conversation at one time. Each person can hear or talk to all others who are participating.

24. **C** Backing up
    RATIONALE: A backup is a tape or disk for storage of files to prevent their loss in the event of hard drive failure.

25. **E** Future events arranged in chronologic order
    RATIONALE: A tickler file is a chronologic file used as a reminder that something must be done on a certain date. This type of file is frequently used as a follow-up method.

26. **A** Diarrhea
    RATIONALE: CPT is a listing of descriptive terms and identifying codes used for reporting medical services and procedures performed by the physician. All of the choices are procedures except diarrhea.

27. **E** All of the above
    RATIONALE: The receptionist is usually the first person in the medical office with whom the patient has contact. The appearance, professionalism, attitude, and manners of the receptionist as well as the appearance of the reception area as a whole can influence the patient's perception of the entire practice.

28. **C** See also
    RATIONALE: *See also* is the coding convention that gives the direction to the coder to consider another code.

29. **E** All of the above
    RATIONALE: ICD-10-CM includes several new features compared to ICD-9-CM. These include more extensive information related to ambulatory care and managed care encounters, expansion of injury codes, combination of diagnosis and symptom codes which decreases the need for two codes, and more codes that allow for more precise coding of body parts and patient encounters.

30. **D** Letter informing a patient who has missed several appointments to find a new provider
    RATIONALE: Certified mail serves as legal evidence that an item was mailed by the sender with a receipt.

31. **E** All of the above
    RATIONALE: Evaluation and Management (E&M) descriptors include basic diagnostic and treatment services such as office visits and physical examinations. These descriptors are part of the CPT coding system.

32. **B** Medicare
    RATIONALE: A third-party payer is any person, insurance company, or government agent other than the patient or the patient's family who pays the patient's account.

33. **C** A numbered list of present problems
    RATIONALE: The problem-oriented medical record (POMR) system is designed to organize the patient's medical record and the information it contains. The system uses four parts: (1) database, (2) problem list, (3) treatment plan, and (4) progress notes. The database includes the chief complaint, present illness or illnesses, and the patient profile.

34. **D** Ledger card totals and account-receivable balance
    RATIONALE: A trial balance is a method of checking the accuracy of accounts. It should be done once a month after all posting has been completed and before preparing monthly statements. The purpose of a trial balance is to disclose any discrepancies between

the ledger cards and accounts receivable. It does not prove the accuracy of the accounts.

35. **C** Another physician

RATIONALE: The person answering the telephone is expected to screen all incoming calls. Good judgment in deciding whether to put through a call comes with experience. Calls from other physicians should be put through at once if the physician is available to take the call.

36. **E** Diagnosis

RATIONALE: The patient's diagnosis may not be made at an initial visit. At the first visit, the patient may complete a patient information form that includes name, address, telephone number, insurance information, business information, and referral information.

37. **A** 8½ × 11; no. 10 envelope

RATIONALE: A standard-size letter (8½ × 11 inches) is used for general business and professional correspondence. Standard ways of folding and inserting letters are used so the letter fits properly and is easy to remove. A size no. 10 envelope is used for a standard-size letter.

38. **A** The checkbook

RATIONALE: A bank statement is periodically sent by the bank to the customer. It shows the status of the account on a given date. The bank statement balance and the checkbook balance should be the same, or they need to be reconciled (disclosure of any errors in the checkbook or bank statement).

39. **D** Minutes

RATIONALE: The record of the proceedings of a meeting is called the *minutes*. The minutes contain a record of what was done at a meeting, not what was said by the members. Minutes should be signed by the secretary and kept on file according to the procedure of the organization.

40. **D** By classification of disease or condition

RATIONALE: The Tabular List of the ICD-10-CM manual displays the actual codes, arranged in 21 chapters according to the classification of the disease or condition or factor influencing health status.

41. **C** Grouping

RATIONALE: Grouping or clustering allows the provider to make good use of time by seeing patients with the same needs at the same time. For example, a provider may perform complete physical examinations only on Wednesday mornings.

42. **B** W-4 form

RATIONALE: The W-4 form is the Employee's Withholding Allowance Certificate. It is filled out by the employee and allows him or her to determine the number of withholding allowances.

43. **C** Invasion of privacy

RATIONALE: Invasion of privacy is the act of divulging patient information that has been acquired through privileged interaction (provider-patient communication) without the consent of the patient, which is an intentional tort. Information shared between the provider and the patient is confidential. A release of information form must be signed before this information can be shared.

44. **A** Omission of all punctuation

RATIONALE: The US Postal Service attempts to read, code, sort, and cancel all mail electronically. The success of this system depends on the correct format that can be read by the automatic equipment. This format includes all addresses typed in block format in the correct area of the envelope, everything in the address capitalized, all punctuation eliminated, states abbreviated using the standard two-letter code, and the ZIP Code must be included in the last line.

45. **B** A subpoena

RATIONALE: A *subpoena duces tecum* is an order to provide records or documents to the court. Authority to release information from the medical record lies solely with the patient unless required by law.

46. **B** Accounts payable

RATIONALE: Accounts payable are the outstanding bills of a business

47. **B** Enclosure

RATIONALE: The enclosure notation identifies any material that may be accompanying the correspondence. The notation is placed two lines below the signature line. If more than one enclosure is included, specify the number (e.g., Enclosures 2).

48. **A** Insurance claim

RATIONALE: A superbill is a combination charge slip, statement, and insurance reporting form. It is completed and given to the patient at each visit.

49. **E** All of the above

RATIONALE: Complete and accurate records are essential to a well-managed medical practice. Health information management includes not only the assembling of the record but also having an efficient system for saving, retrieving, protecting, transferring, storing, retaining, and destroying these records.

50. **B** *International Classification of Diseases*, 10th edition Clinical Modification (ICD-10-CM)

RATIONALE: ICD-10-CM is the coding system used to code diagnoses or disease conditions. CPT, HCPCS, RVS, and RBRVS are systems used to code medical procedures.

51. **C** Initials come after complete names

RATIONALE: Indexing rules are standardized and are based on current business practices. The rule that applies to initials states "that initials precede a name beginning with the same letter." For example, the chart for M. Johnson would be filed before the chart for Mary Johnson.

52. **C** $250.00

RATIONALE: A participating provider in the Medicare program must bill for the patient, accept assignment of benefits, and accept Medicare's determination of allowable charges for the service.

53. **B** Bit

RATIONALE: A bit is a binary digit. It is the smallest piece of information that can be processed by a computer.

54. **D** Directory

RATIONALE: The directory is the index of files on a disk. It shows the names of the documents that are saved on that disk. The operator can choose a file and open it.

55. E B and C only
RATIONALE: The scheduling system chosen by the facility must be individualized for each specific practice. Important factors that determine the best system include patient need, physician preferences and habits, and facilities available.

56. B Mixed punctuation
RATIONALE: Mixed (standard) punctuation is appropriate for use with block or modified block letter styles. It places a colon after the salutation and a comma after the complimentary closing. It is the most commonly used punctuation pattern.

57. C Operating manuals
RATIONALE: An inventory of all capital items (equipment) should be prepared every year. For each item, the name, serial number, date of purchase, price, and any warranty information are included. Operating manuals should be kept separate and readily accessible.

58. C Preexisting condition
RATIONALE: A preexisting condition is a physical condition of a person that existed before the insurance policy was issued.

59. D Inactive files
RATIONALE: Inactive files generally are files of patients whom the provider has not seen for 6 months or longer. When the patient returns for care, his or her chart is moved to the active file.

60. A Patient confidentiality
RATIONALE: The patient is entitled to complete confidentiality with regard to his or her medical records and release of information. Computer technology allows for the gathering and storage of vast amounts of information. This information can be accessible to a variety of individuals. The monitor displays information and should be positioned away from others who may be at the desk.

61. E All of the above
RATIONALE: All patients should be escorted to the examination or treatment room. All patients are generally more cooperative and less anxious if they understand what is expected of them.

62. B Name of assisting physician
RATIONALE: Surgery is scheduled by type of procedure and availability of facilities. Important information includes the name of the procedure; expected length of the procedure in hours; type of anesthesia; and the patient's name, age, and telephone number.

63. B A copy of the letter is sent to Dr. Jones
RATIONALE: The copy notation (c:) indicates that a copy of the document was sent to a third party or parties. The notation is placed one to two lines below the enclosure notation.

64. B Accept predetermined fees
RATIONALE: Managed care is a type of prepaid health plan. It was developed to provide health care services at a low cost. Managed care includes health maintenance organizations (HMOs) and independent practice associations (IPAs). The traditional HMO builds a group of physicians who agree to be paid on a per-patient basis instead of a fee-for-service basis.

65. D Preferred provider organization (PPO)
RATIONALE: The preferred provider organization uses a fee-for-service concept. Providers agree on a predetermined list of charges for all services. Care is not prepaid. The patient must pay deductibles.

66. B The patient record
RATIONALE: The patient record screen shows the patient information such as demographics and insurance information.

67. E Deposit slip
RATIONALE: Deposit slips are itemized documents of cash, checks, and other funds that a depositor presents to the bank with the items to be credited to an account. All deposits must be accompanied by a deposit slip. A copy of the slip is kept on file.

68. D Patient's surname
RATIONALE: One system of color-coding files is the alphabetic color-coding system. This system uses different-colored tabs to represent a different segment of the alphabet. The chart is coded by the patient's last name (surname).

69. C Times not available
RATIONALE: To develop the matrix in the appointment book, block out the times the physician or physicians will be unavailable. All else revolves around physician availability.

70. B Medicare Part B
RATIONALE: Medicare Part A provides coverage of hospitalization services. Individuals age 65 or older are automatically enrolled in Part A with no premiums to pay. Part B covers physician and other provider services. It must be purchased.

71. A Extensive editing capability
RATIONALE: The computer, as a document production tool, permits efficient preparation and editing of written documents. Spell-check and column layout are simply added benefits. Storage capacity relates to the computer as a whole and is not specific to word processing.

72. A Insurance coverage is available
RATIONALE: Certified mail requires the receiver's signature as proof of delivery and receipt. Any mail in which first-class postage is paid can be accepted as certified mail.

73. D Place of employment
RATIONALE: Demographic information is statistical information of a population. It is used to identify and provide necessary information about the patient. It includes name, age, address, occupation and place of employment, Social Security number, and name of closest relative.

74. E The estate is billed
RATIONALE: Estate claims are made against the estate of a deceased patient. When the office receives notification of the patient's death, the office must submit a claim for the unpaid balance to the administrator of the estate. Each state has different rules and regulations concerning the filing of estate claims.

75. A Immediately
RATIONALE: Endorsement is a signature or writing on the back of a check by which the endorser transfers

all rights of the check to another party. All checks received as payments should be restrictively endorsed (for deposit only) immediately to safeguard against loss or theft.

76. **E** Andrew Stephen

RATIONALE: In alphabetic filing, a person's name is indexed with the surname as unit 1, the given name as unit 2, and the middle name as unit 3. Names are alphabetized according to the first unit letter by letter.

77. **E** David Roberts, M.D.

RATIONALE: The inside address includes the name, title, and address of the receiver. When addressing a letter to a physician, omit the courtesy title, and type the physician's name followed by his or her academic degree.

78. **B** NE

RATIONALE: The use of standard two-letter abbreviations aids in the reading, coding, sorting, and canceling of the mail. The US Postal Service has issued a list of two-letter state abbreviations to be used with ZIP Codes. None of the other choices is a US state abbreviation.

79. **C** Full block style

RATIONALE: The full block style places all lines flush at the left margin. The other choices vary indentation of the margins.

80. **C** Complimentary close

RATIONALE: A memorandum is a written communication among persons within an office or organization. It uses guide words that indicate the date, sender, receiver or receivers, and subject.

81. **C** Name, page number, and date

RATIONALE: The second and continuous pages of a letter or report are placed on plain paper that matches the letterhead in weight, color, and fiber content. The heading of the subsequent pages must contain the name of the addressee, page number, and date.

82. **A** Two

RATIONALE: The complimentary close is placed on the second line below the last line of the body of the letter.

83. **D** Physician charges

RATIONALE: A fee profile is established by compiling and averaging the usual charges for services of the physician over a given period. This profile is used to determine the amount of third-party liability.

84. **B** Date of birth

RATIONALE: Demographics relate to the statistical characteristics of a population. It includes the name, date of birth, marital status, children, occupation, education, and social information of the patient.

85. **D** Irritable bowel syndrome

RATIONALE: ICD-10-CM assigns numeric codes to diseases, illnesses, injuries, and health-related conditions. The coding system is used to establish medical necessity to facilitate payment for health care services and to translate written terminology or descriptions into numbers to provide a universal common language.

86. **B** 1:00 p.m.

RATIONALE: The United States is divided into four time zones: (1) Pacific Standard Time (WA, OR, NV, and CA), (2) Mountain Standard Time (MT, UT, ID, WY, CO, NM, AZ, and parts of ND, SD, NE, and KS), (3) Central Standard Time (MN, WI, IA, MO, AR, OK, TX, LA, MS, IL, AL, and parts of TN, KY, ND, SD, NE, and KS), and (4) Eastern Standard Time (all others). Central, Mountain, and Pacific Standard Time zones are 1 or more hours behind Eastern Standard Time. Pacific Standard Time is 3 hours behind Eastern Standard Time; when it is 1:00 Pacific Standard Time, it is 4:00 Eastern Standard Time.

87. **B** Third ring

RATIONALE: If possible, the telephone should be answered on the first ring and always by the third ring.

88. **E** At the next scheduled billing after the insurance has paid

RATIONALE: If a patient has insurance, a bill is usually not sent until the insurance company has paid its portion of the bill. The statement for the balance would be sent with the next billing cycle.

89. **D** CMS-1500

RATIONALE: The CMS-1500 is a universal claim form developed by the Health Care Financing Administration (HCFA) that standardizes the data required by most insurance carriers to process insurance claims.

90. **D** At the end of the day

RATIONALE: Patients who are habitually late for appointments should be scheduled at the end of the day so as not to disrupt the workflow.

91. **C** Draw a single line through the error, write the word "error," make the correction, and date and initial the entry

RATIONALE: Corrections are made in the medical record by drawing a single line through the error, writing the word "error" next to it, making the correction, and dating and initialing the correction (SLIDE rule).

92. **D** Problem-oriented progress notes

RATIONALE: SOAP is an organized way of charting progress notes. *SOAP* stands for *s*ubjective, *o*bjective, *a*ssessment, and *p*lan.

93. **A** A referral to another physician

RATIONALE: The physician must notify the patient of his or her intention to terminate the relationship to protect the physician against abandonment. The physician is not required to refer to another physician.

94. **E** Should be squeezed in for a brief visit so the physician can decide what the next treatment step should be

RATIONALE: If the patient requires immediate attention, he or she should be accommodated. If the patient does not need immediate care, a brief visit with the physician and a scheduled appointment at a later date may be the best policy. The patient should be told that the office runs on an appointment basis.

95. **B** Immediately offer a new appointment time

RATIONALE: An attempt should be made to reschedule the appointment while the patient is on the telephone. Patients with advance appointments may fill canceled appointments.

96. **B** Low-pitched and expressive voice
    RATIONALE: The telephone voice should be warm, friendly, and natural. Pronunciation and enunciation should be clear and distinct. A normal tone of voice carries best. Variance in tone brings out the meaning of words and adds vitality to what is said. The other choices present opportunities for disconcertion, confusion, or miscommunication.

97. **B** To deal with the collection agency
    RATIONALE: After an account has been released to a collection agency, the medical office makes no further attempts at collection. No more statements are sent. The patient's ledger is marked so that the office knows it is in the hands of an agency. The patient should be referred to the agency if he or she contacts the office in regard to the account. Any payments should be reported to the agency.

98. **D** Word processing
    RATIONALE: Word processing is the system used to process written communications. It is a document production tool. Telecommunications involve verbal communication; documentation, interfacing, and formatting are not types of computer systems.

99. **B** Enclosed packing slip
    RATIONALE: All orders received should be compared with the original purchase order and the invoice included with the shipment. The order should be checked for correct items, sizes, styles, and amounts.

100. **C** The patient pays in advance
    RATIONALE: A credit balance is the amount of advance payment or overpayment on an account. The amount of receipts exceeds the amount charged.

Pretest 3 Answer Key

Clinical

1. **A** Washing hands
   RATIONALE: Hand washing is the process of cleansing or sanitizing the hands. It is considered the most important medical aseptic practice for preventing the spread of infection. Hand washing reduces skin bacteria by the use of friction, soap, and running water.

2. **C** All patients
   RATIONALE: Standard precautions apply to the handling of all potentially infectious body fluids and tissues. Health care workers should take nondiscriminatory precautions to protect themselves.

3. **B** In the ear
   RATIONALE: Aural pertains to the ear (auris). An aural temperature is taken in the ear canal.

4. **E** B and C
   RATIONALE: Gloves are considered to be a barrier precaution and should be used when contact with blood or other body fluids is anticipated.

5. **C** 98.6°F
   RATIONALE: Normal adult oral temperature is between 97°F and 99°F.

6. **B** 14 to 20 breaths per minute
   RATIONALE: Normal adult rate can be 14 to 20 breaths per minute.

7. **E** B and C
   RATIONALE: Temperature, pulse, respiration, and blood pressure are considered to be the vital signs. They are the measurements that indicate a patient's state of general health.

8. **B** Usually higher in children than in adults
   RATIONALE: The normal pulse rate for a child is between 80 and 120 beats per minute. Normal values for an adult are between 60 and 80 beats per minute.

9. **E** All of the above
   RATIONALE: The pulse rate is decreased by conditions such as depression, chronic pain, central nervous system disorders, and hypothyroidism.

10. **A** The difference between the systolic and the diastolic blood pressure
    RATIONALE: The pulse pressure is the difference between the systolic and the diastolic blood pressures. It reflects the volume of circulating blood. Less than 30 mm Hg or more than 50 mm Hg is considered abnormal.

11. **B** 99
    RATIONALE: To convert kilograms to pounds, multiply the number of kilograms by 2.2 (45 kg × 2.2 = 99 lb).

12. **A** 6 feet
    RATIONALE: Height is measured in inches. Using the conversion factor of 12 inches equals 1 foot, divide 72 inches by 12 inches (72 ÷ 12 = 6).

13. **A** Chest and back
    RATIONALE: Percussion is the use of tapping or striking the body to elicit sounds, usually done with the fingers or a small hammer. Percussion aids in the determination of the size, position, and density of the underlying organ or cavity.

14. **D** Social history
    RATIONALE: The social history gives information regarding the patient's lifestyle, hobbies, education, occupation, sleeping habits, methods of exercise, sex life, and coping skills.

15. **D** All of the above
    RATIONALE: Subjective findings (symptoms) are perceptible only to the patient or known only to the patient.

16. **E** All of the above
    RATIONALE: The temporal artery thermometer is gently and slowly moved across the patient's

forehead. The procedure is noninvasive, quick, and accurate on all patients.

17. **E** Clearness of vision

RATIONALE: Visual acuity using the Snellen eye chart is a common distance acuity screening test.

18. **B** 0–10

RATIONALE: Numeric pain rating scales ask the patient to choose a number that rates the level of pain with 0 being no pain and 10 being the worst pain.

19. **C** Rectum

RATIONALE: Proctoscopy is the use of a scope to examine the rectum and the distal portion of the colon.

20. **B** Left side and chest, with right leg flexed

RATIONALE: In the Sims' position, the patient lies on the left side with the right knee and thigh drawn up toward the chest. It is sometimes called the lateral position and can be used for rectal examinations and some pelvic examinations.

21. **D** Prone position

RATIONALE: In the prone position, the patient is lying face down on the table.

22. **A** Ophthalmoscope

RATIONALE: The ophthalmoscope is an instrument used to inspect the inner structures of the eye. It has a handle containing batteries and an attached head equipped with a light and magnifying lenses.

23. **A** Glucose and protein

RATIONALE: On all visits after the initial visit, a urine sample is obtained and tested for the presence of sugar (glucose) and albumin (protein). The presence of glucose might be a warning sign of a prediabetic state or diabetes. The presence of protein might be an early warning sign of toxemia. Both of these conditions would require careful medical supervision and treatment.

24. **A** 1 week after her period

RATIONALE: A monthly breast self-examination can detect early signs of breast cancer. The examination should be performed once a month approximately 1 week after the menstrual period because the breasts are usually not tender or swollen at this time.

25. **A** Acute

RATIONALE: Disease is a pathologic process that in some way alters the normal function, structure, or metabolism of an organism. An acute disease process or acute infection begins abruptly with sharp intensity and subsides after a short period.

26. **C** 21 to 28 days

RATIONALE: Double-wrapped sterile packs are considered sterile up to 28 days from the date of sterilization. They should be stored in a clean, dry, and dust-free place. When a pack expires, the contents must be reprocessed.

27. **E** Unwrap the pack, rewrap the pack, replace the indicator, and resterilize

RATIONALE: A sterilization indicator shows that the proper combination of steam, time, and temperature has been achieved. It does not prove that the contents are sterile. Failure of an indicator to change color might indicate that an error has occurred in the sterilization process. The pack should be reprocessed to correct any problem that may have caused the improper sterilization.

28. **E** All of the above

RATIONALE: Postoperative care includes the total recovery period. The patient needs to be taught how to care for himself or herself at home after surgery. These instructions should include signs of infection, how to care for the wound, information about medications prescribed, and when to return for follow-up. These instructions should be given in writing, and the patient or caregiver should acknowledge the receipt of the instructions.

29. **B** Sanitization

RATIONALE: Instruments and other items used in the office must be carefully cleaned before proceeding with disinfection or sterilization. This cleaning process is sanitization. It is used to remove microorganisms, blood, and debris that might interfere with the sterilization process.

30. **C** Acquired active

RATIONALE: Immunity is the body's resistance to pathogenic microorganisms. It is classified as either natural or acquired. Natural immunity is a genetic feature specific to a person's race, sex, and ability to respond. Acquired immunity means that the body has developed an ability to defend itself. Acquired immunity can be active or passive. Active immunity results when a person has been exposed to or has had the disease. Passive immunity is gained from receiving immune substances, bypassing the body's immune system.

31. **E** 8-0

RATIONALE: The size or gauge of most sutures is labeled in terms of zeros; 0 is the thickest, and the number of zeros decreases up to 10-0, which is the thinnest. (The more zeros, the thinner the material.)

32. **D** Forceps

RATIONALE: Forceps are instruments of varied sizes and shapes used for grasping, compressing, or holding tissues and objects. They are two-pronged instruments with either a spring handle or a ring handle with a ratchet closure.

33. **C** Iodine

RATIONALE: Betadine is an antiseptic solution often used to disinfect the skin before a minor surgical procedure. It contains iodine, and a patient who is allergic to iodine would have a reaction to the solution.

34. **E** Purulent

RATIONALE: When a dressing is changed, it and the wound must be inspected for the amount and character of drainage. Drainage that is described as purulent consists of or contains pus.

35. **A** 10 to 15 degrees

RATIONALE: The objective of an intradermal injection is to inject a minute amount of solution between the layers of the skin. The needle is inserted at a 10- to 15-degree angle to deliver the solution to the correct area. When given correctly, the injection produces a wheal on the skin surface.

36. C Sublingual

RATIONALE: With the sublingual route of administration, the drug is placed under the patient's tongue to dissolve and be absorbed.

37. B 1½ inch, 21 gauge

RATIONALE: The main objective when administering an intramuscular injection is to inject the medication into deep muscle tissue for gradual and optimal absorption. The longer length of the needle allows this level of administration to occur. The gauge allows for thick medications to be injected easily.

38. B Diuretic

RATIONALE: Diuretic medications promote the formation and excretion of urine. They can be prescribed to reduce the volume of extracellular fluid in the treatment of many disorders, including hypertension, edema, and congestive heart failure.

39. A 0.5 mL

RATIONALE: Use the following formula:

$$\frac{\text{dose ordered}}{\text{available strength}} \times \text{dose form} = \text{dose given}$$

$$\text{Example: } \frac{250\,\text{mg}}{500\,\text{mg}} \times 1\,\text{mL} = 0.5\,\text{mL}$$

40. E All of the above

RATIONALE: Cholesterol is a substance produced by the liver and found in animal fats. Aerobic exercise can lower cholesterol levels. Diets high in fat and calories add to cholesterol levels. Hypercholesterolemia can run in families.

41. E 1.010 and 1.025

RATIONALE: Specific gravity is the weight of a substance compared with the weight of an equal volume of distilled water. In urinalysis, specific gravity is the rough measurement of the concentration of substances dissolved in urine. Most urine samples are between 1.010 and 1.025. This reading indicates the ability of the kidney to concentrate the specimen, and a reading outside this range might indicate kidney disease.

42. D All of the above

RATIONALE: A complete blood count (CBC) is one of the most common laboratory tests ordered on blood. It provides a complete look at the blood components, giving a wealth of information about a patient's condition. Tests performed in a CBC include red blood cell count, white blood cell count, hemoglobin and hematocrit, differential, platelet number estimation, and red blood cell morphology.

43. D Glucometer

RATIONALE: A glucometer is a palm-sized device used to test blood glucose levels. Glucometers require very small amounts of capillary blood and display the results in seconds.

44. A From a skin puncture

RATIONALE: Capillary or peripheral blood is obtained by performing a skin puncture on the fingertip, earlobe, or great toe or heel of an infant. This method allows for a minimal amount of blood to be collected but is sufficient for many laboratory tests.

45. C Gallbladder

RATIONALE: A cholecystogram is an x-ray of the gallbladder. It is made after the ingestion or injection of a radiopaque substance. The test is useful in diagnosing cholecystitis (inflammation of the gallbladder), cholelithiasis (gallstones), and tumors.

46. A Dilates blood vessels

RATIONALE: Thermotherapy (application of heat) produces local vasodilation and increases circulation. These results of heat application speed up the inflammatory process, promote local drainage, relax muscles, and relieve pain.

47. E All of the above

RATIONALE: Physical examination of a urine sample is the first part of a complete urinalysis. The urine is assessed for color, clarity, specific gravity, odor, and pH.

48. A P

RATIONALE: Electrocardiography is the procedure that records the electrical activity of the heart. The electrocardiogram records a series of waves or deflections above or below a baseline. Each wave or deflection corresponds to a particular part of the cardiac cycle. The P wave reflects contraction of the atria.

49. D 12

RATIONALE: The standard electrocardiogram consists of 12 separate leads or recordings of the electrical activity of the heart from different angles. Each lead must be marked or coded for the physician to know which angle has been recorded. The 12 leads include leads I, II, and III (standard or bipolar leads); leads aVR, aVL, and aVF (augmented leads); and leads V_1, V_2, V_3, V_4, V_5, and V_6 (chest or precordial leads).

50. D 25 mm/s

RATIONALE: The paper used in an electrocardiographic machine is a specialized graph paper with internationally accepted increments for measuring the cardiac cycle. As the paper advances, the heat-sensitive stylus moves along the horizontal line and intersects with a vertical line. The paper advances at a speed of 25 mm/s.

51. D SpO_2

RATIONALE: The pulse oximeter measures the oxygen saturation of the peripheral capillaries. The abbreviation SpO_2 (saturation of peripheral oxygen) is used to record the reading as a percentage.

52. A Prothrombin time

RATIONALE: The drug Coumadin is an anticoagulant and keeps the blood from clotting. The prothrombin time (PT) is a test for detecting coagulation deficits. A prolonged PT can indicate a deficiency in the normal blood clotting mechanism and can help monitor anticoagulation therapy.

53. C Catgut

RATIONALE: The purpose of sutures is to hold the edges of a wound together until healing can occur. Absorbable sutures, usually used on deeper tissues, do not have to be removed because they are absorbed or digested by body fluids and tissues during the healing process. An example of this type of suture material is surgical gut (catgut). Nonabsorbable sutures used on outer skin surfaces are removed after the wound is healed.

54. **C** Strep test
RATIONALE: At a well-child visit in a pediatric office, the provider evaluates the growth and development of the child. These visits can include an examination, guidance, and vaccinations. A child presents with signs and symptoms of disease at a sick-child visit.

55. **C** To prevent urinary incontinence
RATIONALE: The patient should be asked if he/she needs to void before the examination. An empty bladder makes the examination easier and more comfortable for the patient. A urine specimen is then available if needed for testing.

56. **C** 30%
RATIONALE: Hemoglobin and hematocrit values are related. Each 1% hematocrit contains 0.34 g of hemoglobin. The hematocrit should equal three times the hemoglobin within 3%.

57. **D** Erythrocyte sedimentation rate 30 mm/h
RATIONALE: The normal value for an erythrocyte sedimentation rate (ESR) is 0 to 20 mm/h. An increased ESR might indicate inflammation.

58. **A** Gram stain
RATIONALE: Because bacteria are small and possess little color, staining is necessary to observe them under the microscope. Gram stain is used most often. The dyes in the stain are taken up differently in each type of bacterial cell, and they stain different colors. Bacteria are identified as gram-negative (stain red) or gram-positive (stain purple).

59. **B** Alkaline
RATIONALE: pH expresses the degree of acidity or alkalinity of a solution. Usually, freshly voided urine is acidic. After sitting, bacteria contaminate the sample and cause it to become alkaline.

60. **D** Red-stoppered (topped) (serum separator tube [SST], tiger)
RATIONALE: Blood collection tubes are color-coded, depending on the additive a tube contains or does not contain. Red-stoppered (SST, tiger) tubes contain no additives, and so the blood collected in these tubes clots, and serum can be removed.

61. **E** All of the above
RATIONALE: The medication record can tell at a glance what medications and dosages the patient is taking. Prescription medications and over-the-counter (OTC) medications, including vitamins and herbals, must be recorded.

62. **E** All of the above
RATIONALE: Spirometry is a pulmonary function screening test that measures how much air is pushed out of the lungs. It is noninvasive. Patients with lung disease can be monitored with spirometry.

63. **A** Assess the victim's airway
RATIONALE: Check the victim for responsiveness. If the victim is unconscious, assess the ABCs—airway, breathing, and circulation.

64. **D** Pelvic
RATIONALE: Equipment and supplies needed for a pelvic examination include lubricant, cervical spatula, ThinPrep container, vaginal speculum, and uterine sponge forceps.

65. **D** Liver
RATIONALE: After a drug is absorbed into the body and transported to the cells or tissues for which it is intended, it is again picked up by the bloodstream and transported to the liver, the site of metabolism or biotransformation or both. In the liver, the drug is broken down and prepared for elimination from the body.

66. **C** Tests for color-blindness
RATIONALE: Color-blindness is tested using Ishihara plates. The Ishihara color test uses a series of plates on which round dots are printed in various colors and patterns. Patients with normal color vision are able to discern specific patterns on the plates. Patients with a deficiency in color perception cannot do so.

67. **A** Forceps
RATIONALE: Hemostatic forceps are a type of clamping instrument used to stop bleeding, clamp severed vessels, and hold tissue.

68. **C** 1:4
RATIONALE: A fairly constant ratio of four pulse beats to one respiration exists. As a general rule, both pulse and respiration rates normally respond to exercise or emotional upsets. Normal pulse rate for an adult is 60 to 80 beats per minute. Normal respiratory rate for an adult is 14 to 20 breaths per minute.

69. **E** All of the above
RATIONALE: Insulin shock is caused by too much insulin intake, decrease in food intake, or excessive exercise. It is characterized by sweating, trembling, chills, nervousness, irritability, hunger, hallucinations, and pallor. If uncorrected, it can progress to convulsions, coma, and death. Treatment requires an immediate dose of glucose.

70. **C** Antidepressant
RATIONALE: Drugs can be classified according to their actions in the body. An antidepressant medication is used as a mood elevator and is used to treat depression. Fluoxetine (Prozac) is an example of an antidepressant.

71. **B** Friction and running water
RATIONALE: Hands must be washed, using the correct technique, before and after each patient is examined or treated. Proper hand washing depends on two factors: (1) running water and (2) friction. Friction is the firm rubbing of skin surfaces to loosen debris. Running water washes away the debris.

72. **D** 12 months
RATIONALE: For vaccinations for mumps, measles, and rubella, it is recommended that the first dose be given between 12 and 15 months of age. The second dose is recommended between ages 6 and 12 years.

73. **B** Migraine
RATIONALE: Migraine headaches are paroxysmal attacks of headaches that may be completely incapacitating. They are frequently characterized by nausea, vomiting, visual disturbances, throbbing pain in one side of the head, and an aura. An aura

is some type of visual disturbance such as lines or spots across the visual field.

74. **E** All of the above

    RATIONALE: Aspirin is a salicylate. It has four therapeutic properties: relieving pain (analgesic), reducing inflammation (antiinflammatory), reducing fever (antipyretic), and prolonging clotting times (anticoagulant).

75. **A** Ensures the accuracy of results

    RATIONALE: Quality assurance is a major component of the Clinical Laboratory Improvement Act of 1988 (CLIA '88) regulations relating to laboratory standards. It is a comprehensive set of policies and procedures developed to ensure the quality of laboratory testing and includes quality control, personnel orientation, laboratory documentation, knowledge of instrumentation, and enrollment in a proficiency-testing program.

76. **B** 48 to 72 hours after it has been performed

    RATIONALE: The Mantoux test is used for routine screening and diagnosis of tuberculosis. The test uses a purified protein derivative from a live tuberculin culture to test for antibodies. The results should be read 48 to 72 hours after the test is performed by intradermal injection. The extent of induration is measured and recorded.

77. **C** ABCDE rule

    RATIONALE: Malignant melanoma is a cancerous skin growth composed of melanocytes. Early warning signs of melanoma include: *a*symmetry (A), *b*orders (B), *c*olor (C), *d*iameter (D), and *e*levation (E).

78. **D** O

    RATIONALE: Patients with type O blood are considered to be universal donors. Type O blood contains no antigens on the red blood cells; it does not agglutinate in the presence of anti-A and anti-B antibodies in the plasma.

79. **E** Colon

    RATIONALE: A lower gastrointestinal series (barium enema) is an x-ray examination of the colon. Contrast medium (barium) is instilled into the colon through an enema. The colon can then be visualized by x-ray examination.

80. **B** Computed tomography (CT) scan

    RATIONALE: A CT scan is a radiographic technique that produces a film that represents a detailed cross-section of a tissue structure. The technique uses a narrow beam of x-ray that rotates in a continuous 360-degree motion around the patient. The images obtained from this method are highly detailed and simulate a three-dimensional appearance.

81. **A** Cancer

    RATIONALE: Massive or excessive exposure to radiation can cause tissue damage and various side effects, which can include damage to blood cells, skin cells, eyes, and reproductive cells. Overexposure can result in decreased red and white blood cell counts, burns, and an increased incidence of cancers.

82. **B** Leads I, II, and III

    RATIONALE: The first three leads recorded are the standard or bipolar leads (leads I, II, and III). They each use two limb electrodes to record electrical activity.

83. **B** Chains

    RATIONALE: Bacteria may be classified by morphology (size and shape). Streptococci are bacteria that are spherical in shape and arranged in chains.

84. **D** Increasing age

    RATIONALE: Normal pulse rates vary as a result of a person's gender, age, body size, posture, activity level, health status, nervous system function, and emotional state and the volume and composition of the blood. Pulse normally decreases with age.

85. **D** RL

    RATIONALE: The leads of an electrocardiogram measure the electrical activity from the frontal and horizontal planes of the body. The right leg acts as the grounding as electrical activity is recorded from the right arm, left arm, and left leg.

86. **A** OSHA

    RATIONALE: The Occupational Safety and Health Act (OSHA) was established by the federal government in 1970 to set standards and protocols for occupational health and safety. The regulations must be known and followed. They include hazard exposure plans, medical waste management, personal protective measures, general safety precautions, fire safety, staff development, and bloodborne pathogen regulations.

87. **C** An array of tests for identifying a disease

    RATIONALE: A profile (panel) consists of an array of tests that are determined to be the most specific for identifying a disease state or evaluation of a body system.

88. **E** All of the above

    RATIONALE: An analgesic medication lessens the sensory function of the brain. Analgesics are used for pain relief. They can be classified as narcotic (morphine, codeine, meperidine [Demerol]) or nonnarcotic (aspirin, acetaminophen [Tylenol], ibuprofen).

89. **C** Keep a written record of all daily activities

    RATIONALE: A Holter monitor is a portable monitoring system used to record the cardiac activity of the patient for a 24-hour period. Keeping a written diary of all activities during the day that cause stress is important for the patient. Examples of these activities include driving in traffic, stair climbing, and bowel movements. Symptoms associated with possible heart problems should also be included.

90. **B** 1.0 mL

    RATIONALE: Use the following formula:

    $$\frac{\text{dose ordered}}{\text{available strength}} \times \text{dose form} = \text{dose given}$$

    $$\text{Example}: \frac{50\,\text{mg}}{50\,\text{mg}} \times 1\,\text{mL} = 1.0\,\text{mL}$$

91. C 30%
RATIONALE: Hemoglobin and hematocrit values are related. Each 1% hematocrit contains 0.34 g of hemoglobin. The hematocrit should equal three times the hemoglobin, within 3%.

92. C Staphylococci
RATIONALE: Pathogenic bacteria are classified by their shape and arrangement. "Staphyl/o" means clusters, or bunch (as in bunch of grapes).

93. A Silver nitrate
RATIONALE: Topical silver nitrate ($AgNO_3$) solution or an applicator coated with $AgNO_3$ can be used to stop localized bleeding. The applicator must be kept in light-proof brown containers. The applicators are convenient for use in the mouth and nose.

94. A Alanine aminotransferase (ALT)
RATIONALE: ALT is an enzyme found in highly metabolic tissues such as the heart muscle, liver, and skeletal muscle. Levels increase after a myocardial infarction.

95. A 1 mL
RATIONALE: The cubic centimeter (cc) and the milliliter (mL) are interchangeable units of measure in the metric system.

96. C Gallbladder
RATIONALE: "Cholecyt/o" is the combining form for gallbladder, and "-gram" is the suffix meaning record.

97. C Nonsterile gloves, laboratory coat, and goggles.
RATIONALE: Sigmoidoscopy is used to diagnose polyps, hemorrhoids, and diverticular disorders. The sigmoidoscope is a flexible instrument that allows the physician to complete the examination without much discomfort to the patient. Nonsterile gloves, laboratory coat, and goggles are adequate personal protective equipment for assisting with the procedure.

98. D Eating
RATIONALE: The postprandial blood sugar (2-hour PPBS) is a screening test for diabetes mellitus. A fasting blood glucose level is obtained; if the results are within an acceptable range, the patient eats a meal and is retested after 2 hours.

99. A Rince contaminants from the lip of the bottle
RATIONALE: Pouring a small amount of the solution into a waste receptacle rinses any contaminants off the bottle lip. If the bottle has a double cap, this step can be skipped.

100. A Otitis media
RATIONALE: Otitis media is an inflammation (infection) of the middle ear. Fluid collects behind the tympanic membrane. Otitis media is often associated with an upper respiratory infection. The patient experiences pain and fever. The infected canal and eardrum appear red and swollen, and a purulent discharge may be present. It is treated with antibiotics and analgesics.

Posttest Answer Key

1. **B** Antineoplastic
   RATIONALE: An antineoplastic agent (cancer drug) inhibits the growth of malignant cells.
2. **C** Overbooking
   RATIONALE: Overbooking may result in a prolonged waiting time for the patient to see the provider, and it may cause dissatisfaction with the practice.
3. **D** Delay treatment and inform or consult with the physician
   RATIONALE: A physician must have consent from the patient to treat the patient, even though the consent is usually implied. A patient has the right to refuse treatment at any time.
4. **A** Another physician
   RATIONALE: A call from another physician or professional colleague should always be transferred to the physician immediately.
5. **B** Pulmonary artery
   RATIONALE: Blood that is low in oxygen exits the right ventricle through the pulmonary artery where it enters the lungs and picks up oxygen.
6. **B** Cecum
   RATIONALE: The cecum is the first division of the large intestine. It is connected to the ileum of the small intestine. The appendix (vermiform) is attached to the cecum.
7. **D** All of the above
   RATIONALE: Personality is defined as the composite of the behavioral traits and characteristics by which one is recognized as an individual. A person's age, life experience, heredity, and environment all contribute to the composite.
8. **B** Hyster/o
   RATIONALE: The combining forms for uterus include "hyster/o," "metr/i," "metr/o," "metri/o," "uter/i," and "uter/o."
9. **B** Staying calm when dealing with angry patients
   RATIONALE: Professionalism is defined as exhibiting a courteous, conscientious, and business-like manner in the workplace. It is characterized by the technical and ethical standards of a certain profession.
10. **D** May refuse to accept a patient if he or she chooses
    RATIONALE: A physician has the right to limit the size of his or her practice or the number of patients that he or she treats.
11. **B** Villi
    RATIONALE: The wall of the small intestine forms circular folds with finger-like projections called villi (*sing.* villus). The villi increase the amount of digested food that can be absorbed.
12. **B** Glucagon
    RATIONALE: Glucagon, which is produced in the alpha cells in the pancreas, stimulates the conversion of glycogen to glucose in the liver. Its primary function is to increase blood glucose levels.
13. **B** Invasion of privacy
    RATIONALE: Giving out patient information without the patient's consent is an invasion of the patient's privacy, which is an intentional tort.
14. **A** A physician accidentally amputates the wrong finger from a patient
    RATIONALE: *Res ipsa loquitur* means "the thing speaks for itself." It describes a situation in which the nature of the injury can implicate negligence.
15. **D** "Can you tell me more about that?"
    RATIONALE: An open-ended question requires more than a "yes" or "no" answer. It forces the patient to provide additional detail and expand on his or her thoughts.
16. **A** Aplastic
    RATIONALE: Aplastic anemia results from the failure of the hematopoietic cells (stem cells) in the bone marrow. This condition can be caused by exposure

to toxins, alkylating agents, certain drugs, and
radiation.

17. **A** Survival

RATIONALE: Psychologist Abraham Maslow created
what he called the "hierarchy of needs." This
hierarchy categorizes these needs into five levels.
The most basic of these needs are the physiologic
needs: oxygen, food, water, excretion, shelter, and
sexual expression.

18. **D** Occipital

RATIONALE: The occipital bone is located at the base
of the skull. It contains a large opening (foramen
magnum) where the spinal cord exits the cranium.

19. **B** Seminiferous tubules

RATIONALE: The seminiferous tubules are tightly
coiled structures located in each testis. Sperm are
formed in the epithelium of these tubules.

20. **B** Encouraging nonverbal communication

RATIONALE: With non–English-speaking patients,
the medical assistant may need to use gestures and
more body language to convey messages. Having a
bilingual staff member is always helpful.

21. **D** Lines body cavities that open to the outside of the
body

RATIONALE: Mucous membranes line all body
cavities that open to the exterior of the body. They
secrete mucus, a substance that keeps the membrane
moist and lubricated.

22. **C** Quotation marks

RATIONALE: The chief complaint is a concise account
of the patient's symptoms explained in the patient's
own words. This information is set apart from the
other charting information by placing the words in
quotes.

23. **D** Transient ischemic attack

RATIONALE: Transient ischemic attacks are temporary
episodes of impaired neurologic functioning caused
by inadequate flow of blood to a portion of the
brain. Signs and symptoms may include sudden
weakness, numbness, and tingling on one side of the
body, dizziness, confusion, and vision disturbances.

24. **A** "Please tell me more about those feelings."

RATIONALE: Using an open-ended statement
encourages the patient to open up and expand on
his or her thoughts.

25. **C** Lack of blood flow to tissue

RATIONALE: Ischemia is reduced or lack of blood flow
to tissue that results in impairment of cell function.

26. **A** Fax

RATIONALE: A fax machine saves time and labor in
conveying patient information from physician to
physician or physician to hospital. However,
precautions must be taken to ensure security of the
information arriving by fax. This goal can be
accomplished by telephoning ahead to alert the
receiver that sensitive information will be arriving.

27. **C** Closed-ended

RATIONALE: A closed-ended question asks for specific
information. It limits the answer to one or two
words. A "yes" or "no" answer may be enough.

28. **D** State government

RATIONALE: The MD, DO, or DC degree is conferred
on graduation from medical or chiropractic school.
The license to practice medicine is granted by a state
board, also known as the State Board of Medical
Examiners.

29. **A** Notify the patient that her medical care is being
terminated

RATIONALE: The patient-physician relationship is an
implied contract. Both parties must uphold their
part of the contract. Not following the physician's
orders would be grounds to terminate the contract.
The physician must notify the patient by sending a
certified letter.

30. **B** Ask the patient to calm down

RATIONALE: The medical assistant can help calm an
angry patient by speaking calmly and refusing to
return the emotion. Calmly ask the person to take
a deep breath and stop talking for a few moments.
Gradually lowering the volume of the voice will cause
the angry person to lower his or her own voice so that
he or she can hear what the medical assistant is saying.

31. **B** The patient is human immunodeficiency virus (HIV)
positive

RATIONALE: Even though the physician is charged
with safeguarding patient confidentiality, state laws
require certain disclosures. All states require
sexually transmitted diseases to be reported, including
confirmed cases of acquired immunodeficiency
syndrome (AIDS). Most states, but not all, require
that patients who are HIV positive be reported.

32. **B** Uniform Anatomical Gift Act

RATIONALE: The Uniform Anatomical Gift Act states
that any person of sound mind and age of 18 or
older may give all or part of his or her body after
death for research, transplantation, or placement in
a tissue bank.

33. **B** A retirement complex with individual apartments

RATIONALE: Autonomy is the quality of having the
ability or tendency to function independently. A
community where a senior can interact with
persons of the same age and participate in activities
but keep his or her own apartment would allow
independence.

34. **D** Quarterly

RATIONALE: Every 3 months, the employer must file
an Employer's Quarterly Federal Tax Return (Form
941) with the Internal Revenue Service. This form lists
the amounts withheld from employee paychecks.

35. **C** Draw a single line through the misspelled word

RATIONALE: Correct errors in charting by using the
SLIDE rule: draw a single line through the entry,
write "error" above the entry, correct the entry, and
date and initial the entry.

36. **C** Write-protect

RATIONALE: Write-protect is a process or code that
prevents overwriting of data or programs on a disk.

37. **C** Extremities

RATIONALE: The radial pulses are located in the
wrists (extremities).

38. C Preexisting condition

RATIONALE: A preexisting condition is a condition or disease that was present before an insurance policy was issued.

39. D Accounting

RATIONALE: A spreadsheet is a software program for inputting and manipulating numerical data to facilitate a wide variety of financial activities.

40. D Unemployment tax

RATIONALE: Federal unemployment taxes, based on the Federal Unemployment Tax Act (FUTA), are paid entirely by the employer. The FUTA tax provides unemployment payments to workers who lose their job.

41. A Chief complaint

RATIONALE: The patient's history relates to the patient's clinical picture and depends on the patient for answers to specific questions. The history is composed of the chief complaint or the reason why the patient is being seen. This information is usually in the patient's own words.

42. C Initials come after complete names

RATIONALE: Indexing rules are standardized and are based on current business practices. The rule that applies to initials states "that initials precede a name beginning with the same letter." (M. Johnson would be filed before Mary Johnson.)

43. D All of the above

RATIONALE: Complete and accurate records are essential to a well-managed medical practice. Health information management includes not only assembling the record but also saving, retrieving, protecting, transferring, storing, retaining, and destroying records.

44. B Enclosure

RATIONALE: The enclosure notation identifies any material that may be accompanying the correspondence. The notation is placed two lines below the signature line.

45. A A subpoena

RATIONALE: The physician and medical assistant may never release confidential information without the consent of the patient except when it is legally required. A *subpoena duces tecum* is a legally binding request to provide records or documents to appear in court.

46. D 99

RATIONALE: CPT lists and codes procedures and services performed by the provider. The CPT book is divided into six sections. The E&M section codes are 99200 to 99499.

47. C Photocopier

RATIONALE: Capital equipment is equipment used to generate revenue.

48. C Grouping

RATIONALE: Grouping or clustering allows the provider to use time efficiently by seeing patients with the same needs at the same time.

49. D Minutes

RATIONALE: A record of the proceedings of a meeting is called the minutes. They contain a record of what was done at the meeting. Minutes should be signed and kept on file according to the policy of the organization.

50. D W-4

RATIONALE: The Form W-4 is the Employee's Withholding Allowance Certificate. It is filled out by the employee and allows him or her to determine the number of withholding allowances.

51. B Properties owned by the business

RATIONALE: Anything not owed is an asset. Anything owed is a liability.

52. A A request for a change in appointment time

RATIONALE: A change in appointment time is not, in most cases, directly related to the type or quality of patient care, whereas the other choices are.

53. D The mission statement

RATIONALE: A policy manual describes the office philosophy and goals. The office mission statement reflects the reasons for the existence of the practice.

54. C Numerical

RATIONALE: In the numerical filing system, each file is assigned a number, starting with the lowest number and moving up. Files are organized in numerical order. A cross-reference with the patient's name is kept elsewhere.

55. B Employee's marital status

RATIONALE: The amount of money withheld from each paycheck is based on the information the employee provides on Form W-4. The Employer's Tax Guide includes tables showing how much tax must be withheld based on the pay period and the employee's marital status.

56. C Endocrine

RATIONALE: The thyroid gland is a major gland in the endocrine system.

57. D Future events arranged in chronologic order

RATIONALE: A tickler file is a chronologic file used as a reminder that something must be done on a certain date.

58. A When the patient calls to make an appointment

RATIONALE: As a business, a medical office must charge competitive and fair prices for services and must receive payment for the services in a timely fashion. Patients should be fully informed about a practice's fees and payment policies before they receive treatment.

59. B An OUTguide

RATIONALE: An OUTguide is a heavy guide that is used to replace a folder that has temporarily been removed or moved from a filing space. It should be of a distinctive color for easy identification.

60. C Below the return address

RATIONALE: Any notation on the envelope directed toward the addressee, such as "Personal" or "Confidential," should be typed and underlined on the third line below the return address and aligned with the return address.

61. D Postage meter

RATIONALE: The postage meter is the most efficient way of stamping the mail in a large business office. The machine can be purchased or leased; the postage is purchased from the US Postal Service. The date must be changed daily.

62. **C** Holmes-Mathis, Jennie
RATIONALE: Hyphenated elements of a name, whether first name, middle name, or surname, are considered to be one unit.

63. **A** $5630
RATIONALE: Using the income statement, net income equals revenue minus expenses. An asset is anything of value that is owned, not just revenue.

64. **D** A scanner
RATIONALE: A scanner is a device that reads text or illustrations on a printed page and translates the information on the page into a form that the computer can understand.

65. **B** 1½ inch, 22 gauge
RATIONALE: The goal of an intramuscular injection is to deliver the medication into muscle tissue. The length of the needle can be up to 2 inches, depending on the size of the patient and the consistency of the medication. The gauge of the needle can be from 22 G to 25 G, depending on the consistency of the medication.

66. **A** Anticoagulants
RATIONALE: An anticoagulant agent delays or prevents blood clotting. A diuretic promotes urine output. Vasoconstrictors cause narrowing of blood vessels. A vasodilator increases the diameter of blood vessels.

67. **D** Cytologic fixative
RATIONALE: Vaginitis is an inflammation of the vagina usually caused by a microorganism. It is characterized by an abnormal discharge. A specimen is collected and evaluated for the invading organism, usually with a wet preparation. This slide would not be fixed, so fixative is not needed.

68. **D** V_4
RATIONALE: The chest (precordial) leads are unipolar and designated V_1, V_2, V_3, V_4, V_5, and V_6. These leads measure the electrical activity between six specific points on the chest wall and a point within the heart. Lead V_4 is placed in the fifth intercostal space at the left midclavicular line.

69. **D** 20
RATIONALE: Distance visual acuity is frequently part of a complete physical examination. It is widely used in schools and industry and is the best single test available for visual screening. The procedure uses the Snellen eye chart. The patient is positioned 20 feet from the chart (standard testing distance), either standing or sitting.

70. **A** Forced vital capacity
RATIONALE: The forced vital capacity (FVC) is the amount of air that can be forcefully exhaled from a maximal inhalation. FVC is measured through spirometry (pulmonary function test).

71. **B** Auscultation
RATIONALE: In auscultation, the examiner uses a stethoscope to listen to the sounds made by the body.

72. **D** Measure blood pressure
RATIONALE: The instrument used to measure blood pressure is called a sphygmomanometer. It consists of an inflatable cuff, an inflation bulb with a control valve, and a pressure gauge. ("Sphygm/o" means pulse; "manometer" refers to an instrument used to measure the pressure of a liquid or a gas.)

73. **D** Leukocytes: ++
RATIONALE: The normal range for leukocytes in a sample should be negative. The presence of white blood cells usually indicates a urinary tract infection.

74. **A** EDTA
RATIONALE: The anticoagulant ethylenediamine tetraacetic acid (EDTA) is used for hematology studies. It prevents the aggregation of platelets and allows the preparation of blood smears with minimal distortion of white blood cells.

75. **A** Two drops in both ears every 4 hours as needed
RATIONALE: The abbreviation for drops is gtt, AU is the abbreviation for both ears, q4h is the abbreviation for every 4 hours, and prn is the abbreviation for as needed.

76. **B** 1:10 bleach solution
RATIONALE: Disinfection is the process of killing pathogenic organisms or rendering them inactive. For equipment and countertops, the cheapest and most reliable method is the use of a 1:10 bleach solution.

77. **A** Leads I, II, and III
RATIONALE: An electrocardiogram consists of 12 leads. The standard (bipolar) limb leads are recorded first. These leads each use two limb electrodes to record the heart's electrical activity.

78. **D** Tilt the patient's head forward
RATIONALE: Nosebleed (epistaxis) is a hemorrhage from the nose usually caused by the rupture of small blood vessels within the nose. Mild to moderate bleeding can be controlled by having the patient sit upright and lean forward, and by applying direct pressure to the nose.

79. **A** Intradermal
RATIONALE: An intradermal injection places the medication within the skin layers. The site is used primarily for allergy testing and tuberculin screening (Mantoux test).

80. **C** OU
RATIONALE: The abbreviation OU (*oculus uterque*) means both eyes.

81. **B** Pink or red
RATIONALE: The Gram stain is the method of staining microorganisms that serves as a primary means of classifying and identifying bacteria. Using this method, bacteria are either gram-positive (retaining the purple color of the stain) or gram-negative (retaining the color of the counterstain).

82. **D** Urobilinogen
RATIONALE: Urobilinogen results from the breakdown of bilirubin in the intestines. It travels to the liver where it is sent back to the intestines and excreted in feces. Urine levels may be increased in conditions of the liver.

83. **A** Anisocytosis
RATIONALE: In a diseased state, red blood cells may become altered in appearance. They can vary in size (anisocytosis), shape (poikilocytosis), or color (polychromia, hypochromia, hyperchromia).

84. **C** Do not eat red meat for 48 hours before the collection
RATIONALE: Eating red meat and taking iron supplements and certain medications (e.g., aspirin, vitamin C, steroids, anticoagulants) can cause a false-positive result.

85. **A** Schedule I
RATIONALE: Schedule I drugs have no accepted medical use and a high potential for abuse. Possession of these drugs is illegal. Examples of schedule I drugs include heroin, lysergic acid diethylamide (LSD), mescaline, and amphetamine variations.

86. **D** Bronchodilator
RATIONALE: A bronchodilator is used to manage reversible airway obstruction caused by asthma and chronic obstructive pulmonary disease. It helps relax the smooth muscle of the respiratory tract, resulting in bronchodilation.

87. **C** Ecchymosis
RATIONALE: Ecchymosis is a hemorrhagic skin discoloration commonly called a bruise. The skin is not broken; the wound is closed.

88. **A** Facing away from the examiner
RATIONALE: Audiometry measures the lowest intensity of sound that a person can hear. The patient places headphones over both ears. A single frequency is delivered to each ear. The patient is asked to signal when he or she hears the sound. To reduce human error, the patient should be seated facing away from the examiner so the patient cannot see the examiner push the button to deliver the sound.

89. **C** Reduces the number of contaminants to a safe level
RATIONALE: Sanitization is the cleansing process that decreases the number of microorganisms to a safe level as dictated by public health guidelines. This process removes debris so that later sterilization can penetrate all surfaces of the item.

90. **A** Inflammation
RATIONALE: Inflammation is a tissue reaction to disease or trauma that includes heat, redness, swelling, and pain.

91. **D** Aluminum foil
RATIONALE: The wrapping must be permeable to steam.

92. **B** Grasp
RATIONALE: Forceps are classified as a grasping instrument. They can also be used to hold, manipulate, and retract.

93. **D** Oximeter
RATIONALE: Pulse oximetry is noninvasive and measures both the pulse rate and oxygen saturation of arterial blood using an oximeter.

94. **A** Used and discarded in a sharps container
RATIONALE: Sharps should be discarded in a sharps container only.

95. **B** Not douche
RATIONALE: Douching or use of vaginal ointments and jelly can interfere with normal results.

96. **A** Auscultation
RATIONALE: Auscultation is the listening to body sounds with a stethoscope to assess body organs.

97. **D** Tripled in weight and grown 10 to 12 inches in length.
RATIONALE: By age 1 year, the birth weight should triple and the birth length increased by 50%.

98. **D** MMR and Var
RATIONALE: MMR and Var are administered SC.

99. **B** Can cause an incorrect high blood pressure.
RATIONALE: A blood pressure cuff that is too small can cause an artificially elevated BP reading.

100. **B** Diuretic
RATIONALE: A diuretic promotes or increases urination.